Peer Research in Health and Social Development

Peer research is increasingly used in international academic, policy and practice environments. It engages members of a group or social network as trusted members of a research team working in communities and settings they are familiar with.

Critics, however, point to methodological concerns with peer research. These include the extent to which peer researchers genuinely represent the populations under study; data confidentiality; the emotional burden of enquiring into sensitive issues peers may experience in their own lives; and the reliability and credibility of data collected by people who do not have academic training. The book seeks to counter the marginalisation of research experience and skills derived from close relationships with people and communities, while reflecting critically on the strengths and limitations of peer research. Chapters by a wide range of international contributors illustrate the potential of peer research to facilitate an in-depth understanding of health and social development issues and enhance policy and practice.

This interdisciplinary book provides students and professionals working in health, social science and development studies with a thorough grounding in this new style of research. It will appeal to those interested in research and evaluation; sexual health and public health; mental health, disability and social care; gender and sexuality; conservation and environmental management; migration and citizenship studies; humanitarian issues; and international development.

Stephen Bell is an associate professor in the UQ Poche Centre for Indigenous Health and the School of Public Health at The University of Queensland, Australia. He is a social scientist who has conducted community-based research – in partnership with young people and other marginalised populations – in Africa, Asia, Pacific-Asia and Australia. The focus of his work is on sexual, reproductive and maternal health, HIV and other public health issues. His previous co-edited book (with Peter Aggleton), *Monitoring and Evaluation in Health and Social Development: Interpretive and Ethnographic Approaches*, was published by Routledge in 2016.

Peter Aggleton holds senior professorial positions in the Centre for Social Research in Health at UNSW Sydney, the School of Sociology at The Australian National University in Canberra, the Australian Research Centre for Sex, Health and Society at La Trobe University in Melbourne, and the Centre for Gender and Global Health at UCL in London. In addition to his academic work, Peter has served as a senior adviser to UNAIDS, UNESCO, UNFPA and WHO. He has worked extensively across Africa, Asia and Latin America.

Ally Gibson is a lecturer in the School of Health at Victoria University of Wellington – Te Herenga Waka, New Zealand. She is particularly interested in experiences and responses to cancer; sexual and reproductive health; gender, sexuality and identity; and inequity, marginalisation and vulnerability in health. A key priority in her research is to partner with community organisations to promote enquiry driven by the needs and priorities of individuals and community members.

Routledge Studies in Health and Social Welfare

Peer Research in Health and Social Development

International Perspectives on
Participatory Research

Edited by Stephen Bell, Peter Aggleton
and Ally Gibson

Routledge
Taylor & Francis Group

LONDON AND NEW YORK

First published 2021
by Routledge
2 Park Square, Milton Park, Abingdon, Oxon OX14 4RN

and by Routledge
52 Vanderbilt Avenue, New York, NY 10017

Routledge is an imprint of the Taylor & Francis Group, an informa business

British Library Cataloguing-in-Publication Data
A catalogue record for this book is available from the British Library

Library of Congress Cataloging-in-Publication Data
A catalog record has been requested for this book

ISBN: 978-0-367-32139-0 (hbk)
ISBN: 978-0-367-76663-4 (pbk)
ISBN: 978-0-429-31692-0 (ebk)

Typeset in Goudy
by Deanta Global Publishing Services, Chennai, India

For Sophie Ase, an amazing young woman, friend and colleague, and a talented social researcher who dedicated the last 10 years of her life to work on health inequity and social justice at the Papua New Guinea Institute of Medical Research in Goroka. In all she did, she epitomised the best that research can offer. She will be sadly missed, but fondly remembered, by many.

Contents

Figure

Contributors

Peter Aggleton holds senior professorial positions in the Centre for Social Research in Health at UNSW Sydney, the School of Sociology at The Australian National University in Canberra, the Australian Research Centre for Sex, Health and Society at La Trobe University in Melbourne, and the Centre for Gender and Global Health at UCL in London. In addition to his academic work, Peter has served as a senior adviser to UNAIDS, UNESCO, UNFPA and WHO. He has worked extensively across Africa, Asia and Latin America.

Grace Albert is an Indigenous researcher with the Cobra Collective. She is a Makushi descendant originating from the village of Tiger Pond in the South Pakaraima Mountains, Guyana. Grace's interest in community communication and cinema manifests in her work for the first community radio in Guyana and training in participatory video methods that allow communities to use videos to tell their stories.

Jennifer Allsopp is a postdoctoral fellow with the Immigration Initiative at Harvard (IIH) and Harvard Graduate School of Education, and coordinator of the IIH. She is also a research associate with the Refugee Studies Centre at the University of Oxford, and a regular advisor to the European Parliament's Civil Liberties (LIBE) Committee. Her research explores the relationship between immigration control, welfare and well-being, with a particular focus on gender and ageing.

Sophie Ase was a senior researcher in the sexual and reproductive health unit at the Papua New Guinea Institute of Medical Research, where she worked for 10 years. Her research included studies of sociocultural and biomedical understandings of cervical cancer and the acceptability of HPV vaccination, as well as in the prevention of parent-to-child HIV transmission.

Julie Bates is a sex worker rights activist and principal of Urban Realists Planning & Health Consultants, providing specialist advice, education and training to the sex industry, research institutes and policymakers. She is a lobbyist for the decriminalisation of the sex industry, and co-author and investigator on a number of sex work-related research projects. In 2018, she was awarded an Order of Australia in the Queen's Birthday Honours.

Stephen Bell is an associate professor in the UQ Poche Centre for Indigenous Health and the School of Public Health at The University of Queensland, Australia. He is a social scientist who has conducted community-based research – in partnership with young people and other marginalised populations – in Africa, Asia, Pacific-Asia and Australia. The focus of his work is on sexual, reproductive and maternal health, HIV and other public health issues. His previous co-edited book (with Peter Aggleton), *Monitoring and Evaluation in Health and Social Development: Interpretive and Ethnographic Approaches*, was published by Routledge in 2016.

Ryan Benjamin is an avid farmer and cattle owner. He sees participating in Indigenous research as a way of connecting to people from other Indigenous cultures. Ryan has used his work with COBRA to pass on the lessons learned from the project, and exchange ideas from his own personal experiences and culture.

Andrea Berardi is a senior lecturer in environmental information systems at The Open University in the UK. He has over 20 years' experience teaching, researching and building capacity to enable sustainable communities. He led the establishment, as co-director, of the Cobra Collective, a UK-based social enterprise to support community owned solutions.

Elisa Bignante is an associate professor of political and economic geography at the University of Torino in Italy. Her research interests include social marginalities, well-being and therapeutic landscapes, Indigenous geographies, and the use of participative and creative methods to support local communities.

Linda Birt is a senior research associate in the School of Health Sciences at the University of East Anglia in the UK. As a social scientist, she draws on qualitative methodologies to explore the health and social care experiences of older people and people living with dementia. She works on local and regional inclusive involvement research issues and has published on the ethical dimensions of public involvement in research.

Paul Boyce is a senior lecturer in anthropology and international development at the University of Sussex in the UK. He has worked on issues of sexual and gender diversity, health and well-being both in West Bengal, India, and internationally since the mid-1990s. His recent co-edited book *Queering Knowledge: Analytics, Devices and Investments after Marilyn Strathern*, published by Routledge, won the Ruth Benedict Prize (2020) for an outstanding edited volume.

Elaine Chase is an associate professor in education, health promotion and international development at the UCL Institute of Education in London. She was principal investigator for the ESRC-funded Becoming Adult project. Her teaching, research and writing explore the sociological dimensions of health, well-being and rights of individuals and communities, particularly those most likely to experience marginalisation and exclusion.

Judith Dean is a senior research fellow at The University of Queensland School of Public Health, and a registered nurse/midwife with over 25 years' national and international experience in sexual and reproductive health and HIV. In partnership with community, she has extensive experience in developing and implementing gender, sexuality and culturally appropriate models of care, health education and intervention.

Pawan Dhall has been engaged with queer community mobilisation in eastern and other parts of India since the early 1990s. He leads Varta Trust, a Kolkata-based gender and sexuality publishing, research, advocacy and training non-profit agency.

Anthony DiStefano is a professor in the Department of Public Health at California State University, Fullerton, USA. He conducts research on the social determinants of syndemic health problems, including mental health, violence, suicidality and HIV, mainly in California and East and Southeast Asia.

Ruth Edmonds is a social development consultant at Keep Your Shoes Dirty, an associate researcher in the Centre for Research on Families and Relationships at the University of Edinburgh, and Chair of the Research Expert Forum at the Consortium for Street Children. She is an ethnographer who works to generate local cultural and social knowledge to inform programme design with organisations, including the United Nations, governments, and international charities, trusts and foundations.

Lisa Fitzgerald is an associate professor and public health sociologist at The University of Queensland School of Public Health, with research interests in the health and well-being of people experiencing marginalisation and the social determinants of (sexual) health. Her research has informed service provision and policy in sexual health, HIV services, and sex work, both locally and internationally.

Ally Gibson is a lecturer in the School of Health at Victoria University of Wellington – Te Herenga Waka, New Zealand. She is particularly interested in experiences and responses to cancer; sexual and reproductive health; gender, sexuality and identity; and inequity, marginalisation and vulnerability in health. A key priority in her research is to partner with community organisations to promote enquiry driven by the needs and priorities of individuals and community members.

Liz Gill-Atkinson is a researcher and development practitioner with the International Women's Development Agency in Melbourne, and has expertise in qualitative, disability inclusive, participatory and feminist research across diverse social and geographic settings. Her doctorate thesis will explore how women with disabilities in the Philippines understand and undertake participatory research.

Semhar Haile worked as a project assistant on the ESRC-funded Becoming Adult project. She has experience of working in research, ranging from migration to gender studies and climate change. Semhar's reflections on refugeehood and migration are largely shaped by her own migration trajectory and background, as well as by interaction with members of her community.

Lakeram Haynes has 15 years' experience in community development and environmental management. His work experience in senior management and research and traditional foundation provide a strong base for continued leadership in community-based natural resource management in the North Rupununi, Guyana.

Rebecca Hodes is the Director of the AIDS and Society Research Unit at the University of Cape Town, South Africa. She is the co-principal investigator of the Mzantsi Wakho study, and has worked with Médecins Sans Frontières, the Treatment Action Campaign, Paediatric Adolescent Treatment Africa, the International Treatment Preparedness Coalition, UNFPA, UNICEF and UNAIDS to improve access to essential medicines and sexual health.

Brian Hui is the Director of Research and Evaluation at Special Service for Groups, Inc. (SSG), a non-profit human services organisation in Los Angeles. He conducts research in a variety of fields, including homelessness, behavioural health services, racial and ethnic health disparities, family violence, and democratic governance and power.

Deirdre Jafferally is an independent researcher with an interest in traditional knowledge and its use in community-based resource management and practices using participatory methods. With over 17 years' experience working in Indigenous communities, she uses this knowledge to help with the implementation and management of Cobra Collective projects in Guyana. Currently, she is managing a project on integrating traditional knowledge into national policy and practice in Guyana funded by the Darwin Initiative.

Elena Jeffreys is a sex worker and State Coordinator of Respect Inc, a statewide sex worker-led and run peer education and advocacy organisation in so-called 'Australia'. Elena has a doctorate in political science, criminology, policy and administration. Her research has focused on examining how sex worker organisations maintain political autonomy while also receiving external funding.

Jesse Jones is a peer educator with Queensland-based sex worker organisation Respect Inc. A community health worker and the founding editor of *Pink Advocate* LGBTIQ magazine, Jesse's interests include sexual health promotion and improving awareness of gender diversity.

Georgia Katsikis worked as a psychologist in the Department of Neurology at a major hospital in Greece where she provided assessment, treatment and counselling to patients and was involved in a number of clinical research projects.

A spinal cord injury in 2010 ended her career as a psychologist. In 2016, Georgia returned to the workforce as a community researcher and has since been involved in disability-focused projects as a co-researcher.

Angela Kelly-Hanku is head of sexual and reproductive health at the Papua New Guinea Institute of Medical Research and a Scientia associate professor in the Kirby Institute, UNSW Sydney. She is a social scientist and public health specialist who has published extensively on the social research pertaining to health and development in Papua New Guinea.

Tiff-Annie Kenny is a CIHR Banting Postdoctoral Fellow at the Faculté de médecine de l'Université Laval. She has had the privilege of collaborating with Indigenous communities in northern and coastal regions of Canada for over half a decade on research involving social and ecological determinants of health. Her research is informed by her upbringing gathering wild berries in a mining community in Northern Ontario, as well as by the intergenerational legacy of genocide which persists in her own family.

Santa Khurai is a writer, queer activist with 20 years' experience and champion of transgender rights based in Manipur. She is associated with civil society organisations All Manipur Nupi Maanbi Association (AMaNA) and Solidarity and Action Against The HIV Infection in India (SAATHII).

Ashley Lacombe-Duncan is an assistant professor in the School of Social Work and a member of core faculty in the Center for Sexuality and Health Disparities at the University of Michigan, Ann Arbor, USA. Her research centres on healthcare access and health equity, with a focus on community-based research examining healthcare access for people who experience multiple forms of intersecting oppression.

Randhoni Lairikyengbam is a social work professional with the non-governmental organisation SAATHII in Manipur, India. She is currently leading a European Union-funded action on reducing violence and promoting access to justice for LGBTIQ people in Manipur, Odisha and Telangana states.

Roanna Lobo is a senior research fellow in the School of Public Health at Curtin University in Western Australia, and manager of the Sexual Health and Blood-borne Virus Applied Research and Evaluation Network. Her research partnerships involve stakeholders in all aspects of the research process, and participatory research methodologies including co-design and peer-based research.

Carmen Logie is the Canada Research Chair in Global Health Equity & Social Justice with Marginalized Populations and an associate professor in the Factor-Inwentash Faculty of Social Work at the University of Toronto. Her research focuses on HIV/STI prevention, testing and care with people living with HIV, refugees and displaced youth, LGBT communities, Indigenous youth, and persons at the intersection of these identities.

Jullian MacLean is a registered dietitian and health administration graduate from the University of British Columbia. He works as a project director with the Inuvialuit Regional Corporation (IRC) in Inuvik, Canada.

Kahlia McCausland is a research officer at the Western Australia Sexual Health and Blood-borne Virus Applied Research and Evaluation Network and a doctoral researcher in the Collaboration for Evidence, Research and Impact in Public Health at the School of Public Health, Curtin University. Kahlia has experience conducting mixed-methods research and is particularly interested in how the social determinants of health affect people's sexual health.

Lyndsay McLean is a part-time senior lecturer in Anthropology and International Development at the University of Sussex. She was a core team member of the DFID-funded What Works to Prevent Violence Against Women and Girls programme. She is co-founder and senior associate of The Prevention Collaborative, a global network dedicated to preventing gender violence in the Global South.

Jenevieve Mannell is an associate professor at the UCL Institute for Global Health in the UK. She holds a Future Leaders Fellowship from UK Research and Innovation to improve the evidence base for preventing violence against women in the world's highest prevalence settings. Her research focuses on understanding the role of communities in preventing violence and protecting the mental health of women affected by it.

Agnes Mek is section head of social and behavioural research within the Sexual and Reproductive Health Unit, Papua New Guinea Institute of Medical Research. She is a social scientist who has conducted community-based research in partnership with young people and marginalised populations such as people living with HIV and people affected by resource extraction.

Francesca Meloni is a lecturer in the School of Education, Communication & Society at King's College London. An anthropologist working on migration, age, illegality and non-citizenship, she is interested in the interface between precarious legal status, young migrants and social belonging.

Jay Mistry is Professor of Environmental Geography at Royal Holloway, University of London. Her interests lie in environmental management and governance, participatory visual methods, Indigenous geographies, and fire management, particularly in tropical savannas.

Triphène Mpongo joined the Girl-Led Research Unit in 2015 under the DFID-funded La Pépinière programme, in Kinshasa, Democratic Republic of Congo, and continues working to support girl and women-centred research and programmes.

Alaa Nached is a clinical trial administrator at the Clinical Pharmacology GLP-1 Diabetes & Haemophilia Department, Novo Nordisk. Prior to joining Novo Nordisk, Alaa worked in the education sector and as a research assistant in the

Department of Public Health at the University of Copenhagen, cementing her interest in research and the challenges faced by refugees.

Richard Nake Trumb is an experienced researcher in the sexual and reproductive health unit and the Papua New Guinea Institute of Medical Research. He has more than a decade's experiences undertaking innovative research on issues as diverse as masculinity, medical male circumcision for HIV prevention, the prevention of violence against women, TB control, pregnancy and young people, and people in HIV serodiscordant relationships.

Nalisa Neuendorf is a senior research fellow in the sexual and reproductive health unit at the Papua New Guinea Institute of Medical Research. Trained as a social anthropologist, her work uses ethnographic and qualitative approaches to decolonising research practice. Her research aims to strengthen and integrate cultural, social and gendered understanding of sexual and reproductive health and public health to contribute to inclusive public health initiatives and policy in Papua New Guinea.

Claudia Nuzzo is a professional photographer with a master's degree in photojournalism from Naples' Academy of Fine Arts, Italy. She cooperates with different organisations and research projects to promote the use of photography and video in ways that give voice to marginalised groups. She is an active member of the Cobra Collective, a UK social enterprise, and the co-founder of Partaking, an NGO in Italy.

Bonita Pebam has been engaged in working on social justice for queer communities in Manipur since 2008. She is based in Imphal and associated with transgender community group All Manipur Nupi Maanbi Association (AMaNA) and the non-governmental organisation SAATHII.

Fiona Poland is a sociologist and Professor of Social Research Methodology at the University of East Anglia, UK. She uses, co-produces and innovates qualitative research methods and technologies to address the well-being and participation concerns of older people, people living with dementia, their carers and volunteers so as to support the agency and connectedness of disadvantaged and commonly excluded groups.

Nina Langer Primdahl is a research assistant in the Department of Public Health at the University of Copenhagen. She is especially interested in community-based research which involves the critical analysis of inequalities, stigma and hierarchies as well as the co-creation of solutions to improve the everyday conditions of traditionally overlooked communities.

Habib Rezaie graduated with a master's degree in data analytics from De Montfort University in 2019. He worked as project assistant on the ESRC-funded Becoming Adult project and for the Education of Unaccompanied Asylum-seeking Child project in Leicester.

Rowena Rivera, known to most of her family and friends as 'Weng', was born Deaf and grew up in a Deaf family in Manila in the Philippines. She served for many years with the Filipino Deaf Women's Health and Crisis Center and is a well-known activist in the Deaf community in the Philippines, advocating for access to justice for people who are Deaf and hard of hearing.

Bernie Robertson is a young entrepreneur using the skills learned from the COBRA Project to develop an ICT related business. While conducting participatory video research to identify community owned solutions, Bernie found participatory video provided a useful format for telling stories; videography is now a main element of his business.

Linda Selvey is a public health physician and infectious diseases epidemiologist. She worked for Queensland Health in senior positions, including as Executive Director, Population Health Queensland. She also worked as CEO of Greenpeace Australia Pacific. She is passionate about protecting human health from the impacts of the climate crisis and her research interests focus on translating policy into public health benefit and on research to influence policy.

Geordan Shannon is an Australian medical doctor, lecturer in global health and director of the Global Health and Development Masters' Programme at the UCL Institute of Global Health. Her work focuses on critical approaches to understanding gender and health systems, and transformative, transdisciplinary and transnational approaches to global health with a focus on systems thinking, human-centred design and participatory research.

Laura Sims is an associate professor in the Faculty of Education, Université de Saint-Boniface in Winnipeg, Canada. Her research focusses on learning for sustainability in formal and non-formal learning contexts. She currently teaches courses related to cultural diversity, Indigenous perspectives and education for sustainability.

Morten Skovdal is an associate professor in the Department of Public Health at the University of Copenhagen. He specialises in qualitative and participatory research, focusing on the contextual factors and relational processes that shape engagement with services and promote psychosocial well-being.

Suzanne-Melissa Sumaili joined the Girl-Led Research Unit in 2015 under the DFID-funded La Pépinière programme, in Kinshasa, Democratic Republic of Congo, and continues working to support girl and women-centred research and programmes.

Winta Tewoderos was a project assistant on the ESRC-funded Becoming Adult Project. During her time on the project she completed a college access course in health care. She is now in her second year of her undergraduate degree in psychology and criminology and on her way to becoming a neuropsychologist.

Jennifer Thompson is a postdoctoral fellow in the Center for Public Health Research at the University of Montreal. She has facilitated Photovoice, participatory video and cellphilming research and training in Cameroon, Canada, Ethiopia, Kenya, Mozambique, Myanmar, Sierra Leone and the UK. Her co-edited book (with Casey Burkholder), *Fieldnotes in Qualitative Education and Social Sciences Research: Approaches, Practices and Ethical Considerations*, was published by Routledge in 2020.

Naomie Tshiyamba Kabangele, joined the Girl-Led Research Unit in 2015 under the DFID-funded La Pépinière programme, in Kinshasa, Democratic Republic of Congo. She is currently completing her undergraduate studies while continuing to support girl and women-centred research and programmes.

'Alisi Tulua is the Program Manager of Health at the Orange County Asian and Pacific Islander Community Alliance, a non-profit organisation in Orange County, California, USA. She has participated in various community-based research focused on obesity, tobacco, behavioural health, cancer and diabetes, with a focus on racial and ethnic disparities. She is currently leading efforts to build and sustain health disparities research initiatives in Native Hawaiian and Pacific Islander communities in California.

Cathy Vaughan is an associate professor in the School of Population and Global Health at the University of Melbourne. She co-leads a programme of training and mentoring to build capacity to measure violence against women in Asia and the Pacific. Cathy also co-leads the Melbourne Social Equity Institute's university-wide programme of community-engaged research, and teaches and supervises postgraduate students undertaking community-based participatory research on health equity.

Sonia Wesche is an associate professor in Environmental Studies, Geography and Indigenous Studies at the University of Ottawa, Canada. She collaborates with Indigenous communities in Canada's North on research involving adaptation to environmental change, with an emphasis on food and water security.

Rebecca Xavier is an Indigenous researcher with the Cobra Collective. She is a proud Wapichan woman who was raised in the Makushi culture in the village of Wowetta, Guyana. She works with village elders and young people in the transmission and conservation of traditional knowledge using participatory methods.

Oinam Yambung is a trans man activist and leads Empowering Trans Ability, a support forum for lesbians, bisexual women and trans men in Manipur. He is passionate about karate, and lives with Sonia, his partner of 15 years, in Imphal.

Gul Zada is a service manager for refugee services with the British Red Cross in Leicester and was a project assistant on the ESRC-funded Becoming Adult Project. He is a community support volunteer for Leicestershire police and has worked as an interpreter for people going through the asylum process.

Acknowledgements

We thank our partners, Annie, Preecha and Dave, and children, Rosie and Matty, for their understanding and support while preparing this book. Thanks also go to Sarah Hoile for her editorial support throughout the process of preparing the manuscript for publication.

Section I

Critical perspectives on peer research

1 Peer research in health and social development

Understandings, strengths and limitations

Stephen Bell, Peter Aggleton and Ally Gibson

Introduction

Since the 1970s, there has been growing interest in research that takes inform-ants' perspectives seriously, not only for the sake of understanding but also for the development of policy and practice in tune with people's everyday lives and needs. One increasingly favoured approach is peer research, which describes a cluster of methodologies and methods underpinned by a commitment to recog-nising grass-roots expertise on health and social issues, and to working closely with community members as researchers on studies to enhance health and social well-being.

Despite differences, peer research approaches are based on the idea that 'peer researchers' have privileged access to groups that may be difficult to reach using conventional research methods (Price and Hawkins 2002; Coupland and Maher 2005). They aim to facilitate access to 'insider' or *emic* understandings of the health and well-being issues under study (Mutchler et al. 2013; Lorway et al. 2018). Despite the growing use of peer research approaches, working with lay community researchers is not without its drawbacks. Ethical concerns may arise about the extent to which peer researchers genuinely represent the population(s) under study; how best to manage trust and confidentiality during data collection; and how to cope with the burden of researching sensitive, and possibly harmful, issues that peers may experience in their own lives (Greene et al. 2009; Logie et al. 2012; Kelly et al. 2020). Questions have also been raised about the reli-ability and credibility of the data collected and analysed by people who do not have academic training, and who are required to manage multiple identities – as researcher, friend, family member, confidante and so forth – as part of the research process (Sterk-Elifson 1993; Coupland and Maher 2005; Greene et al. 2009).

This book derives from concern about the use of peer research in diverse sociocultural and institutional settings without critical engagement with funda-mental issues underlying this research approach. At the same time, however, we are keen to challenge the values that privilege the expertise gained through academic training above that derived from personal insight and experience in community settings. In particular, this book seeks to counter the marginalisa-tion of research experience and skills derived from people's local relationships and communities, while reflecting critically on the strengths and limitations of peer research itself. Chapters illustrate the potential for rigorous peer research to facilitate an in-depth understanding of health and social development among diverse populations in international settings, together with its impact on policy and practice, as well as for the individuals and communities involved.

Understanding peer research

Roles and definitions

Peer research seeks to engage with the everyday realities of the individuals, groups and communities under study, positioning members at the centre of the research process (Price and Hawkins 2002; Guta et al. 2013). Generally speaking, peer researchers are members of a group or social network who become trusted, equal members of a research team and work as researchers within their own communities (Price and Hawkins 2002; Greene et al. 2009; Logie et al. 2012; Guta et al. 2013). Peer researchers do not need to have prior research experience. Training is often provided for the demands of their roles, covering issues including recruitment and sampling, data collection, verbal and non-verbal communication, and research ethics (Price and Hawkins 2002; Coupland and Maher 2005; Mutchler et al. 2013; Bell et al. 2021).

Peer researchers typically take responsibility for looking after one or more aspects of research, from research question identification and study design, through participant recruitment and data collection, to data interpretation and analysis, and research dissemination. A range of peer research roles have been identified, and the terminology used to describe them varies across studies. It includes 'peer research associate' (Kaida et al. 2019; Zalazar et al. 2020), 'peer research assistant' (Greene et al. 2009; Logie et al. 2018), 'peer ethnographer' (Mutchler et al. 2013), 'lay researcher' (Nichter 1984), 'co-researcher' (Miled 2020), or 'community researcher' (Mosavel and Sanders 2014; Goodman et al. 2018; Lorway et al. 2018) – depending on the researcher's role and responsibilities.

Different models of peer research exist (Roche et al. 2010). In an 'advisory' model, for example, peer researchers join a steering, advisory or governance committee to provide insight and guidance at specific points in the research cycle, but may not be involved in the day-to-day implementation of research studies. In an 'employment' model, on the other hand, peer researchers are recruited as research staff and trained in skills specific to fulfil their role but may have little input into initial study conceptualisation and design. In a 'partnership' model, peer researchers are more likely to be leaders in a study, fulfilling an active, equitable role across all stages of research.

The origins of peer research

In the 1970s, social research in health witnessed growing interest in interpretive styles of enquiry, complementing earlier more positivist forms of understanding

(Bell and Aggleton 2016). Positivist research tends to be hypothetico-deductive in nature, using quantitative methods to study and develop 'law-like' statements connecting human knowledge, attitudes and behaviour. Interpretive research, in contrast, tends to use qualitative methods with the aim of accessing diverse, locally situated, subjective understandings of social life, recognising that how people see themselves and others is heavily contextual and located in social relationships. This growth of interest in interpretive approaches created space and legitimacy for innovative ways of engaging community members in social, health and international development research.

Peer research emerged from the participatory research paradigm promoted around this same time. This called for grass-roots, community-led problem identification and planning to solve local problems, and was based on recognition that community members are experts on their own lives, with a wealth of 'insider' knowledge and insight that outsiders likely lack (Chambers 1983). Nichter (1984), for example, described an early example of peer research as far back as 1979 in which 'lay researchers' conducted health research in rural communities in South India. The study provides an early illustration of a 'de-professionalisation' of social science research, signalling the ability of study participants to take a leading role in research due to their intimate understanding of local issues and concerns.

Since then, the use of peer research has grown in response to national and international agendas supportive of the right of individuals and communities to participate in planning and decision making that affects their lives. High-profile examples of this tendency can be seen in the 1978 *WHO Declaration of Alma-Ata* on primary health care (WHO and UNICEF 1978), the 1989 *UN Convention on the Rights of the Child* (UN General Assembly 1989), the 1999 UNAIDS statement on the *Greater Involvement of People Living with HIV/AIDS* (UNAIDS 1999), and the 2007 *UN Declaration on the Rights of Indigenous Peoples* (UN General Assembly 2007). Each of these declarations, conventions or statements signals the importance of meaningful participation and involvement by ordinary people and lay or community members in health and social development decision making.

But peer research also has origins of a rather different kind – in sociological and anthropological approaches to enquiry. The 'insider' research much favoured by interpretive sociologists holds that when there is a subjective or cultural proximity between the researcher and the communities, cultures, subcultural groups or institutions under study, more fruitful findings are likely to emerge (Hodkinson 2005). Similarly, the ethnographic approach favoured by anthropologists and some sociologists holds that building relationships of trust and rapport with communities is a prerequisite for good quality research to understand culture. What people say about their lives varies according to the familiarity and trust established between the researcher and the researched over time (Price and Hawkins 2002). Because of this, in anthropology, sociology and related disciplines, 'gatekeepers' may be used to facilitate introductions and support participant recruitment, and 'key informants' may provide advice, insight and interpretation of data.

While late 20th-century moves towards an interpretive paradigm supported a renewed emphasis on socially constructed lived experience, they did little to shift the fundamental 'social relations of research production' (Oliver 1992). A clear distinction between the researcher (as the one with specialist knowledge and skills) and the researched (as relatively powerless research subjects) tended to remain in place, and individual and community participation in some forms of interpretive enquiry could be as objectifying and alienating as involvement in positivist research. In consequence, alongside social movements for patient involvement in health, critical health and social scientists demanded change, to rebalance ownership and involvement and give power to populations who otherwise would remain marginalised, powerless or colonised (Oliver 1992; Kiernan 1999; Tuhiwai Smith 2012). In this way, peer research approaches can become a vehicle for emancipation and self-determination (Oliver 1992; Hecker 1997; Bell et al. 2021), especially when trained researchers work as 'activists' (Kiernan 1999) to support research instigated and led by marginalised peoples, with the goal of overcoming experiences of oppression and colonisation.

Contexts and application

Since their initial development, peer research approaches have been used in diverse contexts in South America (Fortin and Bertrand 2013; Zalazar et al. 2020), Africa (Price and Hawkins 2002; Chappell et al. 2014; Logie et al. 2018; Lorway et al. 2018), Asia (Brown et al. 2017; Lorway et al. 2017), North America (Sterk-Elifson 1993; Greene et al. 2009; Mutchler et al. 2013), Europe (Longfield et al. 2007; Buffel 2019; Hintjens et al. 2020) and Australia (Coupland and Maher 2005; Bell et al. 2021). In such settings, peer research studies have engaged a wide variety of populations. These include younger and older people (Buffel 2019; Bell et al. 2021), Indigenous peoples (Hecker 1997; Mistry et al. 2015; Goodman et al. 2018; Bell et al. 2021), migrant and refugee populations (Hintjens et al. 2020; Miled 2020), and people of diverse sexualities and genders (Longfield et al. 2007; Mutchler et al. 2013; Logie et al. 2018; Zalazar et al. 2020), among others.

Peer research approaches have been used to understand lived experiences of a broad range of health issues including HIV (Fortin and Bertrand 2013; Logie et al. 2018; Zalazar et al. 2020); sexual, reproductive and maternal health (Price and Hawkins 2002; Brown et al. 2017; Bell et al. 2021); autism (Aabe et al. 2019) and other forms of disability (Kiernan 1999; Chappell et al. 2014; Burke et al. 2019); dementia (Stevenson and Taylor 2019); and cancer (Mosavel and Sanders 2014). Social issues examined include sex work (Collumbien et al. 2009; Lorway et al. 2017; Lorway et al. 2018), housing and homelessness (Greene et al. 2009), natural disasters (Kita 2017), drug use (Sterk-Elifson 1993; Coupland and Maher 2005; True et al. 2017) and religious persecution (Vassadis et al. 2015; Miled 2020). In each of these fields, the aim has been to instigate and facilitate change informed by the life circumstances and experiences of those involved.

A range of research techniques has been used in peer research. They include participant observation (Mutchler et al. 2013; Lorway et al. 2018; Northcote and Phillips 2019), in-depth interviews (Price and Hawkins 2002; Bell et al. 2021; Hintjens et al. 2020), focus group discussions (Burke et al. 2019), Photovoice (Miled 2020) and participatory film (Mistry et al. 2015), among other visual techniques.

Strengths of peer research

Enhanced access

One of the main advantages of peer research is that it provides access to people and communities that may be hard to reach using conventional research methods (Elliott et al. 2002; Coupland and Maher 2005; Greene et al. 2009; Vassadis et al. 2015; Porter 2016). For instance, using purposive and snowball sampling, peer researchers can gain access to otherwise difficult to reach settings (Price and Hawkins 2002; Coupland and Maher 2005; Logie et al. 2012; Vassadis et al. 2015; Logie et al. 2018). These include nightlife settings – such as pubs, clubs, house parties and outdoor festivals – in which young people consume alcohol at harmful levels (Northcote and Phillips 2019), and locations in which drug use occurs, which may be intimidating or unsafe to 'outsider' researchers (True et al. 2017).

From the perspective of study participants, peer researchers can provide a 'safe' space in which to talk openly about otherwise difficult issues in a context devoid of serious power imbalances. The enhanced rapport that peer research can create has been reported in studies with people who use drugs in Australia (Coupland and Maher 2005), in research with young people in Ghana, Malawi and South Africa (Porter 2016), and with older people who felt more at ease and emotionally connected with peer researchers when discussing the development of age-friendly communities in England (Buffel 2019).

Insider insight

An enhanced understanding of health and social issues is likely to arise in research that builds on trust, cultural capital and cultural competence, and uses cultural protocols not available to outsiders (Porter 2016; Bell et al. 2021). Engaging peer researchers in study design and the development of data collection tools can ensure the right questions are asked, using appropriate vocabulary (Coupland and Maher 2005; Burke et al. 2019). Enabling respondents to engage in research on their own terms and using their own language can elicit fuller, more reflective accounts during data collection (Aabe et al. 2019).

Peer researchers' familiarity with the vocabulary, terminology and language that respondents use is a key benefit of insider status (Elliott et al. 2002; Northcote and Phillips 2019; Bell et al. 2021). For instance, peer researchers were able to use 'street jargon' with adults who used illegal drugs in one study in England (Elliott et al. 2002) and were able to explain in-jokes or novel rules in drinking games in research involving young people in Australia (Northcote and Phillips 2019). Being able to share accounts of lived experiences – especially behaviours and practices considered taboo, stigmatised or illegal – and referring to 'us' or 'we' in communication helped peer researchers make evident the cultural capital they shared with interviewees with disabilities in Senegal (Burke et al. 2019) and people who use drugs in six cities in the USA (Sterk-Elifson 1993).

Through such connections and relationships, peer researchers can generate a 'thick description' of participants' and communities' practices and experiences, which may not be accessible to outsider researchers. For instance, in one study, fieldnotes composed by female sex workers recruited and trained as peer researchers to work in teahouses in China provided detailed information about the social interactions in these leisure spaces; financial and condom negotiation between sex workers and clients; and the power relations between bosses and sex workers (Lorway et al. 2017). In another study in South Africa, young people with disabilities recruited as co-researchers uncovered and documented the secret language young people with disabilities use to discuss love, sex and relationships in front of adults (Chappell et al. 2014).

Facilitating impact and change

Through dialogue and the co-production of knowledge (Greene et al. 2009; Guta et al. 2013; Porter 2016) peer research can support the transition from community member to researcher, from researcher to advocate, and then to changemaker in policy and practice. Peer research practices not infrequently bring community members into relationships and dialogue with governmental and non-governmental agencies, making them partners in the development of community-focused policies and practices.

Internationally, peer researchers have worked with practitioners and policymakers to identify new ways of delivering programmes and services. Examples include the peer-led distribution of condoms and sexual health information in Zambia (Price and Hawkins 2002), the design of an incentives programme to enhance clinic-based STI testing among young Indigenous people in remote Australia (Bell et al. 2021), the development of an online training course for HIV service providers working with transgender women in Argentina (Zalazar et al. 2020), and enhanced awareness of the support needs of diverse male and transgender sex workers in Pakistan (Collumbien et al. 2009).

Specific examples of socio-structural change can be linked directly to the work of peer researchers. For example, working as peers, Aboriginal health workers in South Australia co-led a participatory action research study in the early 1990s which catalysed their inclusion in health service committee meetings (Hecker 1997). The work also stimulated the South Australian Department of Technical and Further Education to provide the first accredited training course for Aboriginal health workers (Hecker 1997). In a study in Sierra Leone, young women working as peer researchers set up a community-based organisation to provide other young women with sexual, reproductive and maternal health support, and income generation activities for young mothers (Otoo-Oyortey et al. 2016).

Pursuit of social justice

The (re)distribution of opportunities, responsibilities and resources in research, decision making and action to overcome experiences of injustice and oppression is key to social justice outcomes. Peer research can be social justice-focused, offering meaningful employment and capability-building opportunities, and showing respect for the expertise and knowledge that community members bring to research, while building social and community solidarity (Logie et al. 2012; Guta et al. 2013; Bell et al. 2021).

Participation in peer research can also provide meaningful income earning opportunities (Northcote and Phillips 2019; Bell et al. 2021) and the acquisition of new research skills (Logie et al. 2012; Aabe et al. 2019; Hintjens et al. 2020). It can result in the development of practical, soft skills such as creativity, social interaction, negotiation and collaboration with co-researchers (Aabe et al. 2019; Miled 2020). These in turn can enhance future employment opportunities. In a study focusing on early child development in rural Swaziland, translating research documents and data provided opportunities for co-researchers to use and further develop their bilingual fluency, an important technical skill required in many cross-cultural research, policy and practice settings (Brear et al. 2020).

Peer researchers report feeling a sense of accomplishment, pride and confidence when they reflect on the new skills gained, how their work has been valued by others, and being seen as capable and doing good (Coupland and Maher 2005; Logie et al. 2012; Bell et al. 2021; Miled 2020). Beyond these personal feelings, involvement in peer research can generate a sense of togetherness and solidarity within communities. A group of young Muslim refugee women in Canada explained how working together as co-researchers enabled them to hear other peers' voices and experiences, giving them the chance to reflect on their lives, journeys and identities, and creating strong connections between them (Miled 2020).

Strengthened solidarity networks, and a broader, more inclusive understanding of the diverse lived experiences of health and social issues within peer communities has, on occasion, also nurtured peer-led action for change (Kelly et al. 2020; Miled 2020). For example, a Somali woman, who sought refuge in England during the civil war in Somalia and whose first-born son has autism, co-led research with an academic researcher about culture-specific issues in autism service delivery in England with wide-ranging effects (Aabe et al. 2019). Findings from the study were shared via a support network she established for Somali families in her local community; with regional practitioners in health, education and social care in a film; with national policymakers via a presentation to the All Party Parliamentary Group on Autism at the House of Commons, London; and with general populations internationally through coverage on the BBC World Service (Aabe et al. 2019).

Limits of peer research – critical reflections

Methodological rigour and credibility

Concern has sometimes been expressed about the validity and credibility of data collected and analysed by people who are not formally qualified academically and have little research experience (Smith et al. 2002; Stevenson and Taylor 2019). Examples include a lack of rigour in the use of discussion guides in research practice, (Buffel 2019), lack of recall and notetaking expertise during participant observation (Mutchler et al. 2013; Northcote and Phillips 2019) and difficulty ensuring consistency in data collection undertaken by large teams of peer researchers (Smith et al. 2002; Northcote and Phillips 2019). Social desirability bias (Mutchler et al. 2013; Zalazar et al. 2020) can arise when study participants share experiences with peer researchers they see as coming from the same cultural or religious community. Criticism has also been directed at a lack of rigour in purposive, snowball sampling when peer researchers recruit friends, or friends of friends, into studies (Hintjens et al. 2020; Zalazar et al. 2020), while possibly overlooking other means of recruitment.

While there are recognised processes for establishing rigour in qualitative research (Bryman 2016), these are not always described in accounts of peer research studies. Without academic training, investigators using peer research approaches may not be aware of these issues in the first place. Transparent accounts of peer research document efforts to ensure rigour and credibility in study design and data analysis. These are based on principles of consistency of findings as a measure of reliability in qualitative research, and internal validity with respect to offering a convincing account of lived experiences in a specific setting (Coupland and Maher 2005; Collumbien et al. 2009). It is also important to explain how strategies such as rapport building, careful sampling guided by local expertise, triangulation of findings across different methods and researchers, and reflexive accounts of peer researcher positionalities (Price and Hawkins 2002; Collumbien et al. 2009; Ryan et al. 2011; Bell et al. 2021) can enhance the credibility and rigorous conduct of peer research practice.

Ethical concerns

A variety of ethical issues related to peer research exist. They include anxiety about the potential for coercive rather than voluntary recruitment of interviewees by peer researchers (Flicker et al. 2010), and the confidentiality of data collected by peer researchers from people they know well and see in everyday life (Coupland and Maher 2005; Flicker et al. 2010; Buffel 2019; Kelly et al. 2020). Concern has also been expressed that peer researchers are not always adequately compensated for their time and expertise and may be subject to exploitation (Elliott et al. 2002; Greene et al. 2009; Logie et al. 2012; Greene 2013; True et al. 2017; Hintjens et al. 2020).

Ethical questions are regularly raised about the safety of peer researchers. For instance, peer researchers leading drug studies in US cities have documented threats to their physical safety when spending time in public and private spaces where drugs were sold or consumed (True et al. 2017). Peer researchers in HIV research must navigate the disclosure of their own HIV status through involvement in a study and when sharing information with participants (Greene et al. 2009; Roche et al. 2010; True et al. 2017; Kaida et al. 2019). In contexts where minority sexual identities are stigmatised or sexual practices illegal, unwanted disclosure can have severe implications for peer researchers.

Emotional labour to cope with stressful feelings in the context of employment (Hochschild 1983) is frequently reported by peer researchers. In a study of young people's difficult transitions from social care in Northern Ireland, peer researchers noted how distressing it was to listen to interviewees describing similar experiences to their own, reawakening feelings of trauma (Kelly et al. 2020). Similar responses were described by African-American peer researchers involved in research about surviving cancer in the USA (Mosavel and Sanders 2014) and by HIV peer researchers in Canada, where one researcher described reading interview transcripts being 'like reading a thousand pages of tears' (Greene 2013, p. 146). These and related concerns should be taken seriously by the institutions and research team leaders who work with peer researchers (Greene 2013).

Navigating changing relationships and identities

Peer research can sometimes overstate the commonalities between peer researchers and study participants, and the ability of peer researchers to use 'insider' status to tap into existing networks of trust and rapport (Greene et al. 2009; Roche et al. 2010; Ryan et al. 2011). Simplistic conceptions of peer researchers' 'insider' positionality may hide a reality that such identities are fluid, intersectional and constantly negotiated across relationships and contexts (Kita 2017).

Such issues are rarely discussed other than in more critical analyses of peer research approaches. In a study with young Muslim peer researchers in England, a peer researcher described having to regularly clarify his religious and ethnic identity with participants, who perceived him as an outsider based on his physical appearance and dress which differed from theirs (Ryan et al. 2011). In a different study in the USA, a peer researcher described how through his own history of injecting drug use, he felt at home in contexts where injecting drug use occurred but found it difficult to relate to and undertake research with those who smoked crack cocaine (Sterk-Elifson 1993).

Insider relationships can also change as community members transition into peer researcher roles. During a study of young Muslim people's identities and experiences of belonging in Melbourne and Brisbane, Australia, the relationships peer researchers were expected to maintain with 'outsider' researchers and the formality of the interviews they were asked to undertake, caused difficulties (Vassadis et al. 2015). These constrained what interviewees were willing to say during recorded interviews, in contrast to what was communicated more freely between them as friends outside interview conditions (Vassadis et al. 2015).

These and other examples highlight the need for critical reflexive relationships and identities throughout the research process.

Power relations

There are numerous accounts of unbalanced power relations in peer research. Many of these reflect unequal power relationships between lead investigators, study coordinators and field researchers. Examples include community researchers in Canada feeling excluded from research decision-making processes (Greene et al. 2009; Guta et al. 2013); Indigenous researchers feeling unsupported to meet the needs of academics in Guyana (Mistry et al. 2015); community researchers lacking the power to cope with emotional burnout and stress in the USA (True et al. 2017); lack of involvement in study development and agenda setting by young Muslim peer researchers in Australia (Vassadis et al. 2015); and exclusion from authorship of a final report in the Netherlands (Groot et al. 2020).

Pre-conceived ideas about roles and responsibilities can inhibit the more equal distribution of power. In a study with people who use drugs in Australia, peer researchers' involvement depended on the extent to which health service collaborators were willing to accept and adjust to working with injecting drug users as colleagues rather than clients (Coupland and Maher 2005). Involvement of peer researchers who are young, illiterate or living with a form of disability in data analysis can sometimes occur only after academic researchers have already undertaken an initial analysis of data, seeking input once findings have already been sorted into predetermined themes (Vassadis et al. 2015; Brown et al. 2017; Burke et al. 2019).

Other factors affect the potential of peer research to become a means of professional development. There is a predominance of part-time, short-term, contract-based employment for peer researchers in universities and research institutes (Northcote and Phillips 2019; Kelly et al. 2020), and a lack of time to support team building, research mentoring, training and support (Logie et al. 2012; Greene 2013; Kaida et al. 2019; Brear et al. 2020; Kelly et al. 2020). Too often, peer researchers are expected to contribute to a single project only, with inadequate commitment to career development through contributions to multiple studies using different designs (Greene et al. 2009; Northcote and Phillips 2019; Bell et al. 2021). Opportunities to secure academic or technical qualifications through peer research work are similarly constrained despite the fact that many peer research studies take place in institutions with certificate, diploma and degree awarding powers.

Summary of contributions

Building on these insights, chapters in this book seek to problematise the uncritical use of peer research while illustrating its potential to aid understanding and contribute to policy and programme change in international health and social development. Authors begin by sharing current perspectives on peer research, raising critical questions about its development and application. The focus then shifts to work with 'hard to reach' participants and populations on particular health and social development themes. Following the discussion of the ethical issues that peer research raises, contributors show how this style of research can influence policy and practice.

With these goals in mind, the first section, titled *Critical perspectives on peer research*, offers perspectives on critical contemporary challenges. In Chapter 2, 'From the researched to the researcher: decolonising research praxis in Papua New Guinea', Angela Kelly-Hanku and colleagues from the Papua New Guinea Institute of Medical Research draw on their collective research experience to discuss the importance of Papua New Guinean researchers leading peer-involved research of local and international importance. The authors reflect on the changing nature of the relationships that have been part of their long-term commitment to decolonising research practices, processes and institutions – in Papua New Guinea and beyond.

In Chapter 3, 'Principled tensions when working with peer researchers: community-based participatory research with five Pacific Islander communities in Southern California', Brian Hui and colleagues explore the multiple dimensions of peer identity present in collaborative research. They show how tensions between principles of equity and scientific rigour manifest in the implementation of community-based participatory research, including in community-based organisations and in assumptions about peer insider and established outsider roles in research.

In Chapter 4, 'The limits of peer research? Reflecting on analytic challenges during health and social development programme research in Rwanda, Nepal, Ecuador and Uganda', Ruth Edmonds draws on work with non-governmental organisations in Rwanda, Nepal, Ecuador and Uganda to explore some of the limitations of peer research approaches. She highlights the challenges that can arise when using certain interpretive analytic approaches with peer researchers. These may inhibit the production of local knowledge about young people's experiences and perspectives for the purpose of evidence-based programming.

In the second section of this book, *Working with hard to reach participants*, attention shifts to the use of peer research approaches to enable engagement with difficult-to-reach groups to generate in-depth understandings of their experiences. In Chapter 5, 'People with dementia as peer researchers: understanding possibilities and challenges', Linda Birt and Fiona Poland illustrate some of the practical and theoretical challenges of involving those with dementia as peer researchers in data analysis processes, but show how involving people with dementia in data analysis has yielded positive outcomes.

In Chapter 6, 'Gender diverse equality and well-being in Manipur, North East India: reflections on peer-led research', Paul Boyce and colleagues focus on gender and sexual minority peoples' experiences of exclusion and prejudice in contexts of employment, education and welfare in the North Indian state of Manipur. Close work with members of community groups run by and for transgender people elicited perspectives grounded in lived experiences that it would not have been possible to access otherwise because gender and sexual minorities are so often excluded by more 'orthodox' research approaches.

In Chapter 7, 'Co-constructing knowledge about the well-being outcomes of unaccompanied migrant children becoming "adult"', Semhar Haile and colleagues provide an account of how peer research – involving a team of migrant young people of mixed legal status – was central to the design of a longitudinal study that investigated the different trajectories of former unaccompanied migrant children as they made the transition to adulthood. The authors reflect on peer researchers' own positionality and subjectivity within the research process.

In Chapter 8, 'Participation and power: engaging peer researchers in preventing gender-based violence in the Peruvian Amazon', Geordan Shannon and Jenevieve Mannell explore the power dynamics present when working with peer researchers in a participatory action research approach to preventing gender-based violence in remote communities in the Peruvian Amazon. By highlighting gender relations in their work, the authors signal the value of feminist approaches to participatory action research, which includes marginalised voices, values local epistemologies and looks closely at knowledge production and dissemination.

Chapters in the third section, *Understanding diverse issues*, offer examples of the diverse range of health and social development themes that peer research can tackle. For example, in Chapter 9, 'Participatory visual research exploring gender and water in Cameroon: a workshop model', Jennifer Thompson reflects on work with 130 community members in media-making and analysis workshops on water governance in Cameroon. She explores methodological and ethical challenges related to peer recruitment, supporting women facilitators, co-facilitation and engaging with structures of power.

In Chapter 10, '"I am the bridge": peer research with women with disabilities in the Philippines and Australia', Liz Gill-Atkinson and colleagues use the notion of reflexive solidarity to explore what researchers without disability should do to support peer researchers, acknowledging the emotional labour undertaken by peer researchers. Their chapter details how peer researchers have contributed to social change to concretely improve the circumstances of women with disabilities.

In Chapter 11, 'Reflecting on the role of peer researchers in collaborative Indigenous food security research in the Inuvialuit Settlement Region, Canada', Tiff-Annie Kenny, Sonia Wesche and Jullian MacLean discuss the evolving relationships between university-based researchers, a regional Inuit organisation, and the female, Indigenous residents of remote Inuit communities working as peer researchers during a participatory food costing project. They illustrate how engaging peer researchers can enhance the richness, rigour, nuance and local relevance of enquiry while affirming the importance of Indigenous perspectives on health and social research.

In the fourth section, *Ethical considerations*, contributors reflect on some of the ethical challenges arising in peer research approaches. In Chapter 12, 'Socio-ethical considerations in peer research with newly arrived migrant and refugee young people in Denmark: reflections from a peer researcher', Nina Langer Primdahl, Alaa Nached and Morten Skovdal highlight the different roles that

Alaa, a Syrian peer researcher, adopted in the study – as a fellow Syrian, a 'sister' and a researcher. The authors stress the importance of instigating dialogue about these different positions, and how they were negotiated, for socio-ethical research practice.

In Chapter 13, 'The ethical dilemmas of working safely with community researchers: lessons from community-based research with lesbian, gay, bisexual, transgender and queer communities', Ashley Lacombe-Duncan and Carmen Logie discuss the ethical challenges encountered by community researchers in multi-method community-based research studies in Canada, Jamaica, Swaziland and Lesotho. These include negotiating the conflicting identities adopted by community researchers, and the stigma associated with being a community researcher investigating 'taboo' issues of sexuality, gender and race, in socially conservative settings.

In Chapter 14, 'Blurred lines: treading the path between "research" and "social intervention" with peer researchers and participants in a study about youth health in South Africa', Rebecca Hodes describes the interplay between formal study protocols intended to ensure safe and ethical research conduct, and peer researchers' real-world adaptations when these protocols are put to the test in neighbourhoods and healthcare facilities. She highlights the imperatives of insight and negotiation, jointly with peer researchers and participants, to allow for urgent departures from formally agreed protocols.

In the final section of this book, *Influencing policy and practice*, contributors focus on the lasting impact of peer research approaches that seek to effect change in health and social policy. In Chapter 15, 'Farmer-led change: addressing environmental and health problems caused by widespread pesticide use in Costa Rica, Nicaragua and Honduras', Laura Sims examines the role of farmers in collaborative research in Costa Rica, Nicaragua and Honduras that aimed to bring about change in agricultural practices and policies regarding the harmful use, handling and storage of pesticides.

In Chapter 16, 'Using empowering methods to research empowerment? Peer research by girls and young women in Kinshasa, Democratic Republic of Congo', Lyndsay McLean and peer research colleagues describe the establishment and achievements of a Girl-Led Research Unit. The authors describe the benefits and challenges of a peer research approach in a context in which girls and young women navigate precarious circumstances to survive economically and socially, and discuss the longer-term impact of these research experiences on policy and practice within the Democratic Republic of Congo.

In Chapter 17, 'Lessons learned from Australian case studies of sex workers engaged in academic research about sex worker health, well-being and structural impediments', Roanna Lobo and colleagues consider the elements required for successful research partnerships between funding organisations, academic teams and sex workers employed as peer researchers. They argue that it is unethical to conduct sex work research without sex workers' involvement and a dedicated commitment to supporting changes to practice and policy that benefit sex workers.

Finally, in Chapter 18, 'The lasting impact of peer research with Indigenous communities of Guyana, South America', Jayalaxshmi Mistry and colleagues draw on their experiences of using participatory video and photography to identify community-owned solutions to environmental challenges in the Guiana Shield region of South America, as a means to further Indigenous empowerment and self-determination. They document the lasting impact of peer research for peer researchers, individuals and communities, as well as policy and practice, beyond project implementation.

In bringing together these different contributions, we have worked hard to illustrate how high-quality peer research can strengthen contemporary community-led qualitative and participatory research practice. Throughout this book, contributors highlight the importance of using peer research to ensure that local people meaningfully contribute to and lead research that emphasises emic insight and local expertise in the production of impactful knowledge to enhance policy and practice at community, national and international levels.

Rigorous peer research holds the potential for academics, practitioners and policymakers to learn more about the lived experiences of others. More importantly, a commitment to peer research approaches can initiate long-term, equitable, emancipatory research collaborations in which the researched become researchers, using their skills, expertise and knowledge to determine the need for – and lead – research studies to identify meaningful solutions to health and social development challenges.

We hope the contributions in this book inspire you to try out some of these methods and approaches for yourself and to document their application in additional contexts. Please join us, as we work towards securing a step-change in the critical and careful use of peer research in relation to social development and health.

References

Aabe, N.O., et al., 2019. Inside, outside and in-between: The process and impact of co-producing knowledge about autism in a UK Somali community. *Health Expectations*, 22 (4), 752–760.

Bell, S. and Aggleton, P., 2016. Interpretive and ethnographic perspectives – Alternative approaches to monitoring and evaluation practice. In: S. Bell and P. Aggleton, eds. *Monitoring and Evaluation in Health and Social Development: Interpretive and Ethnographic Perspectives*. London: Routledge, 1–14.

Bell, S., et al., 2021. Working with Aboriginal young people in sexual health research: A peer research methodology in remote Australia. *Qualitative Health Research*, 31 (1), 16–28.

Brear, M.R., Hammarberg, K., and Fisher, J., 2020. Community participation in health research: An ethnography from rural Swaziland. *Health Promotion International*, 35 (1), E59–E69.

Brown, E., et al., 2017. Men's perceptions of child-bearing and fertility control in Pakistan: Insights from a PEER project. *Culture, Health and Sexuality*, 19 (11), 1225–1238.

Bryman, A., 2016. *Social Research Methods*, 5th ed. Oxford: Oxford University Press.

Buffel, T., 2019. Older coresearchers exploring age-friendly communities: An "insider" perspective on the benefits and challenges of peer-research. *Gerontologist*, 59 (3), 538–548.

Burke, E., et al., 2019. Experiences of being, and working with, young people with disabilities as peer researchers in Senegal: The impact on data quality, analysis, and well-being. *Qualitative Social Work*, 18 (4), 583–600.

Chambers, R., 1983. *Rural Development: Putting the Last First*. New York, NY: Longman.

Chappell, P., et al., 2014. Troubling power dynamics: Youth with disabilities as co-researchers in sexuality research in South Africa. *Childhood*, 21 (3), 385–399.

Collumbien, M., et al., 2009. Understanding the context of male and transgender sex work using peer ethnography. *Sexually Transmitted Infections*, 85 (Suppl. 2), ii3–ii7.

Coupland, H. and Maher, L., 2005. Clients or colleagues? Reflections on the process of participatory action research with young injecting drug users. *International Journal of Drug Policy*, 16 (3), 191–198.

Elliott, E., Watson, A.J., and Harries, U., 2002. Harnessing expertise: Involving peer interviewers in qualitative research with hard-to-reach populations. *Health Expectations*, 5 (2), 172–178.

Flicker, S., Roche, B., and Guta, A., 2010. *Peer Research in Action III: Ethical Issues*. Toronto: Wellesley Institute.

Fortin, I. and Bertrand, J.T., 2013. Drug use and HIV risk among middle-class young people in Guatemala City. *Journal of Drug Issues*, 43 (1), 20–38.

Goodman, A., et al., 2018. "We've been researched to death": Exploring the research experiences of urban Indigenous Peoples in Vancouver, Canada. *International Indigenous Policy Journal*, 9 (2), Article 3.

Greene, S., 2013. Peer research assistant ships and the ethics of reciprocity in community-based research. *Journal of Empirical Research on Human Research Ethics*, 8 (2), 141–152.

Greene, S., et al., 2009. Between skepticism and empowerment: The experiences of peer research assistants in HIV/AIDS, housing and homelessness community-based research. *International Journal of Social Research Methodology*, 12 (4), 61–373.

Groot, B., Haveman, A., and Abma, T., 2020. Relational, ethically sound co-production in mental health care research: Epistemic injustice and the need for an ethics of care. *Critical Public Health*. doi:10.1080/09581596.2020.1770694.

Guta, A., Flicker, S., and Brenda Roche, B., 2013. Governing through community allegiance: A qualitative examination of peer research in community-based participatory research. *Critical Public Health*, 23 (4), 432–451.

Hecker, R., 1997. Participatory action research as a strategy for empowering Aboriginal health workers. *Australian and New Zealand Journal of Public Health*, 21 (7), 784–788.

Hintjens, H.M., Siegmann, K.A., and Staring, R.H.J.M., 2020. Seeking health below the radar: Undocumented people's access to healthcare in two Dutch cities. *Social Science & Medicine*, 248. doi:10.1016/j.socscimed.2020.112822.

Hochschild, A.R., 1983. *The Managed Heart: Commercialization of Human Feeling*. Berkeley, CA: University of California Press.

Hodkinson, P., 2005. 'Insider Research' in the study of youth cultures. *Journal of Youth Studies*, 8 (2), 131–149.

Kaida, A., et al., 2019. Hiring, training, and supporting Peer Research Associates: Operationalizing community-based research principles within epidemiological studies by, with, and for women living with HIV. *Harm Reduction Journal*, 16 (1), 47.

Kelly, B., et al., 2020. "I haven't read it, I've lived it!" The benefits and challenges of peer research with young people leaving care. *Qualitative Social Work*, 19 (1), 108–124.

Kiernan, C., 1999. Participation in research by people with learning disability: Origins and issues. *British Journal of Learning Disabilities*, 27 (2), 43–47.

Kita, S.M., 2017. Researching peers and disaster vulnerable communities: An insider perspective. *Qualitative Report*, 22 (10), 2600–2611.

Logie, C., et al., 2012. Opportunities, ethical challenges, and lessons learned from working with peer research assistants in a multi-method HIV community-based research study in Ontario, Canada. *Journal of Empirical Research on Human Research Ethics*, 7 (4), 10–19.

Logie, C.H., et al., 2018. Marginalization and social change processes among lesbian, gay, bisexual and transgender persons in Swaziland: Implications for HIV prevention. *AIDS Care*, 30 (Suppl. 2), 33–40.

Longfield, K., et al., 2007. Men who have sex with men in Southeastern Europe: Underground and at increased risk for HIV/STIs. *Culture, Health and Sexuality*, 9 (5), 473–487.

Lorway, R., et al., 2017. Sex work in geographic perspective: A multi-disciplinary approach to mapping and understanding female sex work venues in Southwest China. *Global Public Health*, 12 (5), 545–564.

Lorway, R., et al., 2018. Ecologies of security: On the everyday security tactics of female sex workers in Nairobi, Kenya. *Global Public Health*, 13 (12), 1767–1780.

Miled, N., 2020. Can the displaced speak? Muslim refugee girls negotiating identity, home and belonging through Photovoice. *Women's Studies International Forum*, 81. doi:10.1016/j.wsif.2020.102381

Mistry, J., et al., 2015. Between a rock and a hard place: Ethical dilemmas of local community facilitators doing participatory research projects. *Geoforum*, 61, 27–35.

Mosavel, M. and Sanders, K.D., 2014. Community-engaged research: Cancer survivors as community researchers. *Journal of Empirical Research on Human Research Ethics*, 9 (3), 74–78.

Mutchler, M.G., et al., 2013. Using peer ethnography to address health disparities among young urban Black and Latino men who have sex with men. *American Journal of Public Health*, 103 (5), 849–852.

Nichter, M., 1984. Project community diagnosis: Participatory research as a first step toward community involvement in primary health care. *Social Science & Medicine*, 19 (3), 237–252.

Northcote, J. and Phillips, T., 2019. Getting up close and personal: Using peer research assistants for participant observation in a youth alcohol project. *Qualitative Research Journal*, 19 (2), 132–145.

Oliver, M., 1992. Changing the social relations of research production? *Disability, Handicap & Society*, 7 (2), 101–114.

Otoo-Oyortey, N., King, E.G., Norman, K., 2016. Designing health and leadership programmes for vulnerable young women using participatory ethnographic research in Freetown, Sierre Leone. In: S. Bell and P. Aggleton, eds. *Monitoring and Evaluation in Health and Social Development: Interpretive and Ethnographic Perspectives*. London: Routledge, 110–124.

Porter, G., 2016. Reflections on co-investigation through peer research with young people and older people in sub-Saharan Africa. *Qualitative Research*, 16 (3), 293–304.

Price, N. and Hawkins, K., 2002. Researching sexual and reproductive behaviour: A peer ethnographic approach. *Social Science & Medicine*, 55 (8), 1325–1336.

Roche, B., Guta, A., and Flicker, S., 2010. *Peer Research in Action I: Models of Practice*. Toronto: Wellesley Institute.

Ryan, L., Kofman, E., and Aaron, P., 2011. Insiders and outsiders: Working with peer researchers in researching Muslim communities. *International Journal of Social Research Methodology*, 14 (1), 49–60.

Smith, R., Monaghan, M., and Broad, B., 2002. Involving young people as co-researchers: Facing up to the methodological issues. *Qualitative Social Work*, 1 (2), 191–207.

Sterk-Elifson, C., 1993. Outreach among drug users: Combining the role of ethnographic field assistant and health educators. *Human Organization*, 52 (2), 162–168.

Stevenson, M. and Taylor, B.J., 2019. Involving individuals with dementia as co-researchers in analysis of findings from a qualitative study. *Dementia*, 18 (2), 701–712.

True, G., Alexander, L.B., and Fisher, C.B., 2017. Supporting the role of community members employed as research staff: Perspectives of community researchers working in addiction research. *Social Science and Medicine*, 187, 67–75.

Tuhiwai Smith, L., 2012. *Decolonising Methodologies: Research and Indigenous Peoples*, 2nd ed. London: Zed Books.

UN General Assembly, 1989. *Convention on the Rights of the Child*. Available from: https://www.refworld.org/docid/3ae6b38f0.html [Accessed 1 October 2020].

UN General Assembly, 2007. *United Nations Declaration on the Rights of Indigenous Peoples*. Available from: https://www.un.org/development/desa/indigenouspeoples/wp-content/uploads/sites/19/2018/11/UNDRIP_E_web.pdf [Accessed 29 October 2020].

UNAIDS, 1999. *From Principle to Practice: Greater Involvement of People Living with or Affected by HIV/AIDS (GIPA)*. Geneva: UNAIDS.

Vassadis, A., et al., 2015. Peer research with young Muslims and the politics of knowledge production. *Qualitative Research Journal*, 15 (3), 268–281.

WHO and UNICEF, 1978. *Declaration of Alma Ata: International Conference on Primary Health Care, 6–12 September 1978*.

Zalazar, V., et al., 2020. Ethics and the treatment as prevention strategy among transgender women living with HIV in Argentina. *Culture, Health and Sexuality*. doi:10.1080/13691058.2020.1720821.

2 From the researched to the researcher

Decolonising research praxis in Papua New Guinea

Angela Kelly-Hanku, Agnes Mek, Nalisa Neuendorf, Sophie Ase and Richard Nake Trumb on behalf of the Social and Behavioural Research Team, Sexual and Reproductive Health Unit, PNG Institute of Medical Research

Introduction

Papua New Guinea is the largest of all Pacific Island nation states and territories and, like others within the region, was colonised by different peoples. Papua, known then as British New Guinea, and later called the Australian Territory of Papua, was colonised by the UK in 1883. New Guinea, known then as German New Guinea, was colonised by Germany in 1884. After World War II, the Commonwealth of Australia, as mandated by the League of Nations and United Nations Trust Territory, administered Papua and New Guinea as a single country until independence in 1975. Despite independence, the history of the countries remains marred by the practices of colonial rule – in research and other ways.

Research, to paraphrase the Māori academic Linda Tuhiwai Smith (2012), is dirty, marred by colonial practices and institutions, and Papua New Guinea has and continues to be researched, objectified and othered. Despite this, Papua New Guineans are becoming research leaders in increasingly equitable relationships with national and international collaborators and research partners. We are a group of Papua New Guinean researchers who comprise the Social and Behavioural Research Team in the Sexual and Reproductive Unit in the Papua New Guinea Institute of Medical Research, a national institute in the Pacific. Using examples and generated over 15 years, it is the transition from the researched to the researchers that we want to explore. Our work and praxis have been significantly different from the small-scale, short-term peer research practices and approaches that are becoming more prominent in health and social development research. Here we reflect on the changing nature of peer relationships that have been part of our long-term commitment to a bigger project: namely that of decolonising research practices, processes and institutions in Papua New Guinea.

Breaking the traditions of research in Papua New Guinea

There is a story – its truth is irrelevant – that once upon a time anthropology students from all over the world would put a pin on a map of Papua New Guinea to identify somewhere that had not yet been studied and make it the site for a new anthropological quest; the next frontier to be discovered and conquered by Western knowledge of the Orient. They would learn the language, do fieldwork, draw maps of hamlets, unpack complex local belief systems, extract information and then return to their home countries where an 'ethnography' would be crafted, far removed from the site where the study participants continued to live, often oblivious to how they were being represented and talked about. Time in the field was, and is still, sometimes recorded in years and months, as if to validate the authenticity of the academic account. Using such an approach, countless researchers have established stellar careers, many never returning to the field, or at least not for many years.

In this type of research praxis, the 'native' was/is essential to knowledge production, acting as porters, security, translators, gate keepers and 'local families'. For a minority of researchers, these relationships are genuine and authentic ones fostering reciprocity over many decades. In most scenarios, however, the work of these assistants is relegated to an acknowledgment rather than a co-producer of knowledge and co-author, with failure to recognise their contribution to and essential role in research.

Anthropology (like many disciplines) continues to be overdetermined by its colonial heritage and the study of the other (Morton 2010). This is the consequence not of the individual researcher per se, but a systemic outcome of the hierarchy of knowledge production in the disciplines and institutions which govern research. Partnering with the anthropological gaze has been medical research, also a system of power historically steeped in hierarchy over those who are studied, with the study of Kuru in Papua New Guinea providing an illustrative example in living memory (Anderson 2008). Examples of this power and its misuse provide the cornerstone for why decolonisation of research is so critical.

How then can we seek to decolonise research praxis, and make it less dirty? In our own work, we seek to move beyond the disciplinary practices that position Papua New Guineans as little more than research assistants – peers on short-term projects – and servants to outside researchers, instead supporting them to become the researchers. We do this from a position that values Papua New Guineans as peoples linked by language(s), communities, cultures, religions and relationships, by prioritising their role in leading meaningful research of local and international importance.

Our relationship and fit with 'peer research' is a complex one. Not all of us position our approach as part of peer research practice; some of us see our work as contributing to capacity building and international development, for example. In reality, the truth is probably somewhere in the mix. Our programme of research on HIV and sexual, reproductive and maternal health issues pressing to Papua New Guinea and its peoples relies on a smorgasbord of long-term relationships based on trust, respect and longevity. Unlike fly-in-fly-out researchers and consultants who have little regard for the maintenance of relationships, we are here to stay.

The value of the 'other' in knowledge production

In recent decades, peer research approaches have become more prominent as a means to increase the contribution of those with insider or *emic* perspectives on health and social development issues (Mutchler et al. 2013; Bell et al. 2021). Peer research has been defined as a process by which community members design studies and collect data from other people like themselves – i.e. peers – already known to them through membership of significant social networks associated with friendship, neighbours, work or kinship (Price and Hawkins 2002). This transformation in research praxis to include those who are usually 'othered' in knowledge co-production bring with it debates about the benefits and challenges of this model of research inquiry (Kelly et al. 2020). Concerns include doubts about the validity of research because of peers' inadequate research skills and an over-reliance on personal experience. Other writers more invested in a peer research approach value reflection on one's own experiences and the importance of reflexivity and voice in the co-production of research between peers and academics (Kelly et al. 2020).

In our own work, we use peer research approaches similar to Price and Hawkins' (2002) definition, but only for strategic purposes and with certain adaptations. Two recent biobehavioural studies with sex workers, gay and other sexually diverse men and transgender women – *Askim na Save* (Lit: Ask and understand) (Kelly et al. 2011) and *Kauntim mi tu* (Lit: Count me too) (Kelly-Hanku et al. 2018) – are noteworthy in this respect. During initial consultations, community members were reluctant to be interviewed by their peers. Instead, sex workers, gay and other sexually diverse men, transgender women and people with HIV were involved strategically in key roles associated with respondent-driven sampling methods used in biobehavioural surveys. These peers were equitable team members fulfilling vital roles, indistinguishable from others in the research team.

We write this as a team of professional researchers undertaking research that has led to change in programmes and policy in Papua New Guinea and which has contributed to new bodies of knowledge. Excluding Angela, the only non-ethnic Papua New Guinean, this team of Papua New Guinean researchers live in Papua New Guinea and can relate culturally to their fellow citizens in ways often different from the way in which the term 'peer researcher' is commonly used. Our reflections detail the nature of peer relationships involved in our research praxis. The chapter was envisaged by Angela and draws on long-term research experiences and conversations between us all.

Researching 'at home'

Two of the authors first came together as 'teacher' (Angela) and 'student' (Agnes) in a unique research apprenticeship in Papua New Guinea, funded by the Government of Australia in 2006 to support Papua New Guineans to undertake research on and about HIV 'at home' (Jackson 1987).

We use the term 'at home' here to recognise the work of Indigenous and other marginalised researchers to decolonise the discipline by studying their own people, communities and cultures. Within this apprenticeship, known as the cadet-ship programme, we aimed to establish a cadre of Papua New Guineans who could *work at* home – figuratively as Papua New Guineans, making homes in diverse geographical and cultural communities in our country – and provide the health research workforce needed to guide an evidence-based response to HIV and other health priorities. Ten cadets (of whom nine were graduates) were employed by the Papua New Guinea Institute of Medical Research for two years; three have since completed master's degrees, two are currently enrolled on master's degree programmes and one is undertaking doctoral studies.

Papua New Guinea has a long tradition of oral history and knowledge sharing through seeing and doing. In such a context, learning – as in apprentice-ship in a new trade – is best achieved by seeing and doing. For instance, cadets learned to design and conduct semi-structured interviews by repeated exposure to and involvement in interview studies. Their first investigation – which was conducted collectively – explored beliefs and knowledge about HIV among Year 12 students (Kelly et al. 2008). After that, we collectively designed and implemented the first study in the Pacific of people in receipt of HIV antiretroviral therapy (Kelly et al. 2009).

Today, four of the initial nine cadets remain at the Papua New Guinea Institute of Medical Research, three of them in our unit. The team has since expanded to include another 20 other Papua New Guinean researchers (three of whom had degrees at the time of their employment). As with the cadets, all team members are encouraged to think critically about and engage with the cultural practices of their communities, which is not always smooth sailing. By doing so, they move beyond being a peer – someone with similar or shared experiences – to look at themselves and others from further away and to question and make sense of practices and beliefs (Kelly-Hanku 2016). Agnes recalls training as a confronting time:

> We found that the world was not just black and white. There were other things. There were layers to our faith system and to our cultural system that we didn't understand. As we developed, did more reading and were exposed, not just in the office but through travel overseas to conferences and present, our experiences and minds broadened. This was awesome and it set us apart from other researchers in PNG.

The cadetship programme has now ended but training by seeing and doing has continued. The cadets who remain with us now share the same training and mentorship given to them as new researchers in the cadetship programme. This transfer of skills is important for the sustainability and local ownership of research. Being given the freedom to lead from within, and build others as one has been built, fosters independencies, not dependence.

It's not simply a matter of being a peer or not

What does it mean to be a peer? Do we all feel like a peer at the same time and in the same way? While each of us brings emic insight to our work, our reflections are varied. An important issue we focus on is how new and existing identities and relationships are shaped and change through research.

Being a peer

Agnes identifies as being a peer to research participants in several ways. Fluent in *tok pisin*, a language spoken throughout most parts of the country, albeit with geographical differences, she is able to communicate and relate to people in a way an outsider cannot. As a storyteller, one of Agnes' favourite reflections relates to contextualising speech and ensuring that metaphoric meanings are captured:

> There was one international anthropologist who came to Simbu Province and he hired a local man to be his assistant and translate for him. They did a study and the participant was asked a question through the researcher to which the participant replied, *'mipela slip wantaim pik'*. In translation, the local interpreter [assistant] said, 'they sleep with the pigs'. Leaving PNG and the local context in which the response was given, the international consultant wrote [up] his research paper and described the people with whom he met in Simbu as people who have sex with their pigs. So, you see the layer of translation for a Papua New Guinean. If we don't present people's stories and interpret well, and we don't explain clearly to the international consultants or researchers that come into our country … the meaning of the story changes. Literally, the translator was wrong. The context was missed in the first place, thinking that the researcher would understand what he was talking about. What the participant had said was, *'mipela slip wantaim pik'*, which meant 'we are living – sharing accommodation – with the pigs in the same house'. They did not have sex with the pigs! The story became distorted and people were misrepresented …. People use a lot of metaphoric language and we don't speak out direct … because of our cultural barriers …. We beat around the bush and you'll have to uncover the meaning of the story yourself.

Although Agnes is not living with HIV, through her work as a researcher she has developed a rare expertise in issues affecting people and their families who are doing so. She has become a trusted friend and colleague in many communities of people living with HIV around the country. On any one night of the week she will have people visiting her to seek advice on matters ranging from disclosing their HIV status to a child, to supporting a widow being blamed for her husband's infection and subsequent death. On other occasions, she is sent photographs of research participants' graduations and weddings. Since starting research with people living with HIV in 2008, she has re-engaged with local people many times through different projects, developing extensive social networks built on shared experiences. It is through such peer relationships that she is able to undertake new research with participants who she meets through ever-widening networks based on trust.

One leg in and one leg out

There are other members of our professional research team who experience many of the difficulties Papua New Guinea is known for having – problems with alcohol, violence and abuse, oppressive and damaging family expectations, and HIV. Some researchers try to separate their personal and professional lives more fully than others, but for some boundaries are more blurred. In this way, they are much like the people we study.

Richard has worked at the Papua New Guinea Institute of Medical Research since 2009. While originally trained as a draftsman he came looking for work and is now one of our unit's most experienced and valued interviewers. He lives and operates on the fringes of society and can access people, often men, whose practices are illegal, morally bereft (e.g. involved in the torture of women) or who form part of a subculture. For example, in one study on sorcery and violence in the Eastern Highlands, Richard was able to locate and interview men who had raped and tortured women accused of sorcery. In another study conducted in Kimbe, West New Britain, we struggled to identify men who had engaged in foreskin modification such as through the insertion of ball bearings. Richard said:

> Seeing first-hand the lack of progress we were making via the project coordinator I was requested to go out alone and mingle with the community and found these 'hidden' men. Everyone else in the team stayed back at the guest house. Several hours later a small group of men and myself turned up. From there more [came].

Richard is a very special member of our team. He thrives in the field, not in an office. He prides himself in being able to adapt to different communities by his actions (drinking, playing cards, chewing betel nut) and the way he dresses to suit the field. He has blurred the boundaries between being a peer and researcher for a long time, making him uniquely placed to recruit people into studies and to collect the most touching and rich data. Agnes recalled questioning why Angela had employed Richard in a study she was leading on masculinity:

> [Initially] I didn't want him on my team. When we went out to the field, I thought he was wasting his and my time. I thought he was not contributing at all. But then when I went through the interviews that he had done, it was another story. In his own way he can blend into a community when we are out in the field. It's very true he was not trained as a researcher and he doesn't have a degree or have exposure to research. But when we are out in

the field, I can trust him without reservation, and he can come back with the best data.

When employing researchers whose lives reflect those we study, some team members can find the apparent lack of professionalism and accountability in the office wearisome. While office-based tasks are an important part of research, we are reminded by Agnes of the importance of being a field researcher:

> When you keep an eye on him or breathe down his neck and he doesn't have that freedom to do what he needs to do, he doesn't perform. When he is given freedom, that respect and space, he does a marvellous job. A person doesn't have to be a trained social scientist or anthropologist or a professional in order to become a researcher.

An outsider

Sophie was recruited straight from university 10 years ago after experiencing difficulty finding work. Having only received a basic introduction to research at university, the opportunity to work as a transcriber and translator to 'earn money' put her on a research career path she never knew was an option. She was mentored to undertake research and was recently responsible for project management and learning new skills in data analysis and writing.

Importantly, she did not perceive that her relationships, age or identities defined her as a peer in the research she did. Her first projects focused on the prevention of mother-to-child transmission of HIV, and HPV and cervical cancer. An early project concerned sexually transmitted anorectal infection among female sex workers and transgender women. When asked to reflect on whether she was a peer, she said:

> Mum and Dad bought me up really strict …. My first experience leading a study was with the anorectal STI project where we asked about anal sex, willingness to be tested for anal STIs and piloted these diagrams on how to collect anal swabs for STI testing. When Angela took me out to conduct interviews it was my first time doing those types of things. She led the interviews and I watched and learned. The first thing to come to my mind was shock. I couldn't use these words she was using. What she was asking these female sex workers, wow! Honestly, I hadn't known that there was such a thing as anal sex. All I knew growing up was there was just sex!

Even though Sophie was fluent in *tok pisin*, she did not find a sense of sameness with participants as Agnes did. In the communities with which she worked, women used sexually explicit language and Sophie did not feel that she shared a common language or culture with them. But her language repertoire developed over time. This, combined with her youth, meant that we used her skills and identity strategically to engage her in research as a young woman who could speak openly and directly about sexual health and practices – even if she herself did not identify with those whose lives she was enquiring into and studying.

On the periphery

Many Papua New Guineans live outside the country, sometimes taking up citizenship and making a new country home, permanently or temporarily. These voyages are purposeful, often to access education and other opportunities, as well as safety and security. Those who travel away and only return intermittingly or not at all, or those who return after their schooling in other places, can find themselves in a precarious situation with respect to cultural identity. They are Papua New Guinean but not all Papua New Guineans see them as genuine, using phrases such as 'coconut' to describe them as being brown on the outside and white on the inside.

Born in Port Moresby but raised and educated overseas, Nalisa is an Australian citizen whose heritage lies in Kerema in Gulf Province. The opportunity to return home to conduct ethnographic research for her doctorate was an easy decision to make. In Papua New Guinea, she had relatives, a shared history linked to her parents and grandparents, and a commitment to meeting cultural and family obligations from afar. However, while undertaking her doctoral research in the Gulf, Nalisa was associated with the world of the 'white man'.

In Australia, Nalisa was employed as a 'peer' in research about the end-of-life care among Papua New Guineans. She took on this role on the basis of her social connection with study participants who were Papua New Guineans but living in Australia. Yet upon coming 'home' to Papua New Guinea to take up full-time work as a member of our team, Nalisa learned that being a peer was not as straightforward as it had been in Australia:

> It has been challenging coming home; feeling a sense of belonging at times, while also feeling I don't necessarily belong. Working as a researcher in Australia with Papua New Guineans, you get the sense that our connection exists because of shared experiences; we are all away from 'home', we are very much concerned about matters of 'home', while we are also very much immersed in Australian society and life.

Her prior immersion within 'white society' rendered Nalisa an outsider in the local Papua New Guinean community in which she worked – a peer in terms of heritage and shared language cultural understanding, but not in terms of belonging to the same societal group. Her position had to be negotiated with 'peers', in the context of persistent *othering* by peers. Contradictory and competing values regarding self and cultural identity coexist when located on the periphery. The experience for researchers like Nalisa highlights the peripheral position that is projected onto those who are educated and live overseas only to return; they do not belong as much as they should do.

Reflecting on the benefits and challenges of becoming the researchers

Local ownership, trusted relationships, local impact

From inception to completion and dissemination, our research is driven from within Papua New Guinea. We are rarely involved in work that is conceived outside Papua New Guinea or which lacks our engagement and expertise. We understand the limitations of funding rules that determine who can apply for and hold grants in different international settings and acknowledge that good relationships with funders matter. But partnerships matter more, and we respect our reciprocal obligations. We reject being engaged as the 'data collectors', 'research assistants' or a group of 'peer researchers' by other universities and research institutes who are not committed to work with us as equals or leading partners within the research cycle.

There are times when others outside Papua New Guinea have asked for our results before these had been made public or known to the Government of Papua New Guinea and local communities. This occurred when an international non-governmental organisation wanted access to new HIV prevalence data from *Kauntim mi tu* (Kelly-Hanku et al. 2018). By claiming the right to advocate for the needs of sex workers, transgender women and gay and other sexually diverse men, this particular organisation acted in a neocolonial way, disrespecting our research praxis and the accountability we had to communities. More generally, there can be a tendency for international researchers and other organisations to arrive, collect data and then leave. As one participant in a recent study put it:

> Once they come and collect information like this, they go for good. They don't come back with results or even follow-up. Probably they have other research to do. We have a lot of international research on MSM and when they go, they go for good and complete their essays and assignments and say this is what Papua New Guinea is like. This is what the MSM and Transgender are like. They go and get the good out of it. That one thing I don't like. We have to make sure they must bring it back. They must advocate in a way that we feel is acceptable.

In contrast, our team works to ensure that local engagement and ownership is central to all aspects of our work. This was highlighted in *Kauntim mi tu* in the way we engaged with communities throughout the life cycle of the research, particularly in terms of being supported and mentored to design community-specific recommendations which were then included in the study report (Kelly-Hanku et al. 2018).

One of the clearest rationales for working closely with peers lies in the relationships and networks that peers afford (Price and Hawkins 2002). It is these relationships – between researchers and communities – that has made engaging those framed as 'hard to reach' not at all difficult for us. In our work the relationships developed with communities are dynamic and varied. There are several communities – geographical and social – in which and with whom we regularly undertake research. Our history of research with people living with HIV, for example, or with sex workers, transgender women and gay and other sexually diverse men has engendered reciprocal and respectful relationships which continue today, both professionally and personally.

Rich data, interpretation and co-production of knowledge

Many outside researchers come and go from Papua New Guinea, and not all of them have an in-depth understanding of the complex societies in which they work or the multiple languages that may be spoken. *Tok pisin* – one of Papua New Guinea's lingua francas – is sometimes inappropriately described as broken English, but is a vibrant and complex language to understand. We conduct in-house training for staff for whom *tok pisin* is one of their first languages, and English most often a second one. The challenge is not simply one of translation or interpretation. It is important to recognise the nuance and beauty of speech to ensure the cultural significance of modes of description is captured and valued.

Understanding at the stage of analysis and writing up data is a collaborative experience. Being part of a team of Papua New Guineans is essential to both the interpretation and the co-production of knowledge. There may be times when the context or underlying meaning of an event goes unrecognised or not understood. It is common for us to ask each other for help in deciphering what is really going on in a transcript or interview, and we are never afraid to debate meanings and interpretations. Martha and Somu – former research cadets – run advanced classes in interpretation and quality assurance for the team, encouraging lively debate about meanings conveyed in *tok pisin* and how these are best conveyed in English.

The challenge of authorship

A research project is not complete until outputs such as reports, books, films or academic peer-reviewed papers are produced. This is where peer or local researchers are typically acknowledged or simply forgotten. At a bare minimum, all of our publications – and those of collaborators – name the team of researchers involved in knowledge production. The challenge lies in finding the time and support from funders and collaborators – as part of reciprocal obligations and the sharing of expertise – to ensure the team learns how to write for academic publication.

As a national research institute, we are reliant on funding and research grants. The pressure to publish is associated with research performance metrics the world over. Academic culture privileges writing and publishing in English and as the language of the coloniser, this adds another barrier to achieving first authorship in high-quality journals. While we put tremendous effort into other aspects of the research cycle, the development of academic writing skills is a challenging area. There are many reasons for this. One of them is the quality of undergraduate education in the country, where critical thinking is not encouraged and academic writing is weak. A second and more pressing issue relates to how funding is obtained and what staff are paid for. Being dependent on project grants, every moment of our time is accountable to an individual project budget. At any one time, half a dozen projects may be undertaking data collection, while others are at write up stage, or are being developed. Analysis and writing take time. Despite running qualitative analysis and writing workshops, time limitations and the demands of organising numerous projects concurrently have limited the development of expertise in critical thinking, analysis and academic writing.

Having been educated overseas and returned home with a doctorate, Nalisa has acquired many relevant skills and experiences. But without a postgraduate degree, induction into the culture of academic writing and the drive to publish as a first author, others are not so fortunate. Agnes and several others have been the exception. Driven by the deep desire to reach the next stage of her career, she recently wrote a paper from a photovoice study involving young women living with HIV (Mek and Kelly-Hanku 2017) and another on women's experiences of polygyny (Mek et al. 2018). Agnes reflected, 'when it came out, okay, me as a first author, Agnes Kupul Mek as first author, I tell you, I cried'. This aspect of our work is an evolution. It takes time, concerted effort and space away from the demands of data collection and project management to see a publication through to the end. It also relies on the reciprocal obligation of others to support us.

Conclusions

> We love what we do. There have been so many things written about us, about Papua New Guinean cultures and our people. We also believe in what we are doing – we are bringing our people's stories, their lives and contributing to our country's history. We are contributing towards policy, towards programs, to knowledge and we are putting our names on reports and papers. We are presenting at conferences and we are speaking out. I think people in the future will cite what we have done and what we are doing now for our people in order to bring about change.
>
> (Agnes)

Given our investment in the development of long-term, equitable partnerships and research capacity building, reflecting on the issues in this chapter is poignant at a time of heated debate about colonisation, Indigeneity and Black Lives Matter movements. Through daily activities and real-life practice, Papua New Guineans have been exposed to all aspects of the research cycle from conceptualisation to dissemination. While we have not formally conducted the research cadetship programme again, the principles underpinning the programme continue today, through ongoing practices of seeing and doing.

As a collective and as individuals, we are committed to ensuring our approach develops and expands. The long-term engagement we foster underpins concern to undertake the innovative and influential research that we do. Moreover, and perhaps most importantly, it is one of the reasons why our work is highly valued within the country, among those abroad who work in Papua New Guinea, and beyond. For those wishing to work in new, equitable and just ways with communities, individuals and institutes in low- and middle-income countries, we hope this chapter offers reassurance that this is possible and worthy of the effort. For those not yet convinced of this approach, we hope we have challenged them to rethink and work with Papua New Guinean researchers – and local researchers in other international settings – in ways that decolonise the research processes.

If we are to move to a place in which research is less dirty, and where it is owned, effective and impactful in countries such as Papua New Guinea, we must move beyond the limited ways in which 'peer research' has so far been imagined and applied. This means privileging the skills, practices and potentials of researchers and institutions in low- and middle-income countries so as to develop expertise in all aspects of the research cycle. Through our own efforts to do so, we have learned to value how our praxis addresses global agendas of decolonisation; we were and are remain driven by a deep commitment to doing what is just and right, and through this, making a lasting impact.

References

Anderson, W., 2008. *Collectors of Lost Souls: Turning Kuru Scientists into Whitemen*. Baltimore, MD: Johns Hopkins University Press.

Bell, S., et al., 2021. Working with Aboriginal young people in sexual health research: A peer research methodology in remote Australia. *Qualitative Health Research*, 31 (1), 16–28.

Jackson, A., ed., 1987. *Anthropology at Home*. London and New York, NY: Tavistock Publications.

Kelly, A., et al., 2008. *Young People's Attitudes toward Sex and HIV in the Eastern Highlands: Key Findings*. Goroka: PNGIMR and UNSW.

Kelly, A., et al., 2009. *The Art of Living: The Social Experiences of Treatments for People Living with HIV in Papua New Guinea*. Goroka: PNGIMR and UNSW.

Kelly, A., et al., 2011. *Askim na Save (Ask and Understand): People Who Sell and/or Exchange Sex in Port Moresby. Key Quantitative Findings*. Sydney, Australia, and Goroka: PNGIMR and UNSW.

Kelly, B., et al., 2020. "I haven't read it, I've lived it!" The benefits and challenges of peer research with young people leaving care. *Qualitative Social Work*, 19 (1), 108–124.

Kelly-Hanku, A., 2016. The political economy of evidence: A personal reflection on the importance and value of the interpretive tradition and its methods. In: S. Bell and P. Agleton, eds. *Evaluation in Health and Social Development: Interpretive and Ethnographic Perspectives*. Abingdon: Taylor & Francis, 17–31.

Kelly-Hanku, A., et al., 2018. *Kauntim mi tu: Multi-Site Summary Report from the Key Population Integrated Bio-Behavioural Survey, Papua New Guinea*. Goroka: PNGIMR and UNSW.

Mek, A. and Kelly-Hanku, A., 2017. *I Want, I Can, I Will: Photo Stories of Young Girls and HIV in Papua New Guinea*. Goroka: PNGIMR and UNSW.

Mek, A., et al., 2018. "I was attracted to him because of his money": Changing forms of polygyny in contemporary Papua New Guinea. *The Asia Pacific Journal of Anthropology*, 19, 120–137.

Morton, J., 2010. Anthropology at home in Australia. *The Australian Journal of Anthropology*, 10 (3), 243–258.

Mutchler, M.G., et al., 2013. Using peer ethnography to address health disparities among young urban Black and Latino men who have sex with men. *American Journal of Public Health*, 103 (5), 849–852.

Price, N. and Hawkins, K., 2002. Researching sexual and reproductive behaviour: A peer ethnographic approach. *Social Science & Medicine*, 55 (8), 1325–1336.

Smith, L.T., 2012. *Decolonizing Methodologies: Research and Indigenous Peoples*, 2nd ed. London and New York, NY: Zed Books.

3 Principled tensions when working with peer researchers

Community-based participatory research with five Pacific Islander communities in Southern California

Brian Hui, Anthony S. DiStefano, and 'Alisi Tulua

Introduction

Community-based participatory research typically involves close collaboration between a university or universities and community partner organisations (D'Alonzo 2010). Building on the strengths and resources of each partner, key qualities of the approach include a research topic that is perceived as relevant by participating communities; the equitable and respectful involvement of community partners in study design, implementation, data analyses and dissemination; ethical review that accounts for universal and community-specific human subject protections; group reflexivity, credibility and accountability across project partners; co-learning and capacity building at organisational and individual levels; shared decision making and ownership of data; and, when applied to health disparities, social change outcomes to improve community health (Israel et al. 2005; Flicker et al. 2007; Minkler and Wallerstein 2008).

A principal feature of community-based participatory research is a research team partially or wholly composed of members of the community under study (Guta et al. 2013). In research projects, these 'community researchers' (Mosavel et al. 2011) share complex relationships with people defined as peers – either community members who are study participants, or other researchers in collaborating institutions. Negotiating and renegotiating these relationships in the course of a project can contribute to tensions that challenge core community-based participatory research principles. In this chapter, we draw on the experience of our work in a 10-year health-focused community-based participatory research collaborative – Weaving an Islander Network of Cancer Awareness, Research and Training (WINCART) – to examine tensions arising between principles of equity and scientific rigour when working with community researchers.

Peer researcher relations and practices in community-based participatory research

Understanding peer research

We employ a definition of peer research that refers to a type of collaborative, participatory inquiry in which members of a target population participate directly in the research, as peer researchers in the project team (Price and Hawkins 2002; Guta et al. 2013). This type of research offers several benefits. As recognised members of the community being studied, peer researchers can draw on their 'insider' status (Elliott et al. 2002) to gain privileged access to population groups that might otherwise be missed or resistant to participate in studies led by academic and other institutional researchers without such peer credentials (Griffiths et al. 1993). Peer researchers can access their own social networks for participant sampling and recruitment (Price and Hawkins 2002). When more than one peer researcher is involved in a study, the benefit is increased by multiplying the social networks and milieux from which participants are recruited. This, in turn, can improve data validity (Elliott et al. 2002). Other benefits of peer research include relatively rapid data collection (Mutchler et al. 2013); an equilibrium of power between peer researchers and study participants (Kilpatrick et al. 2007); rich understandings of participants' sociocultural lives and practices (Mutchler et al. 2013); insider perspectives and interpretations during data analysis by peer researchers (Price and Hawkins 2002); and the potential for participation in newly empowering experiences and for skills development among peer researchers (Mutchler et al. 2013).

Locating peer research in community-based participatory research

In contrast to more conventional approaches that are typically controlled by university researchers, community-based participatory research aims for an equitable partnership between universities and communities throughout the research process (Minkler and Wallerstein 2008). In particular, these approaches emphasise participation, influence and shared control by non-academic researchers in research processes that lead to the co-creation of knowledge and initiate change (Israel et al. 2003; Flicker et al. 2007). In practice, community involvement can take different forms, from establishing community review panels and advisory groups, on the one hand, to having fully engaged community researchers working as formal members of research teams, on the other (Damon et al. 2017). As community-based participatory research has become more common and better funded, projects have increasingly opted for the latter (Guta et al. 2013). Positioning community researchers as highly participatory members of a research team can be viewed as a hallmark of good practice in community-based research (Greene et al. 2009), helping deconstruct traditional research hierarchies in an effort to reach the ideal of equity (Damon et al. 2017).

When working with community researchers, it is important to consider the nature of peer relationships that exist within research projects. The literature typically emphasises the relationships that exist between researchers on the project team who come from the community being studied (i.e. 'community researchers') and study participants who are members of that same community. This relationship can be defined around the existence of shared social networks (Bell et al. 2020), such as those comprising friends, co-workers or kin (Price and Hawkins 2002), and shared identities based on age, religion or culture (Vassadis et al. 2015). However, the definition of 'peers' can be extended to include the relationships between community researchers and academic researchers within project teams. This enables a closer focus on the ideal of equity that is at the centre of community-based participatory research projects (Roche et al. 2010). Additionally, community-based organisations frequently adopt the role of 'community partner' (Guta et al. 2013), by being the immediate managers or employers of the project's community researchers, either through temporary appointments or using their own permanent staff (Banks et al. 2013). This can create another, complicated layer of peer identity.

Tensions in community-based participatory research practice

There are inevitable tensions between the challenges of ensuring research equity and scientific rigour in community research. Research equity is achieved by full community inclusion in research processes, which have historically been the exclusive domain of university actors (Black et al. 2013). Efforts to create equity resonate with a trend toward decolonising research in the health and social sciences. Decolonising research methodologies challenge hegemonic research approaches that can undermine the local knowledges and experiences of formerly colonised and Indigenous communities. This kind of research is driven primarily by the worldviews and cultural values of the formerly colonised and Indigenous groups with whom the research is undertaken (Keikelame and Swartz 2019) and is thus an expression of community self-determination (Zavala 2013).

Research rigour is achieved through the use of sound scientific methodology and may be tested against indicators of trustworthiness for qualitative data such as credibility, dependability and confirmability, and the equivalents for quantitative data (i.e. internal validity, reliability and objectivity) (Lincoln and Guba 1986; Collins et al. 2018). The ways in which community-based participatory research seeks to improve rigour are well documented. Community involvement and co-leadership can enhance the quality and appropriateness of research questions and data collection instruments, the selection of data collection sites, the recruitment and retention of study participants, and the interpretation of data (Balazs and Morello-Frosch 2013; Nicolaidis et al. 2015; Mayan and Daum 2016). It can also identify accessible research dissemination strategies (Jagosh 2012).

Leveraging the assets of both academic and community researchers bolsters efforts to enhance research equity and scientific rigour (Balazs and Morello-Frosch 2013). However, academic and community partners sometimes prioritise equity and rigour in different ways, which can create tensions within a partnership (Fabrizio et al. 2012). These tensions may be misinterpreted as an irreconcilable conflict between these two core principles at the basic level of theory. Our central argument is that this is not the case. Equity–rigour tensions reflect challenges in enacting theory into practice, but this is not due to flaws in the theoretical framework, and these challenges are not insurmountable.

Researching with Pacific Islanders in Southern California

In 2005, the WINCART collaborative was founded as one of 25 community network programmes funded by the U.S. National Cancer Institute's Center to Reduce Cancer Health Disparities. Serving approximately 100,000 Pacific Islanders living in southern California, the mission was to reduce the disproportionate burden from cancer affecting five of the largest Southern California Pacific Islander populations: Chamorros, Marshallese, Native Hawaiians, Samoans and Tongans. The partnership included two academic partner organisations (California State University, Fullerton; and Claremont Graduate University School of Global Health) and eight community-based partner organisations (Orange County Asian Pacific Islander Community Alliance; Tongan Community Service Center; Samoan National Nurses Association; Guam Communications Network; Pacific Islander Health Partnership; Ainahau O Kaleponi Hawaiian Civic Club; Union of Pan Asian Communities; and Sons and Daughters of Guam).

Between 2005 and 2015, 12 research projects were executed with thematic foci on breast and cervical cancer, HIV, HPV, physical activity and nutrition. The projects used a range of quantitative, qualitative, mixed methods, and quasi-experimental approaches (Schmidt-Vaivao et al. 2010; Tanjasiri et al. 2011, 2019). The overall goal of the work was to address cancer health disparities by developing and implementing programmes to increase cancer awareness; explore community knowledge, attitudes and beliefs regarding risk and protective factors; and enhance culturally competent primary prevention, service access, navigation and survivorship. Working closely with community researchers was central to all the projects, and one specific aim of the programme was to increase the number of trained Pacific Islander researchers through training, mentorship and participatory research experience.

At the start of WINCART, Pacific Islanders in Southern California were already accustomed to different forms of collaboration. For instance, interdependence – which relies on social and community collegiality and cooperation – is a common feature of Pacific Islander cultures (Sripipatana et al. 2010). This manifests itself in cross-Pacific Islander collaboration in local social service provision and pan-Pacific Islander cultural festivals. However, there were also important differences between Pacific Islander groups, not only culturally and historically but also in ways directly relevant to the health disparities research we were doing. For example, Southern California Pacific Islander groups held variable immigration and citizenship statuses affecting health benefits eligibility (e.g. US states versus US territories versus sovereign states; Indigeneity; Compacts of Free Association). There was also unique cancer epidemiology in the source countries of Pacific Islander immigrants. The WINCART projects provided a formal structure in which these diverse Pacific Islander groups could leverage the strength of their shared cultural backgrounds while acknowledging the unique attributes of their communities.

Working with community researchers on WINCART projects

All projects depended on community researchers who were members of local Southern California Pacific Islander communities. In most cases, community researchers were staff members at the Pacific Islander–serving community-based partner organisations; several projects were led by Pacific Islander investigators based at academic institutions. Most community-based partner organisations did not maintain research staff on a full-time basis, so community researchers usually occupied additional roles, such as health educators, health practitioners, case managers, programme staff and administrative personnel.

Nearly all staff at community-based partner organisations had a similar ethnic background to the Pacific Islander communities they served. This was helpful in providing culturally humble services and programming. Shared ethnic identities allowed staff to better navigate cultural norms, expectations and taboos and ensured linguistic competency for monolingual clients. Many staff members also brought other identities and relationships that served service provision and research needs – including access to religious denomination networks, extended family networks, school alumni associations, generational associations and other geographical areas of Southern California. These 'peer' relationships and shared identities were critical in helping project staff fulfil their roles as service providers and community researchers, alike.

Academic and community researcher collaboration

Initially, the role of the academic partners centred on managing the research projects, strengthening the scientific process and maintaining relationships with funding agencies. In contrast, the role of the community partners centred more on engaging communities in study implementation and enriching the process with community insights. With time, however, the collaborative grew beyond those roles. Over the 10-year period, the collaborative invested heavily in building the capacity of community-based partner organisations to respond to emerging research opportunities, establish sustainable research and administrative structures, and train other Pacific Islander scholars to conduct research in the future. Community researchers leveraged their community access to raise awareness about research within their informal relational networks. As a result, over time, communities became increasingly familiar with research processes and associated issues related to power dynamics, expectations about the benefits of research, and meanings of risk to participants and their communities. Building community capacities around research was a collective undertaking by all members of the collaborative, intended to enable community researchers and participating communities to be equitable partners in rigorous research.

Community researchers were partners on, and in some cases led, all parts of the research process – from the identification and approval of research opportunities through to study implementation and data collection, research oversight and governance, and dissemination of findings. They were able to draw upon their community connections and cultural perspectives to make substantive contributions in each of these areas. Formal training was provided to community researchers by representatives from academic and more experienced community-based partner organisations on topics including study design, quantitative and qualitative data collection and analysis, and research dissemination. A mentorship programme for researchers from participating communities – from undergraduate to postdoctoral level – was also implemented to further bridge the gap between academic and community researchers. The project responsibilities of community researchers and community-based organisations subsequently broadened as they strengthened their technical skills through this training and their direct experience on projects. Community researchers presented and co-presented findings at academic conferences and co-authored peer-reviewed publications. In turn, academic research partners received training to enhance their ability to work respectfully, effectively and inclusively with community stakeholders in research. Community stakeholders included not only partner organisations within the collaborative but also elders, religious and social group leaders, local health and social services providers and regular community members who were not part of the research teams. This training typically took the form of informal coaching by other academic partners who were more seasoned in community-based participatory research, but it also offered opportunities for community researchers and community stakeholders to provide guidance on key cultural relationships and dynamics.

Projects undertaken as part of the collaborative were overseen by a collaborative-wide steering committee with a peer researcher majority, and separate project-specific community advisory boards. These committees and boards were responsible for helping all research partners navigate challenging situations, including issues of mutual trust and credibility, managing Pacific Islander religio-cultural taboos, and overcoming fears of community gossip (DiStefano et al. 2013), as well as balancing concerns of research equity and scientific rigour with the aim of maintaining a just and productive research experience.

Critical reflections on implementing peer research

The path to equity: participation vs. inclusion

In the context of the multilayered peer identities and relationships within the collaborative, it is useful to distinguish between concepts of participation and inclusion. Participation practices entail efforts to increase community researcher input and feedback. Inclusion practices entail continuously co-producing processes, policies and programmes for defining and addressing issues of community import (Quick and Feldman 2011). Although participation can provide robust data and support rigorous science, it does not necessarily allow community researchers to contribute in an authentic or fulfilling way. It can thus fall short of establishing full equity among research partners. Inclusive practices emphasise deliberation, discovery and two-way capacity building (Elmore 2005) through which community and academic researchers can both inform the research process (Feldman et al. 2009). In this way, inclusion is a better path to achieving the core principle of research equity.

A number of challenges were experienced when implementing inclusive practices to achieve equity within the WINCART collaborative. First, our approach involved a high degree of collaboration and coordination among academic and community-based partners. An authentically equitable deliberative process obliged partners to dedicate significant time and attention to communicate, educate and build trust to ensure that all partners were well-equipped for collective design, implementation and decision making. For busy academic partners and some of the smaller community-based partner organisations, this level of coordination and active participation compromised other core areas of work, including the delivery of direct services, teaching and publication obligations. These issues led some partners to hesitate about participating in projects and also tempted us to dilute inclusive practices to meet project timelines. Moreover, developing culturally attuned research protocols and materials across multiple Pacific Islander communities was complicated. The more partners that were involved, the more challenging it was to conduct a highly inclusive process, and, thus, the more difficult it was to maintain equity.

A second challenge lay in reconciling conventional research norms with the deliberative processes of co-design, co-implementation and co-ownership in our community-based participatory approach to research. Lengthy decision making processes to ensure equity – which included community and academic researchers adopting practices and processes expected within their associated organisations and community settings – strained the narrow research timelines. In some cases, these deliberative processes led to the adaptation and renegotiation of anticipated scopes of work to ensure that community needs, priorities and expectations were met appropriately.

Third, certain requirements associated with funding impacted inclusion dynamics, and thus equity. As is common with government grants, primary responsibility for the research officially lay with a principal investigator housed in an academic institution, rather than with the partnership collectively. This positionality was reinforced by direct communication between the funder and the principal investigator. It underscored the subcontractor status of community partners and thus many of the community researchers, and the disparity in indirect grant funds received. The effect was to create a partnership in spirit, but with a de facto imbalance of power among academic and community researchers and partners on these specific issues.

Despite these challenges, several actions were taken to enhance inclusion. The steering committee, co-chaired by a community researcher, represented all the constituent communities as well as the academic institutions. This body went to great lengths to maintain transparency among the research partners, regardless of uncomfortable conversations about trust, cultural humility and research competence. Research protocols and materials were co-designed by community and academic researchers and pilot tested jointly. Significant efforts were made to ensure the research funders gained a better understanding of the community-based research practices, processes and actors. For instance, academic partners proactively communicated with programme officers overseeing the grants for the US National Institutes of Health, encouraging funders to participate in regular site visits so that they could develop direct relationships with community partners and better understand the dynamics of these complex collaborative research projects.

Peer insider vs. established outsider researcher

At the inception of the programme, there was an expectation that building trust and understanding with community researchers would lead to higher levels of community engagement and inclusion in research projects. Specific effort was made to find and train Pacific Islander community researchers because they could speak local languages, were familiar with the cultures and had strong pre-existing relationships with their communities. As such, community researchers could contribute as experts in cultural protocols necessary to ensure the authenticity and cultural validity of the data. As subject matter experts and as staff members of community-based partner organisations, community researchers were central to ensuring the implementation of rigorous and equitable research. However, the assumption that as 'insiders' from local participating communities, community researchers employed in community-based partner organisations were better suited to the role of collecting data from communities than 'outsider' academic researchers required deeper examination.

Although in most situations the trust gained from participating communities through working with community researchers proved central to collecting data, in a few instances this was not the case. For instance, some community researchers reported that community-based study participants were less forthcoming with providing data about breast, prostate and cervical cancer, which sometimes involved discussing sexual behaviours deemed taboo to a largely religiously conservative population (DiStefano et al. 2013). Moreover, Pacific Islander communities in study settings had strong internal ties. As a result, individuals were at times reluctant to share information with researchers from their own community out of fear that the data could be used to criticise their familial and cultural relationship networks – upon which community practices, employment and other important customs depended.

These issues affected the work of community researchers in several ways. For instance, study participants sometimes faced greater levels of stress discussing sensitive topics with community researchers who, they knew, shared similar values. Accomplished Pacific Islander researchers were, at times, subject to being treated in accordance with community hierarchies based on family, age and gender. Such situations undermined their ability to conduct formal research activities. Within these community social structures, for example, it would have been inappropriate for a young community researcher to ask, let alone challenge, community elders about subjects of a sexual nature. On several occasions, community resistance to these conversations resulted in low attendance or poor engagement in focus groups. In contrast, there were instances when non-Pacific Islander academic researchers with formal credentials experienced less resistance from community leaders when discussing taboo topics because they were viewed as outsiders to traditional social hierarchies and were thus exempt from following cultural protocol. In this way, the outsider researcher was sometimes advantaged compared to community researchers who were bound up in insider, or community-based, peer relationships.

Such issues were experienced variably throughout the study projects. For instance, some community-based partner organisations did not encounter much resistance to elder participation because the community researchers themselves were considered to be elders, affording them an appropriate place in the cultural hierarchy. The health service training of staff in some community-based partner organisations who fulfilled the community researcher roles was also influential. For example, the Samoan National Nurses Association was staffed mostly by professional nurses, who experienced fewer barriers to discussing health topics. Specific aspects of community researchers' identities – associated with being an elder, health professional or young adult, as well as by religious denomination or ethnicity – afforded a different set of community access points as well as discrete barriers, depending on whom researchers were trying to access for data collection.

These dynamics did not undercut the demonstrated wisdom of engaging community researchers in research. However, they illustrated complex community social dynamics and warned against the uncritical application of undertaking research based on the supposed strengths of peer identities and relationships. The circumstantial presentation of barriers to community researchers (i.e. insiders) versus established academic researchers (i.e. outsiders) further exemplified how challenges encountered during study implementation can challenge assumptions about the benefits of drawing on peer relationships during community-based participatory research. In this case, an uncritical application of the principles of equity and rigour might have led community researchers to more steadfastly guard their role with and access to community participants, to the harm of the project. Yet the reflexivity and trust cultivated by the research collaborative allowed the partners to learn, be flexible and adapt.

Internal tensions within community-based organisations

This community-academic collaboration provided a rare opportunity for small local Pacific Islander organisations to advance and expand their missions through the creation of disaggregated data for, and from, the communities in which they work. In jurisdictions like Los Angeles and California, data regarding individual Pacific Islander ethnicities are typically aggregated into a larger 'Asian and

Pacific Islander' category that is so diverse, it renders the individual character-istics of smaller ethnic groups invisible (Srinivasan and Guillermo 2000). Thus, in some cases, the collaborative established the only available data sets to under-stand specific community needs and support funding applications for future work. Participation in the project also offered community-based organisations a chance to build their visibility and credibility as organisations with research experience, expand the capacity of their staff as community researchers and extend their work beyond direct services.

Nevertheless, whereas some community-based partner organisations had a research focus and did not provide direct services, for other community-based partner organisations, engaging in peer research came at the cost of resources and attention to core support for the communities they served. Such services ensured the immediate health and safety of the community and thus sometimes were more highly valued by the community. Limited time, resources and staff capacity were constraints in the smaller community-based partner organisations, and the prioritisation of commitments was a constant matter of conversation and strat-egy. Shifting the organisational focus to maintaining rigorous research protocols threatened to undermine the work that established and sustained organisations' trusted relationships with the community. This occasionally prompted serious reflection about the community-based organisations' mandate.

This shift in priorities was a particularly difficult transition for community researchers who also fulfilled other formal roles and responsibilities that over-lapped with research activities, such as assisting clients' access to health care or providing advice to families in distress. Pivoting between these different roles, sometimes in the span of a single conversation, was difficult for staff who wanted to perform well in all areas. Community-based partner organisations used sev-eral strategies to manage these competing demands. First, community researcher roles tended to use up enough staff time to warrant hiring additional staff from the community. This afforded partner organisations the opportunity to diversify skills and build organisational portfolios, expand community networks through new community–staff connections and greater community representation, and consolidate complementary staff roles and responsibilities to reduce the number of roles occupied by each individual staff person. Second, research funds in many cases reflected a reliable multi-year source of revenue, offering community-based partner organisations a form of financial stability difficult to establish with service funding alone. Finally, community-based partner organisations used the research findings to raise awareness and support for their work and to pursue additional funding and programme support.

Conclusions

By bringing academic and community perspectives together, community-based participatory research that involves community members as equal members of a research team can leverage the access and insight of community researchers to generate research that is both technically rigorous and inclusive of communities.

The role of partner organisations in maintaining inter-institutional relationships and facilitating the work of community researchers, while their own staff often fill the community researcher positions, adds a layer to and amplifies the contributions of the concept of shared identity. However, in implementation, working with community researchers also introduces new dimensions to the rigour-equity tension, such as advancing from participation to fuller inclusion while balancing robust research protocols, mediating peer insider and established outsider roles, and managing internal tensions and competing priorities at community partner organisations. This could be misinterpreted to mean these core principles cannot be reconciled in practice.

As the WINCART research collaborative demonstrated, making the effort to flatten power dynamics between academic and community researchers and investing in a genuine partnership can produce important research guided by the principles of equity and rigour. The avoidance of compromise and the pursuit of 'fully inclusive' or 'fully rigorous' may play into a divisive impulse to understanding the work through a lens that sees these principles as somehow mutually exclusive. Such an assumption would miss the point of working with community researchers in projects that involve academic and community-based research partner organisations. The aim is to cultivate trusting and durable research partnerships in which community researchers play a central role alongside other research actors and where the complexities of community dynamics and research methodologies can be thoughtfully negotiated to equitably co-produce knowledge.

References

Balazs, C.L. and Morello-Frosch, R., 2013. The three Rs: How community-based participatory research strengthens the rigor, relevance, and reach of science. *Environmental Justice*, 6 (1), 9–16.

Bell, S., et al., 2020. Young aboriginal people's engagement with STI testing in the Northern Territory, Australia. *BMC Public Health*, 20, 1–9.

Banks, S., et al., 2013. Everyday ethics in community-based participatory research. *Contemporary Social Science*, 8 (3), 263–277.

Black, K.Z., et al., 2013. Beyond incentives for involvement to compensation for consultants: Increasing equity in CBPR approaches. *Progress in Community Health Partnerships*, 7 (3), 263–270.

Collins, S.E., et al., 2018. Community-based participatory research (CBPR): Towards equitable involvement of community in psychology research. *American Psychologist*, 73 (7), 884.

Damon, W., et al., 2017. Community-based participatory research in a heavily researched inner city neighbourhood: Perspectives of people who use drugs on their experiences as peer researchers. *Social Science & Medicine*, 176, 85–92.

D'Alonzo, K.T., 2010. Getting started in CBPR: Lessons in building community partnerships for new researchers. *Nursing Inquiry*, 17 (4), 282–288.

DiStefano, A.S., et al., 2013. A community-based participatory research study of HIV and HPV vulnerabilities and prevention in two Pacific Islander communities: Ethical challenges and solutions. *Journal of Empirical Research on Human Research Ethics*, 8 (1), 68–78.

Elliott, E., Watson, A.J., and Harries, U., 2002. Harnessing expertise: Involving peer interviewers in qualitative research with hard-to-reach populations. *Health Expectations*, 5 (2), 172–178.

Elmore, R.F., 2005. Accountable leadership. *The Educational Forum*, 69 (2), 134–142.

Fabrizio, C.S., et al., 2012. Bringing scientific rigor to community-developed programs in Hong Kong. BMC *Public Health*, 12 (1), 1–8.

Feldman, M.S., Khademian, A.M., and Quick, K.S., 2009. Ways of knowing, inclusive management, and promoting democratic engagement: Introduction to the special issue. *International Public Management Journal*, 12 (2), 123–136.

Flicker, S., et al., 2007. Ethical dilemmas in community-based participatory research: Recommendations for institutional review boards. *Journal of Urban Health*, 84 (4), 478–493.

Greene, S., et al., 2009. Between skepticism and empowerment: The experiences of peer research assistants in HIV/AIDS, housing and homelessness community-based research. *International Journal of Social Research Methodology*, 12 (4), 361–373.

Griffiths, P., et al., 1993. Reaching hidden populations of drug users by privileged access interviewers: Methodological and practical issues. *Addiction*, 88 (12), 1617–1626.

Guta, A., Flicker, S., and Roche, B., 2013. Governing through community allegiance: A qualitative examination of peer research in community-based participatory research. *Critical Public Health*, 23 (4), 432–451.

Israel, B.A., et al., 2003. Critical issues in developing and following community based participatory research principles. In: M. Minkler and N. Wallerstein, eds. *Community-Based Participatory Research for Health*. San Francisco, CA: Jossey-Bass, 47–66.

Israel, B.A., et al., 2005. Introduction to methods in community-based participatory research for health. In: B.A. Israel et al., eds. *Methods in Community-Based Participatory Research for Health*. San Francisco, CA: Jossey-Bass, 3–26.

Jagosh, J., 2012. Uncovering the benefits of participatory research: Implications of a realist review for health research and practice. *Milbank Quarterly*, 90 (2), 311–346.

Keikelame, M.J. and Swartz, L., 2019. Decolonising research methodologies: Lessons from a qualitative research project, Cape Town, South Africa. *Global Health Action*, 12 (1), 1561175.

Kilpatrick, R., et al., 2007. 'If I am brutally honest, research has never appealed to me ....' The problems and successes of a peer research project. *Educational Action Research*, 15 (3), 351–369.

Lincoln, Y.S. and Guba, E.G., 1986. But is it rigorous? Trustworthiness and authenticity in naturalistic evaluation. In: D.D. Williams, ed. *Naturalistic Evaluation*. San Francisco, CA: Jossey-Bass, 73–84.

Mayan, M.J. and Daum, C.H., 2016. Worth the risk? Muddled relationships in community-based participatory research. *Qualitative Health Research*, 26 (1), 69–76.

Minkler, M. and Wallerstein, N., 2008. *Community-based Participatory Research for Health*. San Francisco, CA: Jossey-Bass.

Mosavel, M., et al., 2011. Community researchers conducting health disparities research: Ethical and other insights from fieldwork journaling. *Social Science & Medicine*, 73 (1), 145–152.

Mutchler, M.G., et al., 2013. Using peer ethnography to address health disparities among young urban Black and Latino men who have sex with men. *American Journal of Public Health*, 103 (5), 849–852.

Nicolaidis, C., et al., 2015. Community-based participatory research to adapt health measures for use by people with developmental disabilities. *Progress in Community Health Partnerships: Research, Education, and Action*, 9 (2), 157–170.

Quick, K.S. and Feldman, M.S., 2011. Distinguishing participation and inclusion. *Journal of Planning Education and Research*, 31 (3), 272–290.

Price, N. and Hawkins, K., 2002. Researching sexual and reproductive behaviour: A peer ethnographic approach. *Social Science & Medicine*, 55 (8), 1325–1336.

Roche, B., Guta, A., and Flicker, S., 2010. *Peer Research in Action I: Models of Practice.* Toronto: Wellesley Institute.

Schmidt-Vaivao, D.E., et al., 2010. Assessing the effectiveness of breast cancer education workshops among Samoan and Pacific Islander women in Southern California. *Californian Journal of Health Promotion*, 8 (SE), 1–10.

Sripipatana, A., et al., 2010. Talking story: Using culture to educate Pacific Islander men about health and aging. *Californian Journal of Health Promotion*, 8 (Special Issue), 96–100.

Srinivasan, S., and Guillermo, T., 2000. Toward improved health: Disaggregating Asian American and Native Hawaiian/Pacific Islander data. *American Journal of Public Health*, 90 (11), 1731.

Tanjasiri, S.P., et al., 2011. Needs and experiences of Samoan breast cancer survivors in Southern California. *Hawaii Medical Journal*, 70 (11 Suppl. 2), 35–39.

Tanjasiri, S.P., et al., 2019. Design and outcomes of a community trial to increase pap testing in Pacific Islander women. *Cancer Epidemiology and Prevention Biomarkers*, 28 (9), 1435–1442.

Vassadis, A., et al., 2015. Peer research with young Muslims and the politics of knowledge production. *Qualitative Research Journal*, 15 (3), 268–281.

Zavala, M., 2013. What do we mean by decolonizing research strategies? Lessons from decolonizing, indigenous research projects in New Zealand and Latin America. *Decolonization: Indigeneity, Education & Society*, 2 (1), 55–71.

4 The limits of peer research?

Reflecting on analytic challenges during health and social development programme research in Rwanda, Nepal, Ecuador and Uganda

Ruth Edmonds

Introduction

Evidence-based programming, whereby programme decisions are explicitly grounded in evidence in order to increase their efficiency, effectiveness and accountability (Miller and Rudnick 2012), has become prominent in international health and social development sectors (Edmonds 2016). As part of this trend, practitioners have increasingly used peer research approaches to gather local community perspectives to enhance the appropriateness and impact of programmes (DFID 2016). Peer research is sometimes treated as a panacea for the creation of more authenticity in programme research, due to claims that local community researchers ensure better access to insider perspectives (Price and Hawkins 2002) which can be used in evidence-based programming. This chapter reflects on peer research approaches used in partnership with non-governmental organisations to enhance sexual and reproductive health programmes with girls in Rwanda and to address sexual violence and exploitation among street-connected young people in Uganda, Nepal and Ecuador. The aim is to question assumptions that findings generated from peer research provide an adequate or more authentic evidence base for health and social development programmes led by non-governmental organisations. This question is raised on the basis that analytical processes that ground research findings in local ways of making sense of the world may be challenging to incorporate in peer research approaches.

The rise of peer research in youth-focused international development programmes

Peer research

Tapping into established relationships of trust, peer research is an approach in which community members are recruited, trained and supported to undertake research with members of their social networks (e.g. friends, colleagues, kin) or people with whom there is a sense of shared identity (e.g. by gender or sexuality) (Price and Hawkins 2002). Peer research has been characterised as a form of 'co-investigation', in which community members are brought into the research process not simply as respondents who are involved in 'co-production' of knowledge, but as co-researchers with unique community access and insight (Porter et al. 2012).

Peer research has become increasingly popular in the Global South (Porter 2016). This has occurred as part of the participatory research agenda that prioritises community ownership and partnership in order to generate insider understanding about issues and problems and identify locally informed solutions (Chambers 1983). Peer research with children and young people, in particular, reflects a move from viewing children as objects of research to social actors in their own right. It aligns with the children's rights agenda in social research (Johnson and West 2018), in response to children's right to participate, lead and be heard in decision making about their lives, enshrined in Article 12 of the United Nations Convention of the Rights of the Child (United Nations 1989).

Peer research approaches are perceived as beneficial for several reasons. They emphasise collaboration and partnership with local communities (Porter 2016). They position community members as experts on their own lives and social contexts, redistributing status, power and privilege from academically trained researchers and consultants to community members (Porter et al. 2012). They emphasise the capacities of community members to contribute to research and, in enabling skills development, these approaches increase the potential for them to become advocates, activists and transformers within their own communities (McLean Hilker et al. 2016). For such reasons, non-governmental organisations may use peer research approaches to partner with local communities to gather data for use in evidence-based programming for health and social development issues that affect these communities (Edmonds 2016).

However, it should not be assumed that peer research approaches always generate the kind of knowledge needed as a basis for decision making and action in youth-focused health and social development programmes (Lushy and Munro 2015). The inclusion of local researchers does not equate to guaranteeing adequate understanding of health and social development issues specifically in terms of how these are manifest themselves within local cultural systems of meaning and practice. Understanding such 'local knowledge' (Geertz 1983, p. 5) or emic understanding is considered critical to the formulation of locally meaningful evidence-based programming (Edmonds 2019). Local knowledge has been defined as 'understandings of understandings' not our own (Geertz 1983, p. 5). It is distinct from insider perspectives or local voices because it is concerned with knowledge *of* a place, people or practice, as understood by community members *within their own social and cultural frames of reference* (Miller et al. 2010). As such, local knowledge is not generated solely through the gathering of insider perspectives or local voices but through additional interpretive analytic approaches which make use of information about the local cultural system of meaning and practice *from which people formulate and create* their views, attitudes and opinions (Carbaugh 2007). While peer research approaches may be useful for eliciting insider perspectives, they may lack the necessary analytic approaches and skills needed to generate local knowledge about the cultural system for use in responsible evidence-based programming.

Youth-led research in international health and social development sectors

Encouraged by the children's rights agenda (United Nations 1989), academics and practitioners have examined the potential and prominence of youth agency in international health and social development settings (Bell and Payne 2009). More recently, demands for youth leadership in international development have been made due to a large number of young people between the ages of 10 and 24 in the world, the vast majority living in the Global South, with many excluded from decision-making processes that affect their lives both now and into the future (United Nations 2020). By using peer research approaches, non-governmental organisations can demonstrate a commitment to placing control in the hands of young people by involving them directly in attempts to understand their lives and develop programme solutions to the issues that affect them.

Yet such approaches have not been without criticism. Youth participation agendas and youth-led research approaches have been accused of 'collecting voices, rather than achieving change' (Johnson and West 2018, p. 5). The extent to which peer research enables young people to lead research and programme decision-making processes varies. Peer researchers may only be involved in certain activities within the research cycle, including the shaping of research topics and questions; designing data collection methods and tools; leading participant recruitment and data collection; driving data analysis; disseminating research findings with project stakeholders; or governing research processes (Edmonds 2016). They may be less fully involved in policymaking or ensuring research findings influence practice. It is common for youth research agendas to be driven by non-governmental organisations, rather than young people, so the extent to which power is placed in the hands of young people is questionable (Johnson and West 2018). Non-governmental organisations also frequently set research agendas, either implicitly or explicitly, by framing research within their own culturally based preferences and assumptions in terms of programme goals and designs for young people's health and social development which are not, in themselves, local or youth led (Rudnick et al. 2019).

Peer research findings have been used to understand specific issues and as a basis from which to act on local contexts. These critiques raise important questions about the basis for non-governmental organisations' use of peer research approaches and their associated engagement in communities. This is especially the case when organisations undertake research to inform health and social development programmes with vulnerable populations and/or operate in unfamiliar cultural contexts (Edmonds 2019). Given the growing popularity of peer research in the international health and development sectors, it is pertinent to reflect on the potential for – and limitations of – peer research as a basis for evidence-based programming.

The analytic limits of peer research in evidence-based programming

Taking the above issues as a starting point, it is appropriate to reflect on the limitations of peer research approaches in the context of two case study peer research experiences with non-governmental organisations which sought evidence for use in the design of health and social development programmes.

When insider perspectives are not enough

Between 2010 and 2011, I worked with 30 girls, aged 16–18, living in Kigali, Gitarama and Bugasera districts in Rwanda. The girls were recruited and trained as peer researchers to help understand more about girls' lives in urban, peri-urban and rural settings. The aim of the study was to explore aspects of 'girlhood' with a focus on health, education, money, marriage, pregnancy and ambition. Findings from the study were used to inform a range of sexual and reproductive health programmes. The research approach involved peer researchers in a week's training. This included structured sessions to develop the research agenda; craft research methods, tools and questions; practice informal interviewing skills; and learn about their ethical responsibilities (Edmonds 2016). After training, a period of data collection took place during which peer researchers were supported through one-to-one and group mentoring sessions. They were subsequently involved in an analysis week during which they reported back on their interviews and we worked together to generate some preliminary themes in their data. I then used these as a basis for further analysis and completed the final research report for the organisation which commissioned the work.

Additional interpretive analytic approaches were needed to sufficiently ground peer researchers' preliminary themes in an understanding of the local cultural system to enable sense-making of participants' perspectives and experiences in locally meaningful ways. This involved rigorous interrogation of local terms that appeared in interview narratives. For example, a Kinyarwandan term, *agaciro*, was used frequently by peer researchers and interviewees to talk about their lives. *Agaciro* literally translates into English as 'value', is closely connected with the notion of respect (*kwiyubaha*) and inherently connected to decisions and actions which girls make, leading to the gain or loss of *agaciro* (Edmonds 2016). To better understand how this term featured in girls' lives and use it appropriately as an analytic tool for making sense of the data gathered by peer researchers about girls' perspectives and experiences, Cultural Discourse Analysis (Carbaugh 2007) was used to treat the term as a cultural construct and investigate it more deeply. With theoretical origins in the ethnography of communication, where communication is treated as a socially situated practice, I drew on Carbaugh's (2007) model of 'cultural premises'. Cultural premises, described as 'formulations of shared understanding about some of the fundamental dimensions of human experience and expression' (Carbaugh and Boromisza-Habashi 2015, p. 549), include premises of being or personhood (identities), acting (communicative action), relating or sociation (social relations), feeling or emoting (experiencing and expressing affect), and dwelling (living in a place). Applying the model involved listening for local terms related to *agaciro* and exploring how they are manifested through people's practices and what forms and meanings people attach to them. As the peer-led data collection process was iterative in nature, consisting of peer researchers conducting interviews with participants, followed by group reflection sessions to explore what had been learned, the Cultural Discourse Analysis process was conducted alongside these activities.

This additional analysis process depended on the input, expertise and knowledge of peer researchers as key informants (Price and Hawkins 2002). Semi-structured interviews were conducted with several peer researchers to explore how *agaciro* appeared in local discourse and practice amongst girls; how it might be shown or recognised in daily life; how it related to different community identities and behaviours; how it might be obtained or given; and the kind of practices that might be observed in someone with and without *agaciro*, together with examples of it in action. The peer research model used enabled this extra analytic process to happen through opportunities to draw from the relationships I established with peer researchers, as well as their lived experiences growing up in communities in which the research was being conducted and their relationships with other members of their social networks. The peer researchers' intrinsic understanding of *agaciro*, alongside their direct experience of the research topics, gave them a unique position to act as co-producers of local knowledge about *agaciro*.

By relying on girls' dual role as peer researcher and key informant, we worked together effectively to produce the kind of analytic findings which could be used for responsible evidence-based programming (Miller and Rudnick 2012). Our understanding of *agaciro* and, in particular, how girls both gain and lose *agaciro* by engaging in certain behaviours, revealed a disparity between the organisation's goals and girls' goals for programming outcomes relating to sexual and reproductive health initiatives. This was because the concept of *agaciro* helped to show where programming objectives did – and did not – align with girls' perspectives about marriage and pregnancy. For example, organisational goals encouraged girls to have children later in life, while girls were more concerned with making sure they had children only once they were married. This was because they would lose *agaciro* if they had children outside of marriage. By contrast, having children at a young biological age was considered less of a problem by girls because it did not negatively affect their *agaciro* (Edmonds 2016). By understanding the concept of *agaciro*, the organisation was in a better position to develop programme goals and designs which were more relevant and meaningful to girls and more appropriate to the local context.

The unpacking of such cultural concepts and the process of making use of them to ground the data required particular techniques which peer researchers were not equipped to manage themselves. As a result, the project experience highlighted some analytic limits of this peer research approach. While the use of Cultural Discourse Analysis bolstered the analytic process, it diverged from the girl-led approach we had advocated for. Moreover, it exposed some of the limits in terms of what might be expected from peer researchers who have not experienced extensive discipline-based education and training in the theories and methodologies underpinning such ethnographic approaches. However, these experiences also pointed to the importance of integrating additional research techniques, approaches and skills within or alongside peer research processes to fill critical gaps in the generation of local knowledge for use in responsible evidence-based programming.

When meanings get mixed

Between 2016 and 2018, I worked with staff members at three non-governmental organisations in Kathmandu (Nepal), Guayaquilo (Ecuador) and Jinja (Uganda) who were trained as peer researchers to undertake programme research. The aim of the study was to develop resilience-based programming approaches for work with street-connected children affected by, or at risk from, sexual abuse and violence in each of the locations. Within each partner organisation, one social worker took on the role of peer researcher and was responsible for conducting research with other social workers, as well as with the street-connected children they worked with. They were selected as 'peers' predominantly based on their shared identity and experiences with other staff social workers who were involved in the study. However, social workers were also selected on the basis of their use of a 'street work' approach with children (Street Invest 2020). Street work is a child-centred, rights-based approach to supporting street-connected children conducted by trained, adult professionals. It takes place with young people where they are (i.e. on the street) and is characterised by relationships of trust that are established around children's values, issues, experiences and ambitions. Using this approach, the social workers had facilitated deep, long-term relationships with street-connected children, so were able to lead research with them based on the relationships of trust that had been established and which, effectively, positioned them within street-connected children's social networks.

In order to commence the peer research with these three social workers, they were first involved as key informants in an initial phase of data collection to generate cultural concepts of 'resilience' in each location. Cultural Discourse Analysis (Carbaugh 2007) was again used to establish these narratives of resilience which were based on terms for naming and describing resilience in locally relevant ways. These local narratives were used to inform the design of data collection tools. This meant tools could be oriented towards the gathering of stories in relation to perspectives and experiences which were *locally* recognisable as constituting resilience, as opposed to those which reflected hegemonic cultural values of Western societies where the majority of studies on resilience have been conducted (Ungar 2004). In Kathmandu, Nepal, the concept of resilience centred around a person's power and energy to react to difficult situations; in Guayaquil, Ecuador, it was connected to a person's inner strength and determination reflecting an individualised notion of identity; and in Jinja, Uganda, it focused on proactivity in seeking help and advising others, reflecting a relational cultural system which emphasises values and practices of interdependence rather than independence. The narratives of resilience were also used to ground data gathered by peer researchers in locally relevant understandings about what resilience is and how it is observed and felt in each setting.

In-depth interviews were then conducted with each peer researcher to learn about their roles, responsibilities, backgrounds and experiences. This enabled us to tailor group and individual research training sessions to their existing strengths, skills, capacities and needs. This was especially useful because the data collection approach we planned involved gathering stories about resilience and resilience-based programme implementation in each location and so made use of and built directly upon peer researchers' existing social work knowledge and skills in relation to listening and collecting case studies. After this, peer researchers attended a five-day training workshop to learn about the research objectives and the three data collection tools. The first of these took the form of a resilience story game which used a deck of cards developed specifically for each location in collaboration with staff and children to prompt story-telling with pairs of street-connected children. Each card featured a culturally relevant component of resilience drawn from the local narrative of resilience, presented in pictures and words (e.g. internal strength and power – Kathmandu; proactivity in seeking support – Jinja; feelings of determination – Guayaquil). The second tool was a diary entry, gathered through short conversations with individual staff members about their day-to-day decisions, successes, failures and next steps in delivering resilience-based programmes. The third tool was a journey mapping exercise, conducted with small groups of staff, to collect stories about staff experiences of working in resilience-based ways in terms of what happened, who was involved, what outcomes were achieved and what could have been done differently. Written instructions and writing up templates were provided for each to facilitate consistency across data outputs (e.g. interview notes from paired interviews; field diaries; and journey map notes). One template collected together peer researchers' reflexive notes focusing on their research practices, learning and use of the tools. These notes helped the design of additional bespoke training sessions to address the individual needs of the peer researchers and generated feedback to further refine the tools throughout the data collection process.

Once the training workshop had been completed, peer researchers were involved in three 'learning and innovation cycles' based on participatory action research approaches (Chambers 1983) to feed learning into the adaptation and innovation of the non-governmental organisations' respective resilience-based programme approaches. Each cycle lasted between three and five months and involved three phases: *learn* – involving data collection with children and staff to gather information about resilience-based programme experiences; *analyse* – engaging peer researchers in analysis to make sense of the data gathered; and *innovate* – involving the refinement of existing resilience-based programme approaches based on analysis and trialling these innovations in the next cycle. The participatory action research approach emphasised a dynamic, flexible and iterative approach to programme development which centred children's and staff members' experiences and perspectives in programme change. Having the three peer researchers work together also facilitated learning and reflection across organisations and international settings. 'Learning and innovation updates' were produced at the close of each cycle. Once the three cycles had finished, the peer researchers and I worked to produce country reports featuring specific organisational learning and innovation highlights, as well as a comprehensive final report (Consortium for Street Children 2018).

The *analyse* phase proved, once again, to be an area where additional input was required. This study adopted an interpretive thematic analysis approach (Strauss and Corbin 1998) with an emphasis on ensuring that interpretations of data remained rooted in local explanation rather than external frameworks for making sense of the world. Inductive analysis techniques were used to identify themes in the data that were not pre-determined and were recognisable and held some degree of importance to the communities in which the data was generated. To support peer researchers' participation, individual training was provided at the start of the first *analyse* phase. This involved sharing preparatory reading about this analytical approach and the analysis templates to be used during the process (e.g. code log templates to record codes in their data and thematic map templates to help them explore links between codes to identify patterns in their data). Peer researchers were responsible for organising and categorising their data (through a thorough reading and re-reading of data sets and open coding to develop code logs) and finding themes within the data (by reviewing code logs, identifying connections between codes and creating thematic maps), all of which was shared with me during one-to-one analysis sessions with each peer researcher.

However, during the process of thematising, peer researchers tended to attach meanings to the themes by drawing heavily on their own personal experiences, opinions and ideas. As such, they tended to make sense of themes in the research through their own frames of reference, rather than arriving at an understanding *through* the data itself, based on what participants had told them during the research. We used the one-to-one analysis sessions to work closely with the thematised data in a co-dependent way. I brought my interpretive analysis training, experience and approaches to the process, whilst peer researchers contributed their deep contextual and issue-based knowledge to the sense-making process. Together, we developed key learning statements about resilience-based programme practice and outcomes. This experience highlighted the challenges of peer-led interpretive analysis processes but also the benefits of codependent approaches to analysis.

Reflecting on the limits of peer research

Researchers and practitioners have responsibilities in terms of carefully considering what kind of knowledge is needed to address the questions they want to answer. In the context of evidence-based programming, how they choose to employ peer research is a key consideration to ensure research findings constitute a reasonable evidence base for decisions and actions aimed at improving people's lives. It is widely accepted that peer research approaches are beneficial for accessing and gathering local perspectives and experiences of social issues. However, knowledge production also involves data analysis which moves data from 'information' to 'evidence' by 'considering it in relationship to a goal in a systematic and principled manner' (Miller and Rudnick 2012, p. 27). It was the analysis phase of each study presented in this chapter that revealed the most pertinent limitations of peer research approaches.

When international organisations deliver programmes to improve conditions for vulnerable populations in unfamiliar cultural contexts, it is important for them to understand the cultural systems of meaning and practice in which they are operating so this can be used to make sense of people's perspectives and experiences. This is because such contexts may reflect a different set of cultural preferences and assumptions from their own and the meanings attached to decisions and actions in everyday life in local communities may not be clearly or easily understood (Scollo and Milburn 2019). Even when organisations operate within familiar cultural contexts, programme goals and designs may not align with the needs of local communities because these have not been understood from the vantage point of *situated* local experience by making explicit use of cultural phenomena to make sense of people's views, attitudes and opinions.

Such cultural understanding can be revealed through research involving theoretically grounded interpretive analysis processes that reveal systems of meaning and practice which can be used to make sense of perspectives and experiences – people's views, attitudes and opinions (Edmonds 2019). Moving beyond the simple organisation, clustering and description of data, such interpretive analysis, based in ethnographic practice, is both valuable and distinctive, allowing claims to be made that extend the individual stories gathered during data collection to say something about the cultural systems underpinning them. Such an approach requires disciplinary thinking and technical research skills involving interpretive analysis approaches to make sense of data in specific, strategic and situated ways.

Absent particular interpretive approaches and methods, the use of peer research can actually serve to further confuse and obfuscate, rather than reveal and clarify understandings of specific issues. Local people's communication and actions are based on specific assumptions that have normative bases. Whilst these may be shared with those in their own communities, they may not be immediately apparent to others and may be difficult to discern or navigate by those who are not local (Scollo and Milburn 2019). This can result in organisations believing that they understand more than they actually do, simply because they are not aware of what they do not understand when people's experiences and voices are not grounded in cultural phenomena (Edmonds 2019; Scollo and Milburn 2019). Consequently, with the type of evidence about cultural systems that such interpretive analysis yields, organisations are better able to understand appropriate ways of proceeding with health and social development programmes in complex local cultural settings.

Given this, the use of peer research by non-governmental organisations, where this does not involve interpretive analysis process, as a basis for designing and implementing programmes in local communities, is troubling. Responsibilities *towards* peer researchers being able to conduct their research without risk of harm, usually falling within the realm of research ethics, have been widely attended to in the literature (Molyneux et al. 2010). It is time to think about other responsibilities when conducting peer research, such as responsibilities in terms of the production of knowledge itself, to ensure it can be used as a reasonable basis from which, not just to understand, but to act upon lives of others in different local contexts through evidence-based programming.

New directions for peer research

This chapter has explored the ways in which we may have come to expect too much of some peer research approaches and what peer researchers might be expected to achieve in analytic terms. The burgeoning interest in peer research approaches among non-governmental organisations working in health and social development sectors shows little sign of abating. Given such enthusiasm, it is timely to reflect on what might be done to enhance peer research practices and models, as well as to acknowledge the limits of these approaches.

Where peer research approaches are being used, there are good opportunities to involve peer researchers directly in the application of their findings to evidence-based programme design and implementation. Information 'does not apply itself' (Miller and Rudnick 2012, p. 2) and it is not simply through the generation of particular kinds of knowledge that programmes to address social problems and issues are made possible. Rather, the use of such knowledge to inform programme decisions and actions is a strategic process in and of itself, involving specifically designed processes and tools (Miller and Rudnick 2012). Such processes typically fall outside traditional research cycles associated with design, training, data collection, analysis and reporting. One example is 'evidence-based design' (Miller and Rudnick 2012), in which programme design decisions are made by creating or selecting activities on the basis of grounded claims about the value of following a certain course of action in and for a given context. As such, evidence-based design is different to traditional service design or human-centred design processes (which use insights from data as inspiration for design ideas to test); from experience-based or opinion-based programming (which rely primarily on one's judgement) and from negotiation-based programming (in which programme options are created and selected through political negotiation among power holders) (Miller and Rudnick 2012).

However, processes and tools for using evidence in strategic ways to design programmes are rarely adopted by non-governmental organisations or in collaboration with local populations who have been involved in knowledge production either as participants and/or peer researchers. The possibility of incorporating such processes into peer research approaches presents a unique opportunity to create the kind of change that goes beyond 'collecting voices' (Johnson and West 2018, p. 5). This is because peer approaches are built on participatory principles which can facilitate the meaningful involvement of local community members right through the research process to the design of evidence-based programmes.

Greater recognition of the support required to involve peer researchers in all aspects of the research cycle, extending beyond analysis to the translation of evidence into programme design and implementation, is required. Successful experiences of peer researchers leading data collection processes have been widely documented (McLean-Hilker et al. 2016; Porter 2016). However, this chapter has illustrated the challenges with enabling peer researchers to conduct and lead interpretative data analysis. Such involvement requires careful consideration by funders, non-governmental organisations and their partners about what kind of knowledge is needed to answer the questions they have and, therefore, what kind of analytic approaches should be involved in the peer research. Where peer research findings are being used as a basis for decisions about local programming, there is inevitably a cost of inappropriate or inadequate analysis in terms of the extent to which findings can serve the responsible design and implementation of programmes. As the case studies here have shown, by carefully considering the kind of analytic approach needed, which may need to be co-dependent in nature, organisations are able to use peer research approaches which encompass relevant knowledge, skills and experience, as well as associated resources, such as time and funding.

Related to this is the need to encourage long-term commitment to education and training of peer researchers (Porter and Abane 2008) and more sustained relationships with peer researchers which build their skills and experience to undertake and lead analytic processes. This might include the provision of opportunities for peer researchers to build their skills through successive engagements in peer research projects (McLean Hilker et al. 2016) and opportunities to progress their research skills through formal academic qualifications (McLean Hilker et al. 2016). In some research contexts, it may be helpful to consider whether peer researchers who are in receipt of education, training and formal qualifications still retain enough of their insider identity to conduct the research, or whether a threshold is reached when they no longer retain a shared identity, access and trust with their social networks.

The rising popularity of peer research approaches in health and social development has not always been matched by critical thought and reflection about the possibilities and limits of this work. This chapter has illustrated limitations in terms of the extent to which peer researchers can reasonably engage with and lead on some analysis processes without appropriate – and potentially extensive – support and discipline-based training in the theories and methodologies themselves. This is pertinent given that the value of peer researchers' insider identities could be compromised by the inclusion of extensive education and training in some research contexts. The chapter, therefore, raises questions about what peer research models can – and cannot – contribute to in terms of producing knowledge about the cultural system of meaning and practice that can be used to ensure perspectives and experiences are locally situated to enable responsible evidence-based programming. It is time for researchers and practitioners to address such limitations by embarking on new directions which extend the benefits and opportunities of peer research approaches specifically to processes of analysis and its subsequent application in health and social development programming.

Acknowledgements

I am grateful to the Consortium for Street Children and its network members, Juconi Ecuador, S.A.L.V.E. International, Uganda and CWish, Nepal, for inviting me to be part of their research. I extend my gratitude to the Oak Foundation for their collaboration and funding. Finally, I thank Lisa Rudnick for her helpful comments on earlier drafts of this chapter.

References

Bell, S. and Payne, R.E.D., 2009. Young people as agents in development processes: Reconsidering perspectives for development geography. *Third World Quarterly*, 30 (5), 1027–1044.

Carbaugh, D., 2007. Cultural discourse analysis: Communication practices and intercultural encounters. *Journal of Intercultural Communication Research*, 36 (3), 167–182.

Carbaugh, D. and Boromisza-Habashi, D., 2015. Ethnography of communication. In: K. Tracey, ed. *International Encyclopedia of Language and Social Interaction*. Malden, MA: Wiley-Blackwell, 537–552.

Chambers, R., 1983. *Rural Development. Putting the Last First*. Harlow: Prentice Hall.

Consortium for Street Children, 2018. *Resilience-Based Approaches for street-Connected Children Exposed to Sexual Abuse and Sexual Exploitation*. Research Report funded by Oak Foundation. London: Consortium for Street Children.

DFID, 2016. *Putting Young People at the Heart of Development: The Department for International Development's Youth Agenda*. London: DFID Publication.

Edmonds, R., 2016. Generating local knowledge: A role for ethnography in evidence-based programme design for social development. In: S. Bell and P. Aggleton, eds. *Monitoring and Evaluation in Health and Social Development*. London: Routledge, 81–94.

Edmonds, R., 2019. Making agency visible: Towards the localisation of a concept in theory and practice. *Global Studies of Childhood*, 9 (3), 200–211.

Geertz, C., 1983. *Local Knowledge: Further Essays in Interpretive Anthropology*. New York, NY: Basic Books.

Johnson, V. and West, A., 2018. *Children's Participation in Global Contexts: Going beyond Voice*. Abingdon: Routledge.

Lushy, C.J. and Munro, E.R., 2015. Participatory peer research methodology: An effective method for obtaining young people's perspectives on transitions from care to adulthood? *Qualitative Social Work*, 14 (4), 522–537.

McLean Hilker, L., Jacobson, J., and Modi, A., 2016. *The Realities of Adolescent Girls and Young Women in Kinshasa: Research about Girls, by Girls*. Report by Social Development Direct. Available at: http://www.sddirect.org.uk/media/1700/la-pep-glru-full-report-english.pdf [Accessed: 24th August 2020].

Miller, D., Rudnick, L., and Kimball, L., 2010. Designing programmes in contexts of peace and security. SEE Bulletin, 4 (3), 3–7.

Miller, D. and Rudnick, L., 2012. *A Framework Document for Evidence Based Programme Design*. Geneva: United Nations Institute for Disarmament Research (UNIDIR).

Molyneux, S., Kamuya, D., and Marsh, V., 2010. Community members employed on research projects face crucial, often under-recognised, ethical dilemmas. *American Journal of Bioethics*, 10 (3), 24–26.

Porter, G., 2016. Reflections on co-investigation through peer research with young people and older people in sub-Saharan Africa. *Qualitative Research*, 16 (3) (Special Issue: Feminist Participatory Methodologies), 293–304.

Porter, G. and Abane, A., 2008. Increasing children's participation in African transport planning: Reflections on methodological issues in a child-centred research project. *Children's Geographies*, 6 (2), 151–167.

Porter, G., Townsend, J., and Hampshire, K., 2012. Children and young people as producers of knowledge. *Children's Geographies*, 10 (2), 131–134.

Price, N. and Hawkins, K., 2002. Researching sexual and reproductive behaviour: A peer ethnographic approach. *Social Science and Medicine*, 55, 1325–1336.

Rudnick, R., Witteborn, S., and Edmonds, R., 2019. Engaging change: Exploring the adaptive and generative potential of cultural discourse analysis findings for policies and social programs. In: M. Scollo and T. Milburn, eds. *Engaging and Transforming Global Communication through Cultural Discourse Analysis: A Tribute to Donal Carbaugh*. Vancouver and Lanham, MD: Fairleigh Dickinson University, 253–272.

Scollo, M. and Milburn, T., eds., 2019. *Engaging and Transforming Global Communication through Cultural Discourse Analysis: A Tribute to Donal Carbaugh*. Vancouver, BC and Lanham, MD: Fairleigh Dickenson University Press.

Strauss, A. and Corbin, J., 1998. *Basics of Qualitative Research Techniques and Procedures for Developing Grounded Theory*, 2nd ed. London: SAGE Publications.

Street Invest, 2020. *More about Street Work*. Available at: https://www.streetinvest.org/s treet-work-0 [Accessed: 24 August 2020].

Ungar, M., 2004. A constructionist discourse on resilience: Multiple contexts, multiple realities among at-risk children and youth. *Youth and Society*, 35 (3), 341–365.

United Nations, 1989. *The United Nations Convention on the Rights of the Child*. Geneva: United Nations.

United Nations, 2020. *World Youth Report: Youth, Social Entrepreneurship and the 2030 Agenda*. Available at: https://www.un.org/development/desa/youth/wp-content /uploads/sites/21/2020/07/2020-World-Youth-Report-FULL-FINAL.pdf   [Accessed: 24 August 2020].

Section II

Working with hard to reach participants

5 People with dementia as peer researchers

Understanding possibilities and challenges

Linda Birt and Fiona Poland

Introduction

Understandings of the realities of living with complex health conditions are con-textualised and strengthened when we hear directly from those who experience them. This way of knowing is especially important in complex conditions such as dementia. People with dementia experience a syndrome of symptoms including memory loss, decline in language, reduced forward planning skills and changes in behaviour. Symptoms impact in specific ways on the physical, psychological and social well-being of the person affected, their families and wider society (WHO 2014). Societal assumptions about the cognitive capabilities of people with dementia, alongside pragmatic procedural research challenges, have histori-cally excluded those living with dementia from research (Wilkinson 2002). In contrast and in this chapter, we report on how we prepared to work with indi-viduals with dementia as peer researchers, describing the practical analysis activi-ties we undertook before reflecting on the pragmatic and theoretical outcomes of the peer researcher activity. We draw some conclusions about the utility of peer research as a means of enhancing social citizenship.

Background

Since the 1980s, health and social care services in England have focused on seeking input from people who will be affected by service changes or related evidence-producing research (Staley 2009). This activity is called 'patient and public involvement'. In 1996, the English government funded the organisation, INVOLVE, as an advisory group working to 'bring together expertise, insight and experience in the field of public involvement in research ... as an essential part of the process by which research is identified, prioritised, designed, conducted and disseminated' (INVOLVE 2019). Patient and public involvement is now a requirement of many research funding bodies and takes many forms, including lay people reviewing patient information sheets, commenting on acceptability of data collection methods, and inputting into relevant policy and practice out-comes (Boote et al. 2010). A distinctive form of patient and public involve-ment is peer or co-research, where people living with a health condition work alongside the research team, not merely in reviewing materials but in generating research data and results (Hartley and Benington 2000).

In dementia research, the right for people with dementia to be involved in research is frequently curtailed by the negative assumptions of others. Historically, academics and clinicians have felt there is an ethical need to protect the frail and a clinical expectation that the symptoms of the disease render those with dementia incapable of being reliable research informants (Moore and Howlett 2003). Nationally and internationally, there are now specific groups striving to support people with dementia to have a voice in research and practice (Gove et al. 2018). However, there is no policy requirement to include particular categories of people within patient and public involvement; family carers still often represent the experience of the person with dementia. There are major flaws in such a proxy approach to research involvement, as the lived experience of those with dementia may differ from their carers' perceptions of their experience (Charlesworth 2018). Being part of patient and public involvement activities has positive benefits for individuals (Brett et al. 2014); however, there is little empirical evidence on its impact on research theory. Therefore, it is timely to explore both the pragmatic and theoretical realities of involving people with dementia in peer research, as a distinct form of patient and public involvement activity.

Peer research approaches have the potential to address inherent power imbalances often present in 'traditional' research. Peer research respects 'the researched group ... [and] their own views and abilities' (Alderson 2011, p. 241), with peer researchers' experiences 'unmediated by entrenched professional positions' (Clough et al. 2006, p. 5). A particular challenge for implementing peer research in dementia studies is formulated in the societal discourse that positions people with dementia as frail and vulnerable, lacking capability or agency. Such a biomedical lens on capability is counterbalanced both by those living with dementia who have spoken out about their condition (Dementia Action Alliance 2019) and by academic debate that illustrates the agentic abilities of people with dementia to make choices and reflect on how others perceive them (Birt et al. 2017; Birt et al. 2019a).

Being involved in peer research may counteract negative stigmatising attitudes by enabling people with dementia to be, and be seen as, social citizens. Social citizenship recognises that a person has 'rights, history, and competencies' including the right to maintain relationships, participate and have status in their social communities, while also acknowledging that such involvement may need to be facilitated (Bartlett and O'Conner 2010, p. 39). Peer research is an activity that creates a space for reinforcing the history and social status of people with dementia. However, ethical tensions can develop when academics attempt to blur and shift power and roles in a research environment (Banks et al. 2013).

Against this background of historical exclusion and the recent impetus to be more inclusive and respectful of the capabilities and wishes of people with dementia, we decided to include peer research activity in qualitative data analysis within a study exploring ways in which to support independence in people with dementia.

Working with people with dementia as peer researchers during data analysis

The involvement of peer researchers in data analysis activity took place during a five-year programme, called the PRIDE study (Yates et al. 2019). The ethos of the programme was on people being supported to remain as independent as possible in making choices about aspects of their life and living well at home. The tenet of peer research as a means of enabling social citizenship had good fit with the overall study aim.

Our peer research approach was informed by a structured literature review – the review was undertaken in collaboration with the European Working Group for People with Dementia, an organisation comprised entirely of people with dementia – which focused on the use of peer research with people with dementia and other forms of cognitive impairment. Findings from the review emphasised that people with cognitive impairment require a range of practical support to engage in peer research activities. For instance, practical lessons included a careful approach to training (consisting of short sessions to develop confidence in research and peer researchers' new roles); discussing, defining and revisiting people's roles during activities; accessibility of written materials and physical environments; support before and after research activities to deal with emotional consequences for peer researchers; and ensuring that adequate financial resources are available to support payment of peer researchers and facilitators, and venue hire (Tanner 2012; Di Lorito et al. 2016).

Peer researchers were involved in the analysis of a data set collected as part of the qualitative research component of the PRIDE study, which aimed to develop a critical understanding of the social discourses of dementia. Research interviews were undertaken by two academic researchers and three family carer peer researchers (Birt et al. 2019b). All had extensive experience of communicating with people with dementia; the tacit expectations and challenges of working with family carers as peer researchers during data collection have been documented elsewhere (Poland et al. 2019). The data set consisted of 124 in-depth qualitative interviews documenting the fears and realities of aging and aging with dementia. Initially, interviews were undertaken with 124 participants consisting of older people, people with dementia and family carers. Each person participated in a repeat interview at 12 months to record any changes.

Peer researcher recruitment

The recruitment of peer researchers was supported by two NHS Trust research departments. Good relationships with the staff in these departments had been established during participant recruitment for interviews, so they were fully briefed about the aims and ethical commitments of the study. Each NHS Trust made contact with people with dementia who were interested in research, with trust staff acting as gatekeepers between the research team and those interested in adopting a peer researcher role. They contacted potential participants by telephone to discuss the study and following up with an information sheet. One person was recruited through the Alzheimer's Society, via their research advisory group. We also tried to recruit peer researchers directly through public dementia groups and community organisations. However, this was not successful, suggesting that the role was perhaps seen as more authentic, relevant and achievable when information about it was shared by someone already known to the person with dementia. The Health Research Authority ethics committee reviewing the study stipulated the use of participant information sheets and consent forms as part of this recruitment process, even though there was no intent to collect data from them as per more traditional forms of qualitative research.

In total, ten peer researchers were recruited. Two cancelled before the workshop: a relative phoned to explain that one person was 'too confused', and another person was ill on the day. Therefore, eight peer researchers – seven men and one woman; four from each site – participated in analysis workshops. Aged between 60 and 80, peer researchers had been living with dementia for between six months and four years. We did not access medical notes but people appeared to be living with mild to moderate dementia. Some disclosed that they had a diagnosis of Alzheimer's Disease and another had Frontotemporal dementia. All were fully mobile and, other than wearing glasses and hearing aids, none had sensory loss. They described symptoms such as challenges in everyday life associated with planning and short-term memory loss. Adaptions for these symptoms had to be made during the data analysis.

Peer researcher analysis workshops

Peer researcher workshops took place in two locations in England, and in each location four people attended morning workshops over two consecutive days. Mornings were selected as the loss of light towards the end of the day can lead to increased confusion known colloquially as 'sundowning'. Workshop venues, a hotel and a university, were centrally located and fully accessible. Each venue had spaces for 'timeout', either for those with dementia or their carers if they had brought the person in. We requested that carers did not attend the workshop activity as their experience of dementia can differ from that of the individual living with the condition. To help peer researchers engage with the analysis material, two facilitators – an NHS Trust staff member and academic researcher who were known to the peer researchers – attended each workshop.

Each workshop lasted three hours and consisted of seven distinct analysis activities which were planned across the two days. Four activities enabled peer researchers to consider – i.e. interpret – segments of data by commenting on their understanding of others' experience of living with dementia. Three activities enabled the peer researchers to match – i.e. code – data by recognising patterns in such experiences. Each activity was introduced to the group, and then time was given for individual peer researchers to consider the data with support from facilitators, before wider group discussion. Each analysis activity was planned to last for 20–30 minutes, providing ample time for settling in, having breaks and general talk.

The first challenge in planning for the workshops was reducing the large qualitative data set of interviews with 124 participants in preparation for data analysis. To make the peer research analysis practicable, we needed to select and present the data in an accessible way. Although seemingly contradictory to an inclusive participatory approach, the academic research team made decisions on what data to share with peer researchers to enable their useful involvement in the process. Such a process is consistent with decisions that qualitative research-ers make when selecting illustrative quotes – i.e. choosing short statements that most clearly illuminate points or illustrate arguments – for publication (Holloway 2005). Initially we selected data from the 51 participants who were living with dementia, as this more closely reflected the peer researchers' lived experiences. We then selected data that represented the emerging themes in our preliminary analysis of the data. These themes included 'talking about dementia', 'getting a diagnosis', 'talking about friendship', 'living with dementia', 'staying well' and 'using technology'. We produced four short case studies so peer researchers could see data in the context of individual research participants rather than single short quotes. When selecting quotes, we ensured age, length of time living with dementia and sex were represented.

The second challenge related to presenting data for analysis in an accessi-ble way, and we followed guidance on accessibility to do so (Dementia Voices 2013). For example, in preparing the activity on 'talking about friendship,' we revisited preliminary coding and selected approximately 40 extracts of data that included positive and negative accounts of friendship. To enhance accessibility, we selected succinct quotes (the longest extract was 38 words); used quotes that described tangible actions (abstract thinking can be difficult for people living with dementia); and formatted documents to make texts easier to read, using coloured paper or coloured speech bubbles, size 18 sans serif font, 1.5 line spacing, and ensuring large areas of paper without text.

We chose not to offer formal research training before the analysis workshops as short-term memory is often impaired with dementia. Instead, at the start of each workshop, we shared an overview of the research project, the role of the peer researcher and the analysis activities. This information was printed and given to the peer researchers to take home and discuss with family.

Recognising the expertise of people with dementia in data analysis

All peer researchers said that they had enjoyed having a private place to talk about issues affecting their lives, where people did not judge them. There was a shared sense of participating in something that was of value, which reflects Brett et al.'s (2014) findings that public involvement in research processes led to people feeling valued and empowered. The analysis activities supported people with dementia to enact and demonstrate aspects of their agentic selves as social citizens. Bartlett and O'Conner (2010) propose that social citizenship 'recognizes the person with dementia as an active agent with rights, history, and competencies' (2010, p. 39). These activities illustrated the expertise that these people brought to a qualitative data analysis process. Peer researchers drew on their personal histories to compare and contrast their experiences with the data – they were socially active individuals and intellectually capable of considering alternative viewpoints to their own. Here we illustrate some examples of their contribution to interpretation and analysis of data.

Confirming the interpretation of data

Throughout the analysis activities, peer researchers repeatedly confirmed our preliminary analysis and interpretations, stating that participants' stories related closely to their own experiences. While this indicated credibility in our preliminary analysis, we were eager to encourage further interpretation of the meaning of the quotes. To do so, we listened to peer researchers' confirmation of how they recognised their experiences, then challenged them to discuss what they thought the quotes meant about research participants' experience of dementia. For instance, the following quote about receiving a diagnosis generated differing interpretations:

> Bugger! That's the best word I can use to describe it. I was stunned. It was a long time before – I'm not going to say I didn't accept it; it was more, 'Why?'

Peer researchers were asked how they thought the participant had felt about their diagnosis. Two peer researchers focused on the unexpected nature of the diagnosis, indicated by the word 'why'. Another peer researcher said we should focus on the word 'bugger', as this was most pertinent because the interviewee may have expected the diagnosis. This prompted academic researchers to explore, within the main data set, whether an expected or unexpected diagnosis shaped the participants' acceptance of the diagnosis.

There was not always consensus on the meaning of the data. For example, when we shared the following quote in the interpretation activity that focused on 'talking about friendship', one peer researcher emphatically stated that this must be a lie, as he had lost all his friends after his diagnosis:

> We've told people, suddenly everybody comes out of the woodwork and we've had meals in all our friends' houses. We realise that we're surrounded by crowds of friends.

The researcher explained that this was what someone had said in an interview, but this did not reassure the peer researcher who again stated it must be a lie. Meanwhile, other peer researchers agreed that friends were important and that they found people had been helpful since their diagnosis. The peer researcher who thought it was a lie was becoming agitated about the differing views. To help to reassure him that his experiences were valid, while also enabling the rest of the group to provide their interpretations, we shifted the focus of analysis activity from discussing the meaning of this individual quote to asking peer researchers what phrases they thought were important in other quotes. This redirection was successful in moving discussion on, and all then agreed with the sentiment within another quote, that '[You] can't rely on friends. Families are different'. This activity enabled members of the academic research team to review the data for any other non-confirmatory data where participants might have experienced a loss of friendship. The event highlighted the need to be alert to, and have respect for, multiple views during analysis. The aim of working with peer researchers – who have become experts through lived experience – is not to seek a 'truth' or validate findings (Clarke et al. 2018), but rather to encourage dialogue in which an exchange of ideas and experiences can extend, compare and contrast with academic researchers' understandings of data.

Bringing new understandings to data analysis

Peer researchers challenged interpretations to bring new understandings to these texts. This was the case in relation to the activities which focused on talking about and living with dementia. To stimulate a coding activity which focused on living with dementia, we shared two theme cards entitled 'positive experiences' and 'negative consequences'. However, peer researchers challenged these coding categories, stating that the pre-selected quotes did not readily fit into the theme cards. For instance, one peer researcher said that two quotes – 'It's not what I would have chosen in life, but it's what life's given me, so you just get on with it' and 'don't feel as secure, I suppose, because you can be out and about doing things and suddenly you've got a blank' – were neither positive or negative, but instead were about 'living within limits'. This generated further discussion about another theme. Peer researchers placed the following quote in a new theme they developed called, 'accepting limits':

> I get frustrated and very down because I think, phew I can't remember that, and there's a little flicker, an expression change, it's like they are trying to understand what I say.

Such interactions led the research team to reflect on how the analysis might not be helpful if it reduced complex life circumstances to dichotomous statements.

In another example, when thinking about living with dementia, peer researchers encouraged us to reconsider our interpretation of the quote, 'the whole village is supportive', which we had initially thought was a positive, supportive response from other community members. However, peer researchers explained that when too many people know about the diagnosis it can make the person feel that 'they are in a zoo', with too many well-meaning people looking in, and so, not necessarily positive. This lived experience insight led to our reviewing the original interview to see if the meaning of the quote had perhaps been changed to overemphasise the positives by taking it out of context. It also sensitised us to the trust a person with dementia might need in order to share a diagnosis.

Identifying alternative lens of analysis

Peer researchers helped us identify an alternative lens through which to explore the data. For example, when looking at data about friendships and receiving a diagnosis, the female peer researcher questioned whether there might be different experiences based on gender. We were looking at two quotes – 'If you are losing your memory people's attitudes change' and 'all my friends have gone' – and she explained that in her experience, female friends seemed to find it harder to acknowledge her diagnosis than her male friends. This prompted us to return to the main data set and explore gender differences. Although we only had a small sample of women living with dementia, it did appear that they struggled to maintain friendships. In contrast, the wives of men with dementia helped to organise their husband's social lives.

Another peer researcher suggested that we explore the different experiences people might have depending on their age, or whether they had accepted their diagnosis or not. While we had already considered these issues in our preliminary analysis, this confirmed peer researchers' abilities to consider theoretical reasons why narratives on dementia may differ.

In qualitative research, coding can often be at single word level, and in discussing the quotations in detail peer researchers challenged some of our interpretations. For example, when focusing on living with dementia, one quote read, 'It's the small things that are a nuisance'. The researcher had focused on the word 'nuisance' as having most importance. Peer researchers explained that the most important words were 'the small things', as it was the gradual build-up of small things that made daily life such a struggle. This interpretation was reconfirmed by peer researchers when we looked at the quote, 'It's small things but they build up and you do feel that you're not in charge'.

Unexpected challenges of working with peer researchers

We sought to mitigate the emotional distress associated with peer researchers engaging with data about other people's similar or more complex lived experiences of dementia. For instance, we ensured workshop facilitators were experienced in supporting people with dementia; created space and time at the end of the activities for people to talk and socialise; provided participants with follow-up contact details and sent them letters a week after the workshops to thank them for their help. However, a number of unexpected challenges arose.

The first of these concerned making transparent the different role of peer researcher and research participant. At several different stages of the recruitment process, we explained that the peer researcher role was not to be a participant in a study but rather to work alongside researchers to understand the research data. During the workshops, people occasionally spoke of enjoying taking part in the research, which led us to reiterate the difference in the roles. In part, this may have been exacerbated by the study's ethical requirement that peer researchers signed consent forms before starting the workshops. Poor understanding of differences between participant and public involvement may also be indicative of the complex definitions and activities which are named as public involvement (Mathie et al. 2014), suggesting a need for increased clarity and equity in roles and subsequent knowledge generation anticipated in peer research partnerships.

When undertaking similar analysis activities, Clarke et al. (2018) noted that in the early workshops peer researchers tended to talk of their own experiences, and different activities were required to move discussion from talking about personal experience with no reference to data, to linking personal experiences to the data, to finally discussing data extracts without reference to personal experiences. With support from facilitators we were able to have discussions which focused on comparing and contrasting their lived experiences with the data. The most effective technique at moving discussion from personal experiences to the meaning of the data was a coding activity that asked peer researchers to make a decision about placing quotes on particular theme cards.

A second challenge lay in making data fully accessible so that people with cognitive impairment could engage and contribute effectively. Despite our efforts, a couple of peer researchers struggled with activities, particularly when needing to remember information to make a judgement on its meaning. For example, during the coding activity that focused on talking about dementia, one man repeatedly picked the card up and looked at it, explaining he needed to do this because each time he lay the card down, he forgot what it said.

A third challenge occurred prior to the data analysis workshops and was associated with the influence of gatekeepers on peer researcher recruitment. Initially we had intended to work with people with dementia as peer researchers in both interviews and analysis. To raise awareness of the opportunity and initiate recruitment of peer researchers, we provided information to gatekeepers, including health professionals and family carers. After three months, we had received only one expression of interest from a person with dementia, but the family withdrew the person due to concerns about travel. To enable some representation of those with a lived experience of dementia in the data collection phase, we worked with family carers who undertook the interviews. Gatekeepers were concerned about the 'appropriateness' and 'emotional safety' of people with dementia being a peer researcher (Waite et al. 2019). Our success in recruiting peer researchers into the data analysis activities seems to have been based on having established trusting relationships between the health workers – who were attuned to the capabilities of many people with dementia – and the academic research team during data collection.

Discussion

The work described provides new and distinctive insights into the potential contributions a peer research approach brought to the research process and the challenges that arose from involving people with dementia as peer researchers. Identifying and evidencing the positive benefits of peer research activity may help shift societal safeguarding concerns around the potential physical and emotional harm for the person with dementia, towards more openly recognising that, with the right support, it is possible to constructively engage people with dementia in research processes. Such activity can provide benefits to the peer researcher, the research team, and to others through the new knowledge the research produces. Immersion in project processes also led us to consider the distinguishing characteristics of peer research activity and how these differ from other forms of patient and public involvement.

Realising agentic potential in the peer researcher role

Our preparatory work highlighted how peer research with people with dementia had rarely been undertaken, because of concerns for the physical and emotional safety of the individual alongside debate about whether people with cognitive impairment could add anything useful to research outputs. Working from such assumptions restricts a person's right to be a social citizen, and prevents them from being agentic in taking on a social role and responsibility that might enhance their own life and the lives of others with similar lived experiences. In this project, we found that being a peer researcher and being listened to created personal satisfaction and generated a social role as being able to help others. The positive emotions the peer researchers experienced in safe, judgement-free spaces, resonate with Bartlett's (2014) findings, which showed how people with dementia derive personal benefits from the enactment of such citizenship roles. Research is now needed to explore the different components of peer research to better understand which components generate the most positive outcomes: whether this is the intellectual engagement, the sharing of experiences with the aim of helping others, or both of these.

Distinguishing the person with dementia's voice from others

Since we embarked on this project in 2016, several publications have reported on peer research with people *living* with dementia (Mockford et al. 2016; Clarke et al. 2018; Stephenson and Turner 2019). The extent to which the authors justify procedures and the descriptions of activity vary, but one point consistently noted is that family carers are accounted for as 'living' with dementia. However, lived experiences of dementia may differ markedly between the carer and the individual with the diagnosis. Our analysis workshops deliberately did not include family carers as their voices can overshadow the voices of people with dementia. More transparent reporting of peer research and co-production in dementia research will enable us to monitor how frequently, and where explicitly, the voice of the person *with* dementia is heard and prioritised.

Distinguishing between peer research and patient and public involvement

Throughout the study, we questioned how the peer research activity differed from more mainstream patient and public involvement. The expectation of public involvement is that such activity will help to ensure the research meets the needs of people, that information is accessible and the research is ethically sound (Health Research Authority 2016). An overarching intention for involving peer researchers in data analysis is to support the generation of new ways of understanding the data, to build new research knowledge. In this study, involving peer researchers in data analysis went beyond patient and public involvement, as they confirmed, challenged and produced new insights, which underpinned novel interpretations enabling knowledge-building.

Revaluing the practicalities of peer research approaches in dementia research

Our work with peer researchers with dementia highlights the need to be realistic, rather than dismissive, of the extent to which a medical condition affects a person's abilities. Providing clear information on the expectations of peer researchers involved in these workshops enabled gatekeepers to see the potential of the activity. Subsequently, respecting the autonomy of peer researchers enabled them to assert their opinions during the analysis activities. We followed guidelines concerning the pragmatics of venue, transport, payment and accessibility (Di Lorito et al. 2016) and received advice from those living with dementia on how best to involve others in patient and public involvement activities (Gove et al. 2018). By making explicit our rationale on how we selected data to realise research aims, we have aimed to make the analytic processes more transparent. As the benefits of peer research become apparent, so researchers may have increasing confidence in sharing research processes for generating knowledge (Boaz et al. 2016). However, we acknowledge that while sharing power and control may be the ultimate aim in participatory methods, in this peer research, the management of data remained under the research team's control.

Conclusion

In dementia studies there is a growing impetus to involve people with dementia in research activities, as participants and through patient and public involvement. Distinct from simply participating in research and providing commentary on their own lives, people with dementia are able to offer their particular insight and expertise into qualitative data analysis, by interpreting, comparing and contrasting their encounters with research data to extend their understanding and meaning. To facilitate peer researchers' access to and engagement with research data, peer research activities will similarly need to be distinctive, jointly shaped by the needs of those with dementia and the research team's priorities. While peer research activity can support agentic social citizenship roles, it must be acknowledged that the research team may also need to work with gatekeepers on facilitating this activity. Furthermore, it must also be acknowledged that research teams will ultimately retain control over the research data and make the decisions on how to develop findings in ways that enable peer researchers to engage with analyses. Making such accommodations does not mean we should simply avoid peer research approaches but recognise these processes as key if we are to progress the continued development and evaluation of participatory research in dementia studies.

References

Alderson, P., 2011. Children as researchers: The effects of participation rights on research methods. In: P. Christensen and A. James, eds. *Research with Children: Perspectives and Practices*. Abingdon: RoutledgeFalmer, 241–257.

Banks, S., et al., 2013. Everyday ethics in community-based participatory research. *Contemporary Social Science*, 8 (3), 263–277. doi:10.1080/21582041.2013.769618.

Bartlett, R., 2014. Citizenship in action: The lived experiences of citizens with dementia who campaign for social change. *Disability and Society*, 29 (8), 1291–1304. doi:10.1080/09687599.2014.924905.

Bartlett, R. and O'Conner, D., 2010. *Broadening the Dementia Debate: Towards Social Citizenship*. Bristol: Policy Press.

Birt, L., et al., 2017. Shifting dementia discourses from deficit to active citizenship. *Sociology of Health and Illness*, 39 (2), 199–211. doi:10.1111/1467-9566.12530.

Birt, L., et al., 2019a. Maintaining social connections in dementia: A qualitative synthesis. *Qualitative Health Research*, 30 (1), 23–42.

Birt, L., et al., 2019b. Relational experiences of people seeking help and assessment for subjective cognitive concern and memory loss. *Aging & Mental Health*, 27, 1–9. doi:10.1080/13607863.2019.1592111.

Boaz, A., Biri, D., and McKevitt, C., 2016. Rethinking the relationship between science and society: Has there been a shift in attitudes to patient and public involvement and public engagement in science in the United Kingdom? *Health Expectations*, 19, 592–601. doi:10.1111/hex.12295.

Boote, J., Baird, W., and Beecroft, C., 2010. Public involvement at the design stage of primary health research: A narrative review of case examples. *Health Policy*, 95, 10–23. doi:10.1016/j.healthpol.2009.11.007.

Brett, J., et al., 2014. Mapping the impact of patient and public involvement on health and social care research: A systematic review. *Health Expectations*, 17, 637–650. doi:10.1111/j.1369-7625.2012.00795.x.

Charlesworth, G., 2018. Public and patient involvement in dementia research: Time to reflect? *Dementia*, 17 (8), 1064–1067. doi:10.1177/2397172X18802501.

Clarke, C.L., et al., 2018. A seat around the table: Participatory data analysis with people living with dementia. *Qualitative Health Research*, 28 (9), 1421–1433. doi:10.1177/1049732318774768.

Clough, R., et al., 2006. *Older People as Researchers: Evaluating a Participative Project.* York: Joseph Rowntree Foundation.

Dementia Action Alliance, 2019. *The Dementia Statements.* Available from: https://www.dementiaaction.org.uk/nationaldementiadeclaration [Accessed 12 May 2020].

Dementia Voices, 2013. *Writing Dementia Friendly Information.* Available from: http://dementiavoices.org.uk/wp-content/uploads/2013/11/DEEP-Guide-Writing-dementia-friendly-information.pdf [Accessed 12 May 2020].

Di Lorito, C., et al., 2016. A synthesis of the evidence on peer research with potentially vulnerable adults: How this relates to dementia. *International Journal of Geriatric Psychiatry*, 32 (1), 58–67. doi:10.1002/gps.4577.

Gove, D., et al., 2018. Alzheimer Europe's position on involving people with dementia in research through PPI (patient and public involvement). *Aging and Mental Health*, 22 (6), 723–729. doi:10.1080/13607863.2017.1317334.

Hartley, J. and Benington, J., 2000. Co-research: A new methodology for new times. *European Journal of Work and Organizational Psychology*, 9, 463–476. doi:10.1080/13594320050203085.

Health Research Authority/INVOLVE, 2016. *Impact of Public Involvement on Ethical Aspects of Research.* Available from: http://www.invo.org.uk/posttypepublication/public-involvement-in-researchimpact-on-ethical-aspects-of-research [Accessed 9 May 2020].

Holloway, I., 2005. *Qualitative Writing.* In: I. Holloway, ed. *Qualitative Research in Health Care.* Maidenhead: Open University Press, 270–286.

INVOLVE, 2019. *What is Public Involvement in Research.* Available from: https://www.invo.org.uk/find-out-more/what-is-public-involvement-in-research-2/ [Accessed 12 May 2020].

Mathie, E., et al., 2014. Consumer involvement: UK scoping health research. *International Journal of Consumer Studies*, 38, 35–44. doi:10.1111/ijcs.12072.

Mockford, C., et al., 2016. A SHARED study-the benefits and costs of setting up a health research study involving lay co-researchers and how we overcame the challenges. *Research Involvement and Engagement*, 2 (8), 0–10. doi:10.1186/s40900-016-0021-3.

Moore, T.F. and Howlett, J., 2003. Giving voice to persons living with dementia: The researcher's opportunities and challenges. *Nursing Science Quarterly*, 16 (2), 163–167. doi:10.1177/0894318403251793251793.

Poland, F., et al., 2019. Embedding patient and public involvement: Managing tacit and explicit expectations. *Health Expectations*, 22 (6), 1231–1239.

Staley, K., 2009. *Exploring Impact: Public Involvement in NHS, Public Health and Social Care Research.* Eastleigh: INVOLVE.

Stephenson, M. and Turner, B., 2019. Involving individuals with dementia as co researchers in analysis of findings from a qualitative study. *Dementia*, 18 (2), 701–712. doi:10.1177/1471301217690904.

Tanner, D., 2012. Co-research with older people with dementia: Experience and reflections. *Journal of Mental Health*, 21, 296–306. doi:10.3109/09638237.2011.651658.

Waite, J., Poland, F., and Charlesworth, G., 2019. Facilitators and barriers to co-research by people with dementia and academic researchers: Findings from a qualitative study. *Health Expectations*, 22, 761–771. doi:10.1111/hex.12891.

WHO, 2014. *Dementia Fact Sheet*. Available from: https://www.who.int/news-room/fact-sheets/detail/dementia [Accessed 12 May 2020].

Wilkinson, H., 2002. Including people with dementia in research: The methods and motivations. In: H. Wilkinson, ed. *The Perspectives of People with Dementia: Research Methods and Motivations*. London: Jessica Kingsley, 9–24.

Yates, L., et al., 2019. The development of the promoting independence in Dementia (PRIDE) intervention to enhance independence in dementia. *Clinical Interventions in Aging*, 2019 (14), 1615–1630. doi:10.2147/CIA.S214367.

6 Gender diverse equality and well-being in Manipur, North East India

Reflections on peer-led research

Paul Boyce, Pawan Dhall, Santa Khurai, Oinam Yambung, Bonita Pebam and Randhoni Lairikyengbam

Introduction - Gender transition and recognition in India

In this chapter, we reflect on peer research and advocacy led by gender diverse and 'transgender' community organisers in the North East Indian state of Manipur. In the context of the present project, this involved community organisers training other gender and sexual minority participants to conduct research on employment and welfare experiences in their community. These actions were designed to impact on gender and sexual rights, recognition and economic well-being in this region of India especially, although with national and international relevance. The project was a research *and* advocacy initiative; peer researchers were community leaders who had mobilised transgender communities through the years, founded transgender support forums in Manipur and advocated for their concerns with diverse influencers. The peer research did not stop at data collection but also involved developing strategy on the basis of the findings, identifying relevant stakeholders in the region with whom to develop new initiatives aimed at the economic inclusion of gender and sexual minorities.

In reflecting on the process involved, we consider the terms and language via which our work was taken forward. In the North East of India (as in many other settings) the employment of the rubric 'transgender' operates as an especially varied and contested political signifier in research, activism and everyday life. Such complexities have relevance to participatory, peer-led research interventions in contexts of gender and sexual diversity within the wider Indian political and legal context.

One of the ways in which peer-led, community-oriented investigation with gender and sexual diverse persons has been utilised has been to enable the expression of minority voices that might otherwise be silenced. This has included, with respect to policy and welfare actions, anti-violence campaigns and projects aimed at improving transgender people's health and socio-economic circumstances (Collumbien et al. 2009; Ganju and Saggurti 2017; Shears 2019). Such actions can become complex in the context of activist movements, laws and policies wherein the terms of recognition for gender non-binary/non-conforming persons become subject to query. Language can run up against the limits of political representation whereby a term such as 'transgender' is contested or employed as if universally applicable. This may be so, for example, where it is used as a proxy for all gender-diverse experience or when it is assumed that all gender non-binary ways of being lead to transition in biomedical terms. A related issue is that regional and vernacular terminologies for gender and sexual diversity have often come to be cited in research and policies as if straightforward local exemplars of a putatively universal category (i.e. transgender) (Dutta and Roy 2014; Stryker and Currah 2016).

Such concerns have been especially salient in India in recent years where the central government agency NALSA (National Legal Services Authority) judgement of 2014 initiated state of gender as a matter for self-determination. This creates a template for the acknowledgement of the historical marginalisation of 'transgender' and 'third gender' peoples in India. The judgement was followed in 2019 with the ratification of the Transgender Persons (Protection of Rights) Act, which had a prior processual history as the Transgender Bill (2014) and which has been subject to much protest. Non-binary, gender-fluid, queer, transgender, *hijra* and other activists in India have campaigned against ways in which NALSA and the Transgender Act have been implemented, undercutting the very rights supposedly protected (Semmalar 2017). Protesters have, for example, vociferously critiqued governmental insistence on including, in one form or other, a 'screening process' to 'determine' who is transgender or not, as a means of deciding who might avail of the state recognition afforded by law. Recognition in these terms is not based on self-determination of gendered experience but on external judgements made by members of regional-level transgender welfare boards.

One part of the problem described arises from the unexamined use of 'transgender' as if a singular progressive overarching categorisation in law, welfare and policy. In practice, the organising of state action in India around this categorical logic has served to erase gender specificity and diversity before the law and other mechanisms and has impacted on the welfare of gender non-binary persons, who find themselves unable to avail of the welfare measures – such as identity documents, ration cards, progressive employment actions – that the boards are supposedly intended to assist with.

Such issues have been especially prevalent with regards to transgender and other gender-diverse rights and welfare in Manipur in recent years, having been highlighted in our prior research (Dhall and Boyce 2015). In particular this work highlighted the need for contextually specific research and information, based in the lived experience of welfare, work and legislation among transgender and other sexualities and gender diverse peoples. In these terms peer-led research resonates with a very particular ethical commitment in our project. This is not just located in an ethos of inclusive action but as has been taken forward in conjunction with asserting the right to self-determination of gendered experience that is currently both highlighted and erased for many sexual and gender minorities in India.

Against this background the word 'transgender' expresses specificity in that it has acquired a particular intimate and political resonance in the North East of India as used by activists and others in the region. This both connects to and diverges from ways in which the term has come to be more used in South Asian sociopolitical contexts in recent years (Khurai 2019). For example, activists in the North East have explicitly protested against the conflation of transgender categorisation as mobilised in respect of right-wing Hindu nationalism, or a more general assumption of a pan India Hindu culture. In 2019, for instance, transgender activists in Manipur publicly burned the book *Invisible Men* for its portrayal of a national, Hindu, transgender culture, which was seen to erase recognition of (and self-determination in respect of) rich Manipuri gender diverse histories. As such, while we sometimes employ the term 'transgender' in this chapter, the word does not simply dub a universal, or national, categorisation over contextually varied gender expression. Rather, we employ the category as deployed by transgender-identifying activists in Manipur and along with other regional terms of recognition.

Amidst the issues described, this chapter considers the use of peer-led research run with and by community advocates in Manipur to examine experiences of exclusion and prejudice in contexts of employment, education and welfare, on the basis of gender difference and diversity. The choice of Manipur is significant, not only for the current complexities of gender and sexualities activism in the state but also for the region being largely neglected in discourse on development and welfare in India on account of geography, political differences and ethnicity (Dhall and Boyce 2015).

Transgender recognition in Manipur

As in the rest of India and South Asia (Reddy 2005; Dutta 2012; Hossain 2018), a multitude of Indigenous and nominally 'western' terms that might be included under the 'transgender' umbrella exist in Manipur (Dhall and Boyce 2015). As noted, 'transgender' has a particular history in North East India, having gained currency in the region from around the late 2000s, with the emergence of politically prominent activists. An initial motive for this activism was to question the reductionist terminology that had become prevalent in the sphere of HIV interventions with regards to gender and sexual minorities at that time. A particular concern pertained to how a range of 'non-cis-gendered' subjects found themselves included under the rubric of 'MSM' in the health promotion world, whereby the term MSM became used to designate a particular sub-categorisation of men who have sex with men who nonetheless embodied *feminine* self-presentation and were seen to practice 'passive' sexual roles. In other parts of India, the reaction to such actions was a catalyst for the then growth in public recognition of *kothis* as a gender and sexual minority subject category that is oft presented as a core, Indigenous regional identity in health and other research in South Asia. In practice, while *kothi* identification may express rich traditions of gender diversity, the popularisation of the term can also be seen as tied to the influence of HIV prevention actions where in a sense it performed as 'made-up' grouping of gender and sexual difference, a kind of hybrid 'cultural category' – both local and conceived out of the needs of global health paradigms to categorise and typify gendered and sexual 'others' (Reddy 2005; Boyce 2007; Lorway et al. 2009). This was seen by Manipuri activists, as in some other contexts in South Asia, as 'writing-over' far more nuanced gendered and sexual life-projects and histories in insensitive terms.

While contested, such erasures have also acted as important catalysts for activists who have defined and advocated for 'otherwise gendered' terms of identity to be taken up in health promotion and other public sphere actions. In Manipur, such contestations led activists to explore terms that articulated gender diverse experiences that were seen to be *already* part of Manipuri cultures, especially the culture of the Meitei communities in the Manipur valley. This is the numerically dominant ethnic group in the state, with Hinduism and Shanamahism among the main religions followed (while also diverting from the kind of pan Indian Hinduism cited above). At one time, the term *nupi saabi* – derived from the Meitei context – became prevalent as a terminology promoted by activists. This expression came about from the popularity of individuals assigned male at birth cross-dressing and playing female roles in Shumong Leela, a traditional Manipuri theatre form. *Nupi saabi* was a popular reference to these actors and literally implied 'men who were like women'. At one stage, this was seen as a sign of Manipuri society being 'inclusive' of gender diversities (at least among people engaged in the development sector in and outside the Manipur state). However, in the 2010s, transgender activists in the region began highlighting the fact that *nupi saabis* were often subject to exploitation and there were many among them who did not see *nupi saabi* as defining of their genders and sexualities. The expression was also often used in a derogatory sense. So, in parallel to the growing popularity of the term 'transgender' in Manipur, there were activist assertions that a different Manipuri term was needed to convey the experience of 'being transgender' or a 'transgender woman'. *Nupi maanbi* for transgender women and later *nupamaanba* for transgender men were taken by a new generation of activists, where these terms were better seen to convey essential qualities of gender (difference) as opposed to association of simple 'acting like' a gendered type. What it is important to note here is that the use of terms such as *nupi maanbi* does not just express an already present culture or history but rather is too a version of sexual and gendered contextualisation that is re-made in response to the sociopolitical imperatives of the present (Yukhamibam 2020).

Such diversification in the politicisation of gendered and sexual minorities' social action and language in Manipur in turn connects to varied issues that arise in peer-led research. This is especially so as the coordinates of participation (i.e. who takes part in a project and in what terms) reflect complex social and subjective attributes pertaining to inclusion regarding gender in this instance. A key attribute of activism in Manipur has been an imperative to define gender variant recognition beyond the application of external labels or simplified visions of gendered and sexual culture, especially as these might be seen to derive from elsewhere in India (for example, through the recent historical implementation of state-level HIV programmes or current state legislation). The self-understandings of gender and sexualities diverse peers thus became an especially important political act in the region. This in turn connects to the wider politics of the North East region for its marginalisation in many mainstream health and development initiatives in India (Phanjoubam 2019).

Law and transgender advocacy in India and Manipur

Recent civil society debate and actions regarding transgender well-being in Manipur have been provoked by the establishment of the Manipur Transgender Welfare Board (AMaNA et al. 2016). This was set up in concert with similar actions in other Indian states as an outcome of the NALSA judgement. As noted, implementing the judgement (and the evolution of the subsequent Transgender Bill) involved establishing state-level Transgender Welfare Boards in many Indian states. To date, such actions have not led to consistent on-the-ground implementation by government stakeholders.

Amidst such concerns, while larger Indian transgender movements have been conscious of the need to take along anyone who has an identification or affinity to the transgender umbrella, there have been disagreements about such processes that have been manifest in Manipur in particular ways (Bhattacharya 2019). *Hijras* constitute one of the most prominent and recognised sections of Indian transgender movements, their geographical spread more or less correlating with large parts of what the Manipuris often call the 'Indian mainland' – all of northern, western and central India and parts of southern and eastern India, extending up to Assam in the North East. Among the most marginalised sections of gender and sexual minorities, and yet possibly the most visible and vocal, *hijras* occupy a centre space in the public mind, with media and academic representation often conflating *hijra* with 'transgender' in South Asia.

To an extent, heated debate around gender and sexual diversity in India (after NALSA and the Transgender Act) may be read as having become especially '*hijra*-centric' in recent years (with claims that *hijras* are the 'real' transgender in the Indian context; some aspect of the Transgender Act reflect this especially – Boyce and khanna 2020). For some, such claims have been interpreted as reflecting the general tendency of 'mainland India' to forget the specific contexts and concerns of gender diverse communities in the North East, among other regions. This led to a recent social media campaign by activists from the North East region emphasising that all 'transgender' (and *nupi maanbi* and *nupi maanba*) persons (in India) *are not hijras*. Within the scenario described, participatory practice in the present project not only pertained to an ethos of inclusive engagement but also to an important need to attend to complex relations between multiple gender transitioning experiences in Manipur as politicised in divergent ways within and against the mainstream Indian context and the laws and legislation flowing therefrom.

The project

It was against this complexity that work took shape. Our programme of action comprised an economic inclusion advocacy intervention aimed at addressing the needs of transgender persons in Manipur, with a focus on the state capital of Imphal spread over the districts of Imphal East and Imphal West. The project was directly based on a formative qualitative assessment of economic inclusion of gender and sexual minorities in India conducted in 2014–15 by two of the authors of the present case study (Dhall and Boyce 2015). The work was one component of a five-year international programme of work on Poverty, Sexuality and Law funded by UK Aid and implemented via the Institute of Development Studies, UK. The qualitative assessment revealed that a plethora of government poverty alleviation programmes notwithstanding, heteronormative definitions of gender, marriage and family at the social, legal and policy levels continued to exclude people with non-normative genders and sexualities from economic benefits – both welfare and access to employment – in Manipur and elsewhere. To quote from the assessment:

> [When] S. Thounoujam, a 32-year-old trans man in Manipur applied for a job card under the [Mahatma Gandhi National Rural Employment Guarantee Scheme] for himself and his female partner (as a family unit) in 2009, the Gram Panchayat official refused to entertain his request pointing out that they were 'not a normal man–woman married couple'. Or let us take the example of 45-year-old T. Bimola from Imphal, Manipur, who has been in a relationship with another woman since 2001 and works for a small bakery near her home. She wants to plan for old age for herself and her partner, who works as a security guard. But she has only a vague idea about government housing schemes for the poor. She is also uncertain whether she and her partner can apply for a housing loan as a couple, and adds that if required she will apply as an unmarried woman and not reveal the status of her relationship with her partner.
>
> (Dhall and Boyce 2015, pp. 21–22)

What became especially evident was that there were many ways in which gender and sexual minority persons in Imphal found that their socio-economic precarity was compounded because of their gender and sexualities. This was taking place in the context of a sustained period of economic growth in India. As Dhall and Boyce (2015, p. 3) note, although since market liberalisation began in the early 1990s India experienced significant economic growth (from around 5.5% in the early 1990s to a peak of 10.3% in 2010, with lower rates subsequently but still among the highest worldwide), share of wealth became increasingly unequal and income inequality doubled in about 20 years.

Gender and sexual 'difference' align in important ways with such socio-economic inequities, as stigma, fractures in kinship relations (and related economic support) and prejudice in employment and access to welfare have compounded socio-economic precarity for many gender non-conforming persons. These effects take shape across many identity formations and gendered and sexual ways of being that might, in one way or another, be judged as marginal, suspect, or at least unwelcome in respect of normative values and cultures in workplaces or other sites of livelihood or welfare (and which crucially have been poorly expressed and legislated for in the NALSA judgment and latterly the Transgender Act).

With these challenges in mind, the 2014–15 assessment outlined immediate and long-term recommendations for all stakeholders to ensure large-scale economic inclusion for gender and sexuality non-conforming people in India. Some of these recommendations around capacity building for peer and community-led advocacy with education, employment and social welfare stakeholders formed the basis for this work. We particularly wanted to take up challenges and opportunities with regards to creating pathways to enable gender and sexual minorities to advocate for actions that addressed their socio-economic vulnerabilities, as defined by them. We focused, therefore, on generating a dialogue among gender and sexual minorities in Imphal (the capital of Manipur), particularly transgender, *nupi maanbi, nupa maanba* and other community leaders regarding what their issues around economic inclusion were and how we might collectively strategise advocacy. We focused on Imphal as a regional hub for relevant activism and as an employment centre. We identified specific private sector, non-government and government stakeholders who could potentially make a difference to the situation in and around our project area (Imphal) and then set about sensitising activities. Our aim was to catalyse changes in the spheres of education, skills building, employment and media coverage regarding the concerns of transgender people.

Developing peer-led research and advocacy

Working with members of community groups run by and for transgender people in Manipur, we aimed to elicit perspectives grounded in lived experiences that would not have been possible otherwise. This was *not*, however, because transgender persons were particularly inaccessible. In some global contexts peer-led research with gender and sexual minority people has been advocated as a means to achieve connections with an otherwise 'hard-to-reach' population; this has not been the premise of our project. In particular, we have been concerned that conceiving some populations as 'hard-to-reach' places an emphasis on such peoples to make themselves more visible, for example if they want avail of welfare or other 'practical rights'. This is as opposed to focusing on how policies and legislation may render some people invisible, because the terms of recognition employed do not speak adequately to social diversity, among other factors (Boyce 2019). As such, our project was conceived on the basis of already present leadership by gender and sexualities diverse communities. Peer connections, as such, were already factored into the research design, not as a facet of a problem of accessibility to overcome but as a social and material condition that made our project conceivable in the first place.

The project was co-conceived with two main collaborating transgender community organisations – the All Manipur Nupi Maanbi Association (AMaNA), which was set up in 2010 as a peer-led collective of community-based organisations of transgender women (and to some extent men who have sex with men) and Empowering Trans Ability (ETA), a group for trans-masculine individuals, established in Manipur in 2012 (Dhall 2015). SAATHII (Solidarity and Action Against the HIV Infection in India), a national level NGO working on sexualities, health and HIV prevention, and with regional representation in Manipur, comprised the third key partner. Funding for the project came from the University of Sussex Social Science Impact Fund, with support from the Newton Fund, with a remit to support methods and means to improve employment and welfare opportunities for transgender persons in Manipur. The project comprised a number of training, research and advocacy activities conducted over a period of 20 months from August 2016 to March 2018. We aimed to achieve sustained impact, not only by newly informing employment and welfare cultures with regards to sexual and gender diversity but also by equipping local advocates from transgender community groups with skills and strategic connections for ongoing dialogue and programme development with key potential employers in the region. Peer leadership, in these terms, was not only central to the project's goals, it was also an objective in itself, with an aim to better equip local gender and sexual minority peoples to lead changes to work cultures in the region.

Data, stories and training

Four community advocates from Imphal, who were associated with AMaNA and ETA co-led the project. Two of these people (among the co-authors here) had acted as researchers on the prior (2014–15) study that we had undertaken, and they recruited two more colleagues. The idea for the project arose from their experience and was suggested to other co-authors (Dhall and Boyce). In dialogue we all conceptualised issues arising, seeking to translate these into a form of analysis and project outline that we could use so to leverage funding. The project development process was recursive in these terms – arising from our already ongoing dialogues about needs and possible courses of actions at different scales of action. Community organisers in Manipur led day-to-day aspects of the project, once funding was secured.

The training for the community advocates was undertaken over five phases throughout the project period. The idea was to build up on what the community advocates already knew about issues around economic inclusion and exclusion, gender and sexuality rather than to give them textbook knowledge or definitions from glossaries. We wanted them to look at their own understandings of these issues, and to help them articulate them better. We also asked them to look at how they (and other gender and sexualities 'non-conforming' peoples) experience stigma and discrimination, and how this impacted on their educational and employment opportunities, health, security, basic rights – leading to many micro and macro exclusions on a day-to-day basis.

This process helped community advocates to draw out a pathway of how economic exclusion takes place. We began with family and community acceptance or lack of it, moving on to discrimination in nutrition, education, shelter, skills building, employment, social welfare schemes, and then to how such exclusions may also be reflected in the laws and policies. This framing of the issues was more real to participants than jargon-heavy explanations, and as part of the story-telling involved in this process, community advocates talked about examples from their daily lives.

At the end of an initial training period, the second phase began; we documented key elements in the pathway of economic exclusion – in the Manipur context. We planned that this assessment would comprise a mapping of economic inclusion and exclusion of gender and sexual minorities in Manipur. This involved, for example, group work with a larger cohort of gender and sexual minority people wherein participants located sites in Imphal where they might have suffered prejudice or exclusion, such as schools or workplaces. Mapping in these terms was not simply about identifying geographic locations but identifying the (shared) stories associated with such contexts. It also involved the gathering of quantitative information that might be used for purposes of advocacy. For instance, the baseline survey conducted for our project (pulling together existing relevant data) found that the literacy rate among transgender people in the state was 67.5%, far lower than the national rate of 74.04% and Manipur rate of 79.85% (Census 2011 data). These findings helped develop advocacy strategies and tools, including a blog (Rainbow Manipur | Inclusive Manipur) to document stories of, and data about, economic exclusion that emerged from the study. These were developed into a website that documents lived stories of transgender, *nupi maanbi, nupa maanba* and other 'otherwise' gendered peoples.[1]

The documentation of community advocates' stories and those of the larger gender diverse community in Imphal through digital media required community advocates to pick up the basics of storytelling. A third element of training comprised sessions organised on relevant techniques. The resource person for this was a local journalist and feminist writer. She helped the community advocates to identify aspects from their own lives that related to economic exclusion, and then to try and put them down in the form of a story. A key challenge was to enable a group of adults to go back to their younger years. We used children's books, comics and short video clips – everything to encourage participants to start thinking in terms of how to tell a story as it might have evolved over their own lifetime.

The fourth phase of the training took place towards the end of 2017. All the community advocates who had taken part in the project were asked to list the project activities undertaken since August 2016 chronologically. Then they were asked to look back and write down what new things they had learned and how the experience had changed them. Finally, they were asked to share what they would like to do next in terms of advocacy for economic inclusion. They responded with ideas such as writing a book on the subject, submitting memoranda to the government and providing seed money capital to business aspirants among the transgender communities.

The fifth and the final phase of the training focused on community reporting or citizen journalism – an extension of some of the earlier training but with the purpose of keeping the discourse on economic inclusion alive even after the project period was over. Community advocates were provided with tips on identifying stories around economic inclusion, narrating them in the form of news stories, first person stories or feature articles. This involved advice on how to submit them to queer themed webzines and to use them for continued advocacy through mainstream media and with other stakeholders (the project, for example, was featured in regional television news reports).

Once community advocates had been trained, they undertook 10 meetings, consultations, workshops and mass awareness events (including a public dissemination exhibition of the project in Imphal, and consultations in Delhi and Kolkata) – including data and storytelling highlights. In Imphal (our immediate focus area) activities were undertaken primarily with local entrepreneurs (typically with sole proprietorship or partnership businesses not employing more than 50 people), vocational trainers, media persons and government child-protection and social welfare officials in and around Imphal. The aim was to sensitise such people to the life experiences, needs, exclusions and welfare of gender and sexualities diverse peoples, with training involving storytelling and the presentation of strategies for organisational change by community advocates.

We decided to place the emphasis on smaller non-government actors partly because few interventions on gender diverse socio-economic inclusion in India have tapped their potential to promote economic inclusion. Moreover, Manipur state has relatively few large companies that could be engaged in the intervention. Small entrepreneurs, many of whom are part of India's informal and self-employment sector (where the majority of India's workforce is engaged – 80% and above according to different estimates) constitute an untapped potential in terms of sensitisation towards inclusion of transgender people.

Impact and ongoing actions

After 20 months of work, around a dozen entrepreneurs and vocational trainers began to offer training and employment opportunities to gender and sexual minorities in Manipur as a direct result of this work – this training being developed and implemented with the project team of local community advocates (Rainbow Manipur | Inclusive Manipur 2019). Dialogue was also started on guiding these entrepreneurs develop inclusive human resources policies. An information technology firm MOBIMP, for example, based in Imphal, conducted training events developed with our project team aimed at sensitising their staff on transgender diverse recruitment and workplace equality issues. The company also made all of their toilets gender neutral in 2017 after having participated in sensitisation sessions organised under the intervention.

Similarly, Accent & Allied Infotech, a leading vocational training centre in Manipur, decided to allot one of their three toilets for transgender people in line with need. This was done in parallel to making all their training courses gender diverse and transgender inclusive, marking a difference with previous attempts to run special courses exclusively for transgender people.

Further dialogue also began with the Imphal municipal body to develop transgender inclusive public sanitation facilities, which are vital to improved welfare and equality in work and educational contexts as well as in the public domain (Pebam 2018). This in turn has catalysed a wider aspect of our project with the publication of a collaborative article in the journal *Waterlines* (Boyce et al. 2018), which has helped to set out a new agenda for transgender inclusivity in the water, sanitation and hygiene sector and which has already been influential – for example, in informing the UK Department for International Development's public discussion of transgender inclusive development, and in part based on our project (DfID Inclusive Societies 2018).

Beyond the field of employment, the project also included consultation by the Manipur-based project team with district-level government child protection officers in Bishnupur, a town in the neighbourhood of Imphal. This consultation helped list the steps transgender community groups can take in collaboration with government child welfare bodies to ensure gender variant children in schools facing discrimination and bullying do not drop out and their concerns are addressed urgently. Again, the Rainbow Manipur | Inclusive Manipur blog (as developed by AMaNA and ETA) carries stories on the discrimination faced by transgender persons in schools (Hemabati 2017).

Conclusion

Overall, the project aimed to offer a model for peer-led intervention regarding how incremental impact in terms of employment, education and welfare of gender and sexual minority persons might be achieved within a given context. While in some contexts such peer-led processes have been advocated as a means to better insert transgender and other gender diverse voices into policy and programme development processes, we took a somewhat different approach. Instead the aim was to use the priorities of gender and sexualities diverse community advocates and researchers in designing the focus, reach and priorities of the programme and to advance peer-led training to (potential) employers from this basis. This was conversant with the ethos that gender and sexual minorities peoples are not a hard-to-reach group that peer-led research can help to contact. Rather, the *a priori* basis of our research was to start with the reflections of gender and sexual minority peoples and to build our project design on this basis.

We learned many things along the way. We started with a draft work agenda and then discovered what was feasible. For example, government officials were not always easy to access. This informed the collective decision to focus instead on other stakeholders (i.e. small businesses). In addition, the idea of economic inclusion itself had to be 'sold' to many of the stakeholders involved – not necessarily as an issue that they were not already aware of but as something in which they could also participate in, in a truly collaborative sense. This was achieved through dialogue and conversation during meetings and workshops aimed at building rapport between activists, entrepreneurs and business leaders. Such dialogues were the core attribute of our approach; community advocates and local business people came to view one another as peers in an ongoing process as the project went along. This is not to say that all power differentials were erased by the project or that a simple equity was uniformly achieved. Crucially, however, our programme of work involved altering the terrain of peer relations as gender diverse activists, and local business people sought to come up with actions and solutions *together*. The peer-based approach adopted sought not only to improve prospects for employment, and conditions for gender and sexual minorities in workplaces in Manipur, it also aimed to develop a range of new, proactive and equitable alliances that offer scope for ongoing collaborative action, both regionally and nationally.

Note

1 Rainbow Manipur | Inclusive Manipur https://rainbowmanipur.wordpress.com/

References

AMaNA, ETA and SAATHII, 2016. Media Release: MNP: Government Departments to Strategize for Transgender Inclusion in Services, Schemes and Entitlements. *AMaNA, ETA and SAATHII*, 11 August. Available from: https://www.vartagensex.org/download.php?name=admin/document/_1470940240046-mnp-tg-welfare-brd-action-medrel-11aug16.pdf [Accessed 9 October 2019].

Bhattacharya, S., 2019. The Transgender Nation and Its Margins: The Many Lives of the Law. *South Asia Multidisciplinary Academic Journal*, 20. https://journals.openedition.org/samaj/4930 [Accessed 9 October 2019].

Boyce, P., 2007. 'Conceiving Kothis': Men Who Have Sex with Men in India and the Cultural Subject of HIV Prevention. *Medical Anthropology*, 26 (2), 175–203.

Boyce, P., 2019. Properties, Substance, Queer Effects: Ethnographic Perspective and HIV in India. In: P. Boyce, E.J. Gonzalez-Polledo, and S. Posocco, eds. *Queering Knowledge: Analytics, Devices and Investments after Marilyn Strathern*. London: Routledge, 92–112.

Boyce, P., et al., 2018. Transgender-Inclusive Sanitation: Insights from South Asia. *Waterlines*, 37 (2), 102–117.

Boyce, P. and khanna, A., 2020. Subjectivies, Knowledge and Sexual and Gendered Transitions in India. In: C. McCallum, S. Posocco, and M. Fotta, eds. *The Cambridge Handbook for the Anthropology of Gender and Sexuality*. Cambridge: Cambridge University Press.

Collumbien, M., et al., 2009. Understanding the Contexts of Male and Transgender Sex Work Using Peer Ethnography. *Sexually Transmitted Infections*, 85 Supplement 2, ii3–ii7.

DfID Inclusive Societies, 2018. Transgender Inclusive Development. *Medium*, 29 March. Available from: https://medium.com/@DFID_Inclusive/transgender-inclusive-develop ment-5128f899592 [Accessed 9 October 2019].

Dhall, P., 2015. Trans Queens of Manipur. *Varta*, 20 January. Available from: https:// varta2013.blogspot.com/2015/01/trans-queens-of-manipur.html [Accessed 9 October 2019].

Dhall, P. and Boyce, P., 2015. Livelihood, Exclusion and Opportunity: Socioeconomic Welfare among Gender and Sexuality Non-normative People in India. IDS Evidence Report 106. Brighton: Institute of Development Studies.

Dutta, A., 2012. An Epistemology of Collusion: Hijra, Kothi and the Historical (Dis) continuity of Gender/Sexual Identities in Eastern India. *Gender and History*, 24 (3), 825–849.

Dutta, A. and Roy, R., 2014. Decolonizing Transgender in India: Some Reflections. *Transgender Studies Quarterly*, 1 (3), 320–337.

Ganju, D. and Saggurti, N., 2017. Stigma, Violence and HIV Vulnerability among Transgender Persons in Sex Work in Maharastra, India. *Culture, Health and Sexuality*, 19 (8), 903–917.

Hossain, A., 2018. De-Indianizing Hijra: Intra-Regional Effacements and Inequalities in South Asian Queer Space. *Transgender Studies Quarterly*, 5 (3), 321–331.

Hemabati, O., 2017. No Share of Family Property for Me Because I Have a Vagina …. *Rainbow Manipur | Inclusive Manipur*, 3 May 2017. Available from: https://rainbow manipur.wordpress.com/2017/05/03/no-share-of-family-property-for-me-because-i-ha ve-a-vagina/ [Accessed 9 October 2019].

Khurai, S., 2019. Attempts at Erasing Trans Cultures in Manipur. *Varta*, 20 September. Available from: https://www.vartagensex.org/details.php?p=5d84e6848d020 [Accessed 9 October 2019].

Lorway, R., Reza-Paul, S., and Pasha, A., 2009. On Becoming a Male Sex Worker in Mysore: Sexual Subjectivity, 'Empowerment,' and Community-Based HIV Prevention Research. *Medical Anthropology Quarterly*, 23 (2), 142–160.

Pebam, B., 2018. Trans Inclusive Public Sanitation in Manipur Needs a Bigger Push. *Varta*, 28 July. Available from: http://vartagensex.org/details.php?p=5b5c74f1c49de [Accessed 9 October 2019].

Phanjoubam, P., 2019. Why it Matters How Manipur Became a State. *The Telegraph*, 20 February. Available from: https://www.telegraphindia.com/opinion/why-it-matters -how-manipur-became-a-state-of-india/cid/1684958 [Accessed 9 October 92019].

Rainbow Manipur|Inclusive Manipur, 2019. Bulletin – Skills & Jobs. *Rainbow Manipur|Inclusive Manipur*. Available from: https://rainbowmanipur.wordpress.com/ bulletin-skills-jobs/ [Accessed 9 October 2019].

Reddy, G., 2005. Geneologies of Contagion: Hijras, Kothis and the Politics of Sexual Marginality in Hyderabad. *Anthropology and Medicine*, 12, 255–270.

Semmalar, G.I., 2017. First as Apathy, Then as Farce: The Transgender Persons (Protection of Rights) Bill, 2016. *Orinam*, August 14. Available from: http://orinam

.net/apathy-farce-trans-rights-bill-standing-committee-report/ [Accessed 9 October 2019].

Stryker, S. and Currah, P., 2016. General Editors Introduction. *Transgender Studies Quarterly*, 3 (3–4), 331–332.

Shears, K., 2019. "Because of How You Are": Using Participatory Research to Understand Violence against Transgender Women in Latin America and the Caribbean. *Linkages*, 7 January. Available from: https://linkagesproject.wordpress.com/2019/01/07/becaus e-of-how-you-are-using-participatory-research-to-understand-violence-against-tra nsgender-women-in-latin-american-and-the-caribbean/ [Accessed 12 October 2019].

Yukhamibam, R., 2020. The Emergence of Transgender Community in Manipur: The Case of *Nupi Maanbis. Indian Journal of Gender Studies*, 7 (2), 205–225.

7 Co-constructing knowledge about the well-being outcomes of unaccompanied migrant children becoming 'adult'

Semhar Haile, Habib Rezaie, Winta Tewoderos, Gul Zada, Elaine Chase, Francesca Meloni and Jennifer Allsopp

Introduction

The peer research approach discussed in this chapter comes from a three-year ESRC-funded study, *Becoming Adult*,[1] which explored the well-being outcomes of unaccompanied migrant children in the UK making the transition to institutional 'adulthood' (that is, the age of 18) within complex immigration and social care systems. A team of peer researchers was involved in the study from the beginning. In keeping with the definition of 'peer researcher' used throughout this volume, they shared core characteristics with research participants in that they had previously all been unaccompanied migrant children who arrived in the UK and who subsequently made the transition to adulthood.

The project employed a combination of peer and participatory research approaches. Participatory research designs have been informed by feminist and postcolonialist critiques of traditional research in development studies (Pain 2004; Beazley and Ennew 2006; Dentith et al. 2012). They are informed by a conviction that people should actively take part in decisions and processes which affect their lives, and that issues of involvement and participation are fundamental human rights (Beazley and Ennew 2006; Crivello et al. 2009; Fargas-Malet et al. 2010; McCartan et al. 2012; D'Amico et al. 2016). From this perspective, academics and participants are meant to work together not only to describe and interpret social reality, but also to fundamentally change it (Maguire 1987; Cahill 2007; Cook 2012; Dentith et al. 2012). The aim was 'to change social reality on the basis of insights into everyday practices that are obtained by means of participatory research' (Bergold and Thomas 2012, p. 2). Moreover, by acknowledging that 'the learning processes involved have independent merit' (McCartan et al. 2012, p. 4), participatory research should positively affect participants' lives.

In this context, young people are being increasingly involved in participatory research as 'peer researchers' (Boyden and Ennew 1997) and are believed to be better suited than adults at conducting research with their peers, given they speak the same language, can facilitate access to those who may be hard to reach, and, most importantly, have first-hand knowledge and insights into the issues affecting their peers, as well as their likely impact (McCartan et al. 2012). Many scholars have also highlighted that young people tend to 'open up' more and speak more freely with their peers rather than with adult researchers, and that this results in a better understanding of young people's life-worlds (Schäfer and Yarwood 2008).

The ideas discussed in this chapter emerged through reflection on the nature and practice of peer research shared among the team. This included aspects of the approach that have worked well, as well as those that proved to be more theoretically, practically and emotionally challenging. In keeping with the aims of this volume, we seek to unsettle some of the assumptions surrounding peer research and suggest points of reflection for others embarking on peer-led research. In this chapter, we adopt and critically engage with the definition of peer researcher as a recognised member of a community with whom research is taking place and who has a prominent role in the research cycle.

The peer research process was undoubtedly successful in enabling rich and nuanced insights into factors influencing the well-being of former unaccompanied migrant children as they transitioned to adulthood in the UK. Moreover, the approach involved a longitudinal component, which enabled the research team to sustain contact with some young people over substantial periods of time. This was only possible, we would argue, through having the peer researchers embedded within the research process from the start. Nonetheless, there were a number of core issues that arose in the field which require further unpacking. These include the nature of 'community'; hierarchies of power in the research process; issues of sustaining and supporting peer researchers in a complex and highly changeable field; and the emotional labour involved in being close to, yet simultaneously distanced from, the pain experienced by others in more precarious and uncertain circumstances than those of the peer researchers, even though they share other characteristics.

We explore each of these issues with the aim of illuminating how 'some of the good intentions and well-described practices in participatory action research are demanding and challenging to fulfil in the real world' (Borg et al. 2012, p. 9). In doing so, we also hope to exemplify the value in facilitating opportunities for reflection and co-writing on these research experiences and making them available to the wider academic, policy and practitioner communities.

Background

When unaccompanied migrant children arrive in the UK, they are obliged to make a claim for asylum, a process through which, in order to be granted refugee status, they need to demonstrate a well-founded fear of persecution in line with the 1951 (amended in 1967) Refugee Convention. It is notoriously hard to prove persecution or fear of persecution (particularly for children) and, as a result, most children are not granted refugee status but rather time-limited permission to reside in the UK until they reach adulthood. During this time, they are normally supported by local authority social care systems who assume the role of 'corporate parents'.

On reaching the age of 18 without refugee status, young people often lose their right to remain in the UK, along with their eligibility to publicly funded resources such as housing, education or social care. While they can appeal this process, the likelihood of such an appeal being successful is increasingly unlikely. At this juncture, if they are refused the right to remain in the country by the UK Home Office, many become destitute and may be forcibly removed to countries of origin. In order to avoid this outcome, many young people 'disappear' by disengaging from social care and immigration systems. This amounts to being forced to live illegally in the UK or migrating elsewhere to avoid deportation to countries in which they feel unsafe, distanced from and where they are unlikely to be able to secure a viable future for themselves or others.

While this transition at 18 is a critical time for many migrant young people, to date the research and policy focus has remained almost entirely on the unaccompanied child. The current research sought to address this gap and to refocus policy attention on a growing number of young adults about whom very little is known and for whom governments across Europe responsible for their care seem to absolve themselves of all accountability.

The work described here took place between 2014 and 2017 and involved young men and women from three countries of origin: Afghanistan, Albania and Eritrea. The focus was on understanding the nature of certain objective well-being outcomes (such as in relation to care, housing, education, employment, relationships with others) as well as more subjective aspects of well-being, defined by young people themselves in relation to core issues of safety and security; legal integrity; identity and belonging; a state of sound mental health; being able to design and fulfil viable futures; and the ability to sustain ties and connections (including transnational ties) with significant others (see Chase 2019; Chase and Allsopp 2020).

Methodology

In total, ten peer researchers (three young women and seven young men) took part in various components of the research, although a core team of six were able to stay involved with the project for its duration and worked in three cities in England where they were residing. All researchers originated from the countries of origin of research participants (Afghanistan, Albania and Eritrea) and were within the same age range (17–25). Even though some of the team had to cease or cut down their involvement due to other commitments and complications in their lives (including issues related to their own immigration status), they nonetheless made valuable contributions to the research, particularly in the early design phases of the work.

Between them, peer researchers were involved in every aspect of the project including identifying and recruiting research participants; facilitating the setting up of research discussions; maintaining contact with participants over time;

being directly involved in in-depth research conversations in English or inter-preting through other languages such as Tigrinya, Pashto or Albanian; facili-tating research engagement through other arts-based research activities, such as photography, poetry and comedy; and working with other artists to help develop a theatre in education drama production (including sitting on discussion panels as part of these productions). All processes of data collection involved a peer researcher working alongside an established academic researcher. However, between periods of data collection, peer researchers worked independently to maintain contact with research participants and handle the practical logistics of the research planning. Peer researchers were also directly involved in analysis of the findings, taking on differing roles from group discussions and reflections to thematic coding of data, and continue to assume roles in writing up research findings and presenting at conferences.

Training for taking on these various roles took the form of a summer school, team residential meetings, mentoring through working directly with experienced researchers on the team and one-to-one training and support provided on an indi-vidual basis to peer researchers (for example, in conducting qualitative data anal-ysis once data was loaded into the data management and analysis tool, NVivo). In total, peer researchers facilitated the participation in interviews of more than 60 young people in England (taking part in more than 100 interviews since many young people were interviewed on several occasions), and engaged with many other participants through arts-based research activities. Peer researchers were paid for their time on an agreed hourly rate (and contracted through the host academic university), in all cases where they had the right to work in the UK. For those without the right to work, 'in kind' arrangements were applied in recogni-tion of their contribution to the project.

Shared reflections on the strengths and limitations of the peer research approach

Things that worked well with the peer research approach

Discussions revealed many positive aspects to the peer research process beyond meeting the research objectives. These included opportunities to learn about research, have access to academic spaces, develop new skills, challenge oneself, work as part of a team and build strong supportive team relationships over time. These benefits were summed up neatly by one of the peer researchers[2]:

> Despite having no previous experience of participatory peer research, this project has shown me the usefulness of peer research approaches, especially in the ethnographic research field. In this particular context, peer research enabled for better translation of cultural contexts and concepts that are not easy to translate across languages. Thanks to the project there was a good level of trust between interviewees and researchers, as well as within the team.

Researchers spoke about the strong sense of comradery and having mutually supportive teamwork, which had laid the basis for some deep friendships. They valued the opportunity of coming together as an international team, learning about different worldviews, working across different nationalities and languages and coming to know about each other's lives in Eritrea, Afghanistan and Albania. One of the team commented that one of the things they most valued was: 'Building trust between team members and having an open discussion about the issues raised related to the project, as well as supporting each other throughout the project'.

There were reflections on how, through working on the project, peer researchers gained access to support, mentorship and guidance on different aspects of their lives such as in relation to social care support, education and work opportunities (including help with CVs and reference letters). They equally valued opportunities such as public speaking and attending conferences and connecting with other non-governmental organisations working with migrant young people to discuss the key themes of the project and gain knowledge about similar projects in the field.

The team recognised benefits to research participants through their role as peer researchers. At times, for example, they were able to refer participants through the established links of the project to other services and support, which participants otherwise did not know about or how to access. They felt that in many cases young people benefited from open discussions about their migratory experiences with people who had similarly had to transition between very different worlds in terms of culture, religion and language. They felt it sometimes helped research participants articulate how they coped with the fact that their expectations of what it would be like to arrive in the UK and the realities and complexities of what they actually experienced were often very different. One of the peer researchers commented:

> There was a friendly approach to participate, creating safe and friendly environments, where participants feel comfortable to discuss … and building trust between researchers and practitioners and helping participants to overcome culture barriers.

Finally, the flexibility of the research approach was valued by the peer researchers. They liked the fact that there was space to question methods and their underlying assumptions and adapt the approach as appropriate. For example, recognising the limitations of orthodox narrative interviews and the reticence to participate by some young people, such flexibility enabled the exploration of other complementary open-ended forms of engagement, such as use of photography and other arts-based methods (see Meloni et al. 2017).

Aside from the many benefits which, on the whole, affirmed the value of working through participatory and peer-led approaches previously cited in relevant scholarship, there were also important issues raised by the team which required further attention and reflection. These are discussed below around four intersecting and cross-cutting themes.

Sustaining training and support

The team valued the training that was provided throughout the project including residential trainings, meetings with experienced members of the research team and learning through co-working. This is reflected in comments such as

> The training we received was vital to us as a peer researcher, with very relaxed and open environment where everyone was open to the discussion of issues [they were] facing through the project.

Nonetheless, they felt that more time could have been allocated to supporting their roles. This is partly the result of the difficulties in second guessing what issues would emerge in a highly complex research field and the limitations of capacity which meant that experienced research team members were unable to be on the ground all the time to provide training and support accordingly. As a result, peer researchers sometimes described feeling 'out of their depth'. The challenges of adequately equipping young researchers to work in the field have been identified elsewhere. According to McCartan et al. (2012), for example, while young people might be better suited at conducting research with their peers, they may lack the research skills required for such a task and therefore need to be trained in a relatively short period of time.

The *Becoming Adult* project was a multi-site study with a core research team of limited capacity. Moreover, peer researchers had many other things going on in their lives (including study and work commitments, as well as involvement in faith-based or other organisations) and in some cases, as noted earlier, were struggling with their own uncertainties about their immigration status or what was going to happen in their immediate futures. Over the lifespan of a three-year project, as we learned, people's lives can fundamentally change, affecting the extent to which they are able to sustain their research involvement. Respecting people's commitment and being adaptable to these temporal dynamics was vitally important to the intended ethos of the project. Yet, accommodating this diversity may generate a pattern and rhythm to the research which is entirely different to more top-down conventional research projects which tend to adhere to strict project timelines and milestones.

Having a relatively well-funded project over three years enabled some of these irregularities in the rhythm of the project to be ironed out and, over its lifespan, the project was highly successful in meeting its objectives. The challenging dynamics in the field were also partly mitigated through ongoing support in the field and the fact that, for the purposes of data collection at least, young people were not left alone but rather worked in tandem with an experienced researcher. Nonetheless, being embedded in their own communities and engaging in these worlds outside of the research field meant that peer researchers frequently came into contact with young people who were struggling, who they felt powerless to help and who, due to the nature of the research, derived no immediate benefits in terms of their circumstances through their participation (other than recognition of their contribution through gift vouchers and, where appropriate, referral on to other support and advice services). A key learning point would be to allocate further time during both training and fieldwork elements of the project for reflecting on some of the likely challenges raised by the complex dynamics of peer researchers working in these circumstances. In practice, this is likely to mean building in resources for enhanced tailoring of training and support to individual peer researchers in situ (as well as having collective team training) and being able to respond more adequately and spontaneously to emerging issues in the field.

Notions of community and power imbalances

Peer researchers also reflected on some key assumptions which are frequently made when facilitating peer-led research. One of these, which was arguably embedded in the research design, is the idea that because the team members were from the same countries as research participants and had similar experiences, in that they had also migrated alone as children, this was likely to spark a connection between them. While this quite often did happen, having these elements of their lives in common, they stressed, did not automatically mean that interviewees felt more comfortable in the peer researchers' presence to express their feelings, discomforts or personal experiences. Moreover, there were likely to be as many differences as there were similarities between young people in terms of everything from character and outlook to other identity attributes such as gender, ethnicity, cultural experience, whether they had grown up in rural or urban settings, and other socio-economic factors. Moreover, the different lengths of time they had spent living in the UK and their different legal statuses could generate chasms in terms of lack of shared personal experiences of migration. Thus, it was essential not to make automatic assumptions about the nature of 'community'. And even where their experiences were similar, there may be other reasons why it might be more difficult to speak to peers, summed up by one of the team as follows:

> Just because we are from the same country doesn't necessarily mean that the person feels at ease … they still fear the shame and stigma of their situations and it may be harder to admit that to someone from the same background.

A further dilemma for researchers was how they explained their relatively powerful position to others despite their shared experiences. As one team member put it, 'how come we were the ones asking the questions?'; and how do you respond to the questions such as, 'did you come like us?'; or 'or do you get money or support from the government for doing this work?' While such questions could be asked in a 'jokey' way, they still had the same severity behind them and could leave peer researchers feeling uncomfortable and as though they were constantly being 'checked out'. Undoubtedly, working in a context in which the political sensitivities around migration and legality were integral to the research created particular challenges for peer researchers.

A further power and status dynamic emerged as a result of differing legal statuses within the research team. While the majority of the team had a secure legal status which gave them the right to work in the UK, at least one team member was in a situation which was more precarious and very similar to quite a number of the research participants. While the legal situation was resolved by the end of the project, having lasted in total for a period of nine years, it meant differential access to financial resources for working on the project. As noted earlier, peer researchers with a right to work could receive payment on an hourly basis for their labour, but the member of the team with no legal status was not able to be paid in the same way. While alternative ways were found to compensate for his time, this was still limiting and generated a hierarchy of opportunity within the team.

Peer researchers' positionality

Peer researchers spoke about the complex identity of being both researcher and researched in the sense that the focus of the study directly related to their own experiences. Knowing the feelings associated with having previously been unaccompanied migrant children and also recognising that most of them (not all) had a more secure status than the young people they were talking to, left them with multiple mini dilemmas as they carried out their roles as researchers. It is important to note that these same issues arose for the team as a whole. What sorts of questions should or could they ask, and what should they avoid? How could they be sure that they were not re-traumatising young people by asking them to talk about their lived experiences of the past as well as engage with the liminality and uncertainties in their current lives? While it was said to be easier to manage these nuances when research was conducted in English, and when sensitive topics could be gently broached as part of an overarching life course narrative, peer researchers felt it was difficult to do across languages. When they were in the position of interpreting within the research setting, peer researchers often felt an acute language barrier as participants struggled to express their feelings and they were having to interpret such nuances quickly. One of the peer researchers neatly captured the difficulty as follows:

> As a peer researcher, I felt some discomfort to translate some of the correct words that participants wanted to use. This was both a challenge in terms of working across languages and there not always necessarily being any direct translation of concept, words or feelings from one language to another … there was pressure, lots of pressure.

The team also reflected extensively about the processes of facilitating access to research participants from the position of being a friend or confidant. While this worked well in some cases, particularly amongst young men who had established strong networks within local communities with whom they had migrated or whom they met soon after their arrival, it was a very difficult position for some of the team to navigate. They found it hard to understand and respond to the reluctance and sometimes genuine fear some people expressed about participating in the research and felt awkward about asking them to take part. As a result, one or two peer researchers decided that they no longer wanted to help with the recruitment of participants and instead took on alternative roles in the research project. These included helping facilitate arts-based methods such as photography, music and comedy, and taking on core roles in contributing more to the analysis of data and writing up findings.

Peer researchers also had to grapple constantly with questions of how much they should share about their own personal stories when conducting the research. As one of the team commented, 'what do you show or tell of yourself?'. This also emerged as an issue when, on occasion, members of the team were invited to contribute to university teaching sessions or speak at conferences or panel discussions. While some felt relatively relaxed about referring to their past lives and situations, others felt profoundly uncomfortable sharing their personal experiences but felt that there was a tacit expectation that they should do so. Upon occasion, researchers felt that those hearing them speak were either feeling sorry for them or were mistrustful of their intentions of coming to the UK. One of the team reflected on how at one event, there was a person who had extremely strong views on child migration and he felt out of his depth in knowing how to respond. These reflections raised the importance of making the boundaries of participation for peer researchers far more explicit at every stage of the project and also focusing more on equipping the team with further skills and tools in responding to difficult interactions such as those described above. Importantly, it should be added that there were numerous occasions where peer researchers very successfully participated in conferences and also made a clear impact in shifting views and perceptions of migrant young people. One of the researchers on the team spoke about how at one migration conference in Europe she had observed peer researchers completely 'take control of the event, moving from mere tokenistic involvement to owning the situation through telling jokes about, and humanising the policies, that young people were subjected to'.

Emotional labour

A further issue, which we were acutely aware of through previous experience of conducting research with marginalised communities and in relation to sensitive topics, is what has been termed the 'emotional labour' (Dickson-Swift et al. 2009). Emotional labour played out in practice from the perspective of peer researchers in complex ways. Given that, in many situations, participants were recruited to the research through their networks and friendship groups, this sometimes placed peer researchers in an ambiguous position. Besides working hard to help participants feel comfortable about taking part in the research, they often also provided ongoing practical and emotional support outside of the 'field'. For example, some peer researchers took it on themselves to check in with participants on a regular basis to see how they were doing, helped them access services and support when they were struggling, or sometimes helped them out as best they could with food or cash. Often, however, they were unable to provide the level or type of support requested, and there is never an easy response to someone who is desperate to resolve their immigration situation and in constant fear of the real possibility of deportation. Peer researchers described feeling a profound discomfort at being unable to help with immigration matters when asked by participants, even though the fact that we were unable to assist with these matters had been clearly explained early on. These emotional challenges frequently encountered were summed up by one of the team:

> Participating as a peer researcher in projects such as *Becoming Adult*, also comes with emotional and moral burden. Often, there are expectations from interviewees, and often we feel the need to help but we are limited in our capacities. This is particularly difficult to clarify especially with research participants.

Previous work has also highlighted how, when there is a closeness between peer researchers and participants, highly sensitive ethical considerations can emerge (Abebe 2009; Bergold and Thomas 2012). These very much came to light in our own research. Peer researchers sometimes came up against difficult situations in which they felt out of their depth and, on occasion, it transpired that they had felt unable to share some of these dilemmas with those managing the research, due to concerns about breaching confidentiality.

Discussion and conclusion

This chapter set out to capture what emerged through a process of reflective analysis of a set of experiences of conducting peer-led research in the highly complex and politicised field of child and youth migration. It provides a candid appraisal of the potential benefits of peer approaches, but also emphasises its complexities and the sorts of common assumptions we need to be mindful of. Above all, it has illuminated the exacting demands on peer researchers and the importance of fully appreciating these as part of research project design and implementation.

The complexities of asylum and immigration policies in the UK, and how they interact with social care provision for unaccompanied migrant young people, generate a particular set of political and power dynamics which are difficult to navigate in and of themselves. The subjectivities of the peer researchers as former unaccompanied migrant children intensified this complexity and raised a number of research management and ethical dilemmas.

In our discussions about what we might do differently next time, several recommendations emerged from the peer researcher team. The first of these was the importance of always checking the assumption that participants would find it easier to connect with peer researchers due to their shared or similar past experiences. While there were many situations where such connected histories facilitated migrant young people's participation, at other times this was not the case.

Sometimes, it was said, there may be greater trust placed in someone from outside the community, who speaks a different language and is older.

Beyond this, the researchers felt that more attention could have been given to how they negotiated their own positionality in the research. At times they struggled with how best to respond to questions relating to their relative security of status and power vis-à-vis research participants. They were unsure how to deal with the emotional pressures of feeling unable to adequately support the young people they engaged in the research, a dilemma which deeply affected the whole research team. Similar dynamics have been alluded to in other work. Christensen (2004), for example, argues how power relationships are complex and cannot be dealt with only by viewing power as determined by social positions as, for example, the power of adults over young people. Schäfer and Yarwood (2008) have highlighted the often-overlooked power relations between young people and their potentially disempowering effects. Lushey and Munro (2015) also point to the fact that pre-existing relationships between interviewers and respondents might influence the interview process and raise complex concerns about confidentiality, as well as how best to care for participants.

It is, however, important to note that, while there were clear boundaries around not providing information (for example, regarding legal or other matters about which we had no direct expertise or training, as researchers), we were able to signpost young people to available services and support. One peer researcher in particular spoke of the transformative effects this had had on a young woman who, after accessing appropriate advice and information, had a much better understanding of what she was entitled to and how she could access the help she needed. This process was enabled through establishing good connections with local support and non-governmental organisations which, we would argue, is vitally important to relieving some of these pressures from researchers.

It was important to build flexibility into the project in terms of the nature of participation. The team valued the fact that where participants had resisted taking part in orthodox interviews, they were able to engage them in other ways, such as through comedy workshops, photography, music, poetry and other arts-based methods. Leaving space to adjust the research design to the different roles that peer researchers could take on was also appreciated. This allowed them to work to their strengths and remain comfortable within the roles they were taking on. It is worth noting that this variation of peer researchers' roles had not been thought through at the project design phase but became something crucial to address over time. As pointed out earlier, such flexibility does not neatly fit with highly orthodox project plans with strict timelines and milestones. Instead, it requires planning, which allows the research to find its own rhythm and pattern, within the parameters of the research objectives, but which can adapt to the skills, capacities, feelings and emotions of the research team over time.

Finally, there were particular issues emerging with respect to ongoing training and support for peer researchers which, on reflection, required further attention. All the peer researchers said they would value the opportunity to learn how to better handle some of the complex situations they came across, feel more able to respond to sometimes extremely complicated ethical issues, as well as hone new skills such as public speaking and working with the media. This need to strengthen the systems and processes to protect peer researchers has been identified by others too (Lushey and Munro 2015) and is certainly something which in future we would give greater attention to, despite the difficult logistics in terms of people's availability and working across different geographies and time frames.

We end this chapter with a quote from a member of the team, which at once underlines the value of participatory and peer research approaches and the need for critical engagement with them as methodologies:

> A participatory approach is effective in cases where it is used to question the status quo. Thus, it should be used to question approaches, own assumptions and methodologies. This is because participatory and peer research approaches are not more ethical or less top-down by nature, they can reproduce top-down power relations unless there is an active questioning process. They should be flexible and allow for changes in methodologies and provide adequate space for reflections.

Notes

1 www.becomingadult.net.
2 Quotes have not been attributed directly to individuals since peer researchers requested that they be presented as joint reflections.

References

Abebe, T., 2009. Multiple methods, complex dilemmas: Negotiating socio-ethical spaces in participatory research with disadvantaged children. *Children's Geographies*, 7 (4), 451–465.

Beazley, H. and Ennew, J., 2006. Participatory methods and approaches: Tackling the two tyrannies. In: V. Desai and R. Potter, eds. *Doing Development Research*. London: SAGE Publications, 189–199.

Boyden, J. and Ennew, J., eds., 1997. *Children in Focus: A Manual for Participatory Research with Children*. Stockholm: Save the Children Sweden.

Bergold, J. and Thomas, S., 2012. Participatory research methods: A methodological approach in motion. *Forum Qualitative Sozialforschung/Forum: Qualitative Social Research*, 13 (1). doi:10.17169/fqs-13.1.1801.

Borg, M., et al., 2012. Opening up for many voices in knowledge construction. *Forum Qualitative Sozialforschung/Forum: Qualitative Social Research*, 13 (1). doi:10.17169/fqs-13.1.1793.

Cahill, C., 2007. Doing research with young people: Participatory research and the rituals of collective work. *Children's Geographies*, 5 (3), 297–312.

Chase, E., 2019. Transitions, capabilities and wellbeing: How Afghan unaccompanied young people experience becoming 'adult' in the UK and beyond. *Journal of Ethnic and Migration Studies* (Special Issue Unaccompanied Minors in Europe), 46 (2), 439–456.

Chase, E. and Allsopp, J., 2020. *Becoming Adult: The Politics of Wellbeing and Migration*. Bristol: Bristol University Press.

Christensen, P.H., 2004. Children's participation in ethnographic research: Issues of power and representation. *Children and Society*, 18 (2), 165–176.

Cook, T., 2012. Where Participatory approaches meet pragmatism in funded (health) research: The challenge of finding meaningful spaces. *Forum Qualitative Sozialforschung/Forum: Qualitative Social Research*, 13 (1). doi:10.17169/fqs-13.1.1783.

Crivello, G., Camfield, L., and Woodhead, M., 2009. How can children tell us about their wellbeing? Exploring the potential of participatory research approaches within young lives. *Social Indicators Research*, 90 (1), 51–72.

D'Amico, M., et al., 2016. Research as intervention? Exploring the health and well-being of children and youth facing global adversity through participatory visual methods, *Global Public Health*, 11 (5–6), 528–545.

Dentith, A.M., Measor, L., and O'Malley, M.P., 2012. The research imagination amid dilemmas of engaging young people in critical participatory work. *Forum Qualitative Sozialforschung/Forum: Qualitative Social Research*, 13 (1). doi:10.17169/fqs-13.1.1788.

Dickson-Swift, V., James, E., and Kippen, S., 2009. Researching sensitive topics: Qualitative research as emotion work. *Qualitative Research*, 9 (1), 61–79.

Fargas-Malet, M., et al., 2010. Research with children: Methodological issues and innovative techniques. *Journal of Early Childhood Research*, 8 (2), 175–192.

Lushey, C.J. and Munro, E.R., 2015. Participatory peer research methodology: An effective method for obtaining young people's perspectives on transitions from care to adulthood? *Qualitative Social Work*, 14 (4), 522–537.

Maguire, P., 1987. *Doing Participatory Research: A Feminist Approach*. Amherst, MA: Centre for International Education, University of Massachusetts.

McCartan, C., Schubotz, D., and Murphy, J., 2012. The self-conscious researcher- postmodern perspectives of participatory research with young people. *Forum Qualitative Sozialforschung/Forum: Qualitative Social Research*, 13 (1). doi:10.17169/fqs-13.1.1798.

Meloni, F., Haile, S., and Chase, E., 2017. *Walking a Tightrope: Migrant Young People, Transitions and Futures*. London: University College London.

Pain, R., 2004. Social geography: Participatory research. *Progress in Human Geography*, 28 (5), 652–663.

Schäfer, N. and Yarwood, R., 2008. Involving young people as researchers: Uncovering multiple power relations among youths. *Children's Geographies*, 6 (2), 121–135.

8 Participation and power

Engaging peer researchers in preventing gender-based violence in the Peruvian Amazon

Geordan Shannon and Jenevieve Mannell

Introduction

In this chapter, we reflect on our experience using participatory action research to engage community health workers as peer researchers in the development of an intervention to prevent gender-based violence in the Peruvian Amazon. We explore issues of participation and power which emerged over the course of the 'Gender Violence in the Amazon of Peru' (GAP) – or *Violencia de Género en las Amazonas Peruanas* – project. Participatory action research is a collaborative research approach that actively involves community members in research and then seeks to bring about social change on the basis of the insights obtained (Bergold and Thomas 2012). Between 2017 and 2019, we worked with seven peer researchers along the Lower Napo River in the Amazon to research, design and implement activities to prevent gender-based violence in their communities.

By highlighting the complex power dynamics present in relationships established through the project, we uncover a paradoxical relationship between participation and power. Participation in the research process can facilitate a process of 'empowerment' whereby participation engenders a level of critical insight – *conscientização* or 'critical consciousness' (Freire 2000) – and thus enables action. In this way, power is developed through participation. However, this emergence of power is not automatically uniform. Developing collective power through participatory processes means reshaping or negotiating existing power relations, and at worst exacerbating ingrained inequalities. In this way, participation both uncovers and exaggerates complex power dynamics. Here, we discuss some of the issues that arose during the course of the work and highlight the complex challenge of ensuring a participatory and collaborative approach when working with peer researchers.

The challenge of gender-based violence prevention in extreme settings

'Extreme' settings are defined by Campbell and Mannell (2016) as settings where significant poverty coincides with gender inequalities and the widespread acceptance of violence as a normal part of intimate relationships. In such settings, gender-based violence has a significant impact on women's health and well-being. Health impacts may be particularly exacerbated in rural or low-resource settings, where geographic isolation coincides with significant poverty, lack of support networks, the absence of resources to address violence, gender inequalities and a widespread acceptance of violence as a normal part of intimate relationships (Goeckermann et al. 1994; Peek-Asa et al. 2011).

The Peruvian Amazon is an example of an extreme setting. Here, high rates of gender-based violence reflect historical events of colonisation and political marginalisation, intersecting with identities of ethnicity, class and geography, which shape violent behaviours. It has been argued that much gender-based violence in Peru occurs in the context of longstanding political and social violence, from the Spanish Conquest and subsequent colonisation of Indigenous populations, through internal conflict throughout the 20th century, to present-day extreme economic inequity and structural violence (Flake 2005). These factors have coalesced to shape gender-based violence in rural Amazonian settings. Rural Peru has some of the world's highest reported rates of gender-based violence, with a lifetime prevalence of 61% (Devries et al. 2013). Recent figures showed that 79% of women between the ages of 18 and 29 in the Amazonian port town of Mazan reported experiencing sexual violence at some point in their life (Chacaltana 2013). In the context of poverty and geographic remoteness, transactional and commercial sex work leaves many women vulnerable to violence and has been shown to increase risks of HIV transmission (Orellana et al. 2013). Gender-based violence is therefore a complex and burdensome issue linked to deep-rooted historical events.

Over the last 20 years, strategies to address gender-based violence have mainly focused on legislation, justice sector responses, awareness raising and women's shelters, with much less attention being paid to violence prevention (Ellsberg et al. 2015). Promising results have arisen from discrete gender-based violence prevention interventions using participatory community-based approaches to challenge social norms that accept or condone acts of violence in low- and middle-income countries (Jewkes et al. 2008; Abramsky et al. 2016b). One approach called *SASA!* developed by the Ugandan non-governmental organisation (NGO), *Raising Voices*, trained community activists to initiate conversations about power relations as a means of challenging social norms about violence. This intervention reported changes in gender norms including a significant increase in men's likelihood to report greater participation in household tasks and greater appreciation of their partner's work inside and outside the home over a five-year period (Abramsky et al. 2016a). *Stepping Stones* is another participatory education and development package that has led to fewer men self-reporting the perpetuation of intimate partner violence in Uganda (Jewkes et al. 2008), and which has been adapted for Honduras, Guatemala, El Salvador, Nicaragua and Ecuador (Bollinger 2010). In Brazil, an NGO called Promundo has run programmes that target men in communities, which have brought about significant changes in gender-based violence attitudes and a decrease in self-reported use of violence with women partners (Instituto Promundo 2012).

These programmes and interventions highlight the potential for gender-based violence prevention through participatory activities that address social norms within communities. While participatory in their design, they do not generally involve community members in research design and delivery (Cornwall and Jewkes 1995), nor do they use peer researchers as a means of ensuring community participation. In extreme settings which are geographically isolated and lack formal support networks – such as those in the Peruvian Amazon – community needs, and the subsequent nature of participatory gender-based violence prevention strategies, are inherently different. The GAP project has carved out a unique approach in the field of gender-based violence prevention in extreme settings: it specifically worked towards using local resources and building local capacity for primary gender-based violence prevention, with an explicit focus on integrating peer researchers from project conceptualisation and design, to implementation and final evaluation.

Engaging peer researchers in violence prevention using participatory action research

The project aimed to investigate the potential for communities to address gender-based violence as a health issue impacting women's everyday lives. The underlying rationale for using a participatory approach as part of the project was based on our prior experience working with low-resource communities in other countries and a shared conviction that community members have the capacity to address their own health issues.

As researchers, we worked in partnership with DB Peru, a local NGO that provides basic medical outreach services and health training to 25 communities along the Lower Napo River. Each community consists of between 50 and 200 people, many of whom identify as *mestizo* (a person of mixed European and non-European lineage) and live a predominantly subsistence agricultural life. Community members live in severe poverty. Many do not have access to running water or toilets and 83% of women are educated at or below primary level (Instituto Nacional de Estadística e Informática 2011). The issue of violence was first articulated to DB Peru by community members during a previous research study focusing on gender roles and relations in the Napo River and a cervical cancer prevention project conducted in 2015. Government services for gender-based violence response and prevention are concentrated in the capital city of Iquitos, which is over 12 hours by riverboat away from the communities of the Lower Napo River, thus making many of these services inaccessible. Women and men in Lower Napo River communities shared personal or neighbourhood experiences of violence and asked explicitly if there was anything DB Peru could do to address violence locally.

In consultation with community health volunteers, referred to locally as *promotores*, it was decided that collectively they would act to address violence in their communities. DB Peru's model of engagement with the communities has primarily been through *promotores*. There are one or two *promotores* in each community and DB Peru offers regular training to members of this group on a range of health issues. The GAP project was conceptualised to draw on the strong relationship between DB Peru and the *promotores* to iteratively research local perspectives on gender-based violence and design a prevention intervention using a participatory action research cycle of engagement. The *promotores* acted as peer researchers for the project and played an instrumental role in each stage of research.

Participatory action research takes a transformative and emancipatory approach that implicitly involves community members in the identification of common problems using research techniques and then developing and testing potential solutions (Lewin 1946). It combines 'action' research (studies conducted in the course of a particular activity to improve the approach of those involved) and 'participatory' research (an approach that equitably involves community members in all aspects of the research process and in which all partners equally contribute expertise and share decision making and ownership) (Hult and Lennung 1980). As illustrated in Figure 8.1, the GAP project was designed around five stages of participatory action research: engagement, planning, acting, observing and reflecting (Olshansky et al. 2005).

In Stage 1, '*engagement*', community leaders from all 25 communities were invited to a day-long workshop (repeated over three days at different locations along the river) to introduce the project and design local ethical guidelines for community engagement. This process brought together over 80 people from 21 communities along the river, including *promotores*, local political leaders, traditional birth attendants, community agents and other interested individuals. Attendees participated in a group prioritisation exercise using an adapted form of 'nominal group technique' – a semi-structured technique used to elicit group members' opinions, generate group discussion and collate and prioritise ideas (Harvey and Holmes 2012). We used this technique to discuss the moral position of the project and to brainstorm and prioritise ethical concepts to be considered as part of the project going forward. These concepts were then used to develop an ethical framework to guide the project and its activities.

In Stage 2, '*planning*', the research team held a preliminary workshop with 16 *promotores* (3 women, 13 men) from 14 communities. On day 1 of the workshop, we engaged members of the group in role play, theatre and group discussions to develop a shared understanding of gender-based violence and establish expectations for the role of peer researchers in the project. Those who were interested in being involved – eight in total, including seven men and one woman – were then invited to stay for an additional three days of activities. During this time, we worked with the peer researchers to map the realities of gender-based violence in the local communities through in-depth interviews and participatory group activities to explore trends in violence over time (individual lifetime, annual cycle, long-term), identify risk factors and develop 'solution trees' (*árboles de soluciones*) (Anyaegbunam et al. 2004).

At the end of the workshop, we travelled as a group to each of the eight communities where the peer researchers presented the project's objectives and asked for community input. Peer researchers were then given two months to

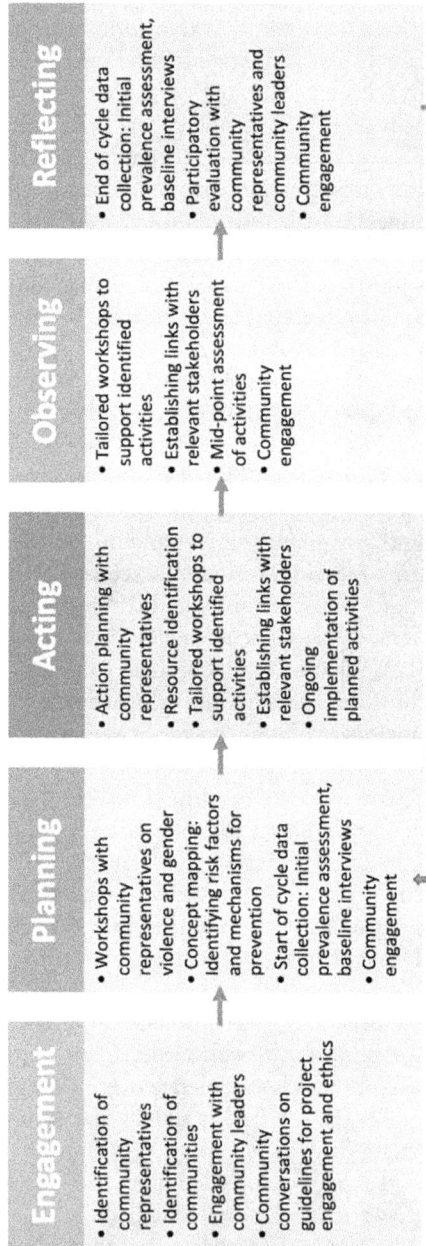

Figure 8.1 Participatory Community-led Intervention Development (PCID) approach for the prevention of gender-based violence.

develop ideas they had for specific activities that could be implemented, consult with community leaders and build support networks. After two months, we met together again as a group to plan specific activities using a 'project planner' (a 15-page activity book developed by the GAP project team) to help define and monitor potential activities within each community. Peer researchers also defined the resources they would need to complete the activities, and a support package (including money for petrol, educational DVDs, pens, chalk, scissors, tape and paper) was provided by the research project.

During Stage 3, '*action*', the peer researchers completed the activities they had designed. A total of 57 activities were carried out across ten communities from March to December 2018, including household visits, community discussions, theatre activities, video presentations and meetings with local authorities about local cases or service provision more broadly. This was completed in parallel with Stage 4, '*observing*', as the peer researchers documented their activities in the project planner, while noting any thoughts they had about their progress in a personal reflection journal.

In the final Stage 5, '*reflection*', the peer researchers participated in a final workshop where we revisited short-, medium- and long-term goals for the project that had been established as part of Stage 2, presented in a 'river of hope' (*rio de esperanza*) diagram. We set up the room in three stations to reflect the original short (e.g. increased knowledge and community support, reducing machismo, less fighting), medium (e.g. small reduction of violence, greater family and community unity, expanded participation in communal activities) and long (e.g. larger reduction of violence, a healthy community without problems, a change in alcohol habits) term goals of the project. At each station, we discussed and reported on whether these objectives had been achieved and then set new objectives for the project going forward. We also used this process to conduct an analysis of the strengths, weaknesses, opportunities and threats that had impacted each of the proposed project goals. The research team also completed final in-depth interviews with each peer researcher about their individual achievements and project experiences.

Participation and power

Our study aimed to involve peer researchers as partners in the design and evaluation of the research as well as its implementation. We conceptualised the *promotores* as 'peers' in the study, with the same (and often more) authority than the research team over decisions about how to understand the issue of violence, what activities should be carried out to addressing violence, and what project success should look like. Our commitment to this goal arose from a deeply held conviction that community members have experiential knowledge that supersedes our own expertise in understanding how to prevent gender-based violence in these local communities (Kovach 2015). In practice, however, we were met with many challenges in achieving this goal, primarily due to existing power dynamics between the various actors involved in the project, including the NGO, the research team, the *promotores* as peer researchers, and the communities themselves. In order to better understand the complex power dynamics in our project, we organised our reflections in a way that allowed us to bring a more nuanced insight to bear upon the notion of power.

Power through participation

Participation and power are closely interrelated. The philosopher and political theorist, Arendt (1963), posited that power was based on relations and communication rather than unilateral domination or force, and that individual interaction with society and politics is a means through which to develop a positive sense of self. Likewise, Freire (2000) articulated how meaningful dialogue and participation in a collective process constituted an opportunity to develop critical consciousness of the social and structural factors influencing one's health and to develop the capacity to act on them, in order to change lived realities for the better. In this view, again, power is developed through participation.

In our project, we were cognisant of how participation in a participatory action research cycle enhanced peer researchers' power to reflect on and address gender-based violence and affect community mobilisation for this purpose. This, we felt, occurred in three key ways: valuing local knowledge, engaging collectively in problem solving, and identifying and mobilising resources beyond the community for gender-based violence prevention.

Our close alignment with the principle that research decisions should be made by peer researchers meant that our research team role was to facilitate and foster promotor-led decision making about violence against women and how its prevention is possible within communities. To generate such discussion, workshops were organised around participatory activities, including having the peer researchers brainstorm what they thought were risk factors for violence and then developing strategies to prevent these risk factors. This peer-led participatory approach generated ideas about violence and its prevention that the research team would not have reached alone. For example, through a number of community mapping activities, peer researchers were able to uncover local networks to help facilitate prevention efforts, including their own family members, local leaders and teachers. Peer researchers shared with each other local strategies to navigate difficult situations or diffuse community tensions. Participation in the GAP project, including being able to speak and act in a space that explicitly valued locally produced knowledge, enhanced peer researchers' value in themselves and of their local resources and networks.

The participatory action research process facilitated open, multidirectional dialogue that helped us collectively problem solve and tackle emergent challenges. For instance, the peer researchers identified children's access to violent films as a major problem in their communities, which they understood to be promoting violent behaviour more broadly. One of the activities organised by peer researchers to address this issue was to hold community film screenings of alternative non-violent and educational films. These activities were well received in

communities and were run independently of external NGO or researcher support. Peer researchers were able to confidently critique the films themselves from
a gender violence perspective. Another example of emergent problem solving
occurred when peer researchers identified that many households experienced difficulties managing household finances, and then strategised the most effective
way of entering households to offer advice in a safe and non-threatening manner.
This part of the research process helped to foster a realisation of collective power
among the peer researchers and their potential to bring about change.

Peer researchers realised their ability to affect change by actively identifying their needs and subsequently linking into resources beyond their communities to enhance local gender-based violence prevention efforts. Peer
researchers felt that many of the activities they identified as potential opportunities to prevent violence – such as couples counselling and enabling men
and women to discuss violence – required specialised support. As a research
team, we responded to requests by pulling specialised resources from a variety
of sources – including connecting with a psychologist in Iquitos, arranging a
visit with regional police officers, and adapting resources from the Ministry
of Health – and training the peer researchers in how to use these resources.
As the project progressed, peer researchers discussed how valuable they found
these resources and continued to ask for new and more diverse resources to
help them with their activities.

However, this last strategy was not without its challenges. By producing these
educational resources, we were in many ways undermining the value of the peer
researchers' local knowledge and affirming their need for training and input
from non-local 'experts'. Structural inequalities have historically undermined
Indigenous epistemologies as part of research practices (Smith 1999), and our
use of participatory action research was intended to challenge these power imbalances. Our participatory approach was meant to surface local Amazonian epistemologies by exposing the power dynamics embedded in knowledge production
and providing space for discussion (Kovach 2015). However, not producing these
educational resources would have also felt as if we were providing inadequate
support to the peer researchers and withholding knowledge about other interventions that had been effective in preventing violence against women. Our process,
therefore, reflected a continual negotiation within the project team to balance
placing value in the local resources of peer researchers with providing external
'expert' resources.

Participation as a tool to reveal power structures

As participatory action research proceeded, we noticed how our presence, and
the project that we were undertaking, meant that local power dynamics were
uncovered and, in some cases, exacerbated. We observed this operating within
communities through low levels of female representation on our project, the
challenges that some peer researchers faced in confronting local power structures, and the way in which peer researchers kept knowledge to themselves. We

also noticed this beyond the community, through the way that peer researchers related with external power structures and resources.

Of the 16 *promotores* who arrived for the first training session (Stage 2: Planning), only three were women. This reflected broader community dynamics and the role of community health workers. Although unpaid, the *promotore* role brings a certain amount of status to individuals within their communities. *Promotores* are provided with specialised health-related training by DB Peru and other NGOs working in the area, which they use to assist members of their community when they are in need. However, the training often means travel to other locations on the river, which requires petrol and can be demanding on one's time. The traditional role of women as caregivers means that they are often unable to travel in this way or to respond to what are often last-minute requests to join training sessions. During the training session, the majority of the women who attended said very little, and only one woman volunteered to become a peer researcher for the project.

The imbalance in women peer researchers affected the project quite significantly. First, it undermined the original identification of violence against women as an issue, originally raised with DB Peru during women's health activities. Women in the communities had therefore been the ones to raise concerns over violence they were experiencing, providing an impetus for the research project as a whole and giving the issue of violence legitimacy as a community concern. However, involving *promotores* as peer researchers served to disconnect this original call for action by women from the project's aims and activities, which were largely carried out by men. Second, the primary involvement of men in the project also influenced the conceptualisation of violence as part of the project. The socially transformative value of participatory action research in theory comes from the ability of participants to reflect on the structural inequalities that shape and define their lives (Ferreyra 2006). In the case of violence against women, these structural inequalities relate to the lower status of women in communities, their absence from leadership and decision-making roles, and social norms that condone violence against women when they step outside of traditional family roles, all of which have been associated with higher rates of violence (Heise 1998; Jewkes 2002). Given that women directly experience the effects of these social norms, it is often much easier for them to reflect on the structural inequalities that guide their behaviour than it is for men. One consequence of mainly involving men as peer researchers, responsible for shaping and defining the project's aims and activities, was that awareness of particular structural inequalities affecting women was often left out of conversations. A prime example of this was in the way in which the peer researchers presented the project back to their communities during Stage 2. In these community conversations, violence against women as a concept was frequently dropped and replaced by the notion of 'family violence', which was often defined as violence by women against children (a risk factor for violence against women, which we had discussed during our workshops with the peer researchers).

The second local challenge that emerged was in navigating local power structures. While all community leaders were initially open to the project, over the course of our work and as the project formed, some leaders expressed resistance to peer researchers' efforts to bring about change in the community. In one such instance, a peer researcher uncovered episodes of violence in the local school perpetrated by a teacher who was a family member of a local leader. As such, their efforts to address this concern were initially thwarted. However, after months of advocacy and action on behalf of the peer researcher, the teacher was removed from the post and there was a change in leadership. The aftermath of these actions meant there was significant community backlash and tension in relation to the leadership change, which manifested as lack of community support and active resistance to the project from some community members. Despite this, the peer researcher perceived there was a positive change in the community's overall condition, and greater awareness of and discussion of violence. This leadership and community resistance highlighted – and possibly reinforced – entrenched local divides and power imbalances.

The third challenge related to knowledge and social capital. The desire for knowledge and expertise was expressed not only by the peer researchers but also by community members. However, in engaging peer researchers in this process we realised that knowledge (as a form of resource and power) was not evenly distributed by peer researchers to the community. In the final stages of the project, we returned to the communities in order to understand more about what the peer researchers had done and how this had been received by community members. We heard frequently about how the peer researchers had done some activities (e.g. holding community meetings or film screenings) but that they had not shared what they had learned as part of the workshops with the broader community. Through these conversations, it became apparent that resources we had developed for the peer researchers were so valuable that they had – consciously or not – kept some of these resources and the knowledge they contained for themselves rather than disseminating them to others in the community. Knowledge, in this way, constituted a powerful resource that established a power differential between community members and the peer researchers.

This speaks to the role of DB Peru, and the research team members by extension, in their interaction with the communities as part of this project. Community members value their relationship with DB Peru, not only because of the medicine and resources they provide, but also because of the educational element of DB Peru's training. DB Peru is perceived as the provider of expert knowledge, which in the ways described above, can also serve to undermine local or Indigenous ways of knowing. The position of the research team as 'experts' on violence against women only served to further emphasise this power dynamic as part of the project. The project was heavily influenced by pre-existing power dynamics that position foreigners as 'knowledgeable others' and locals as needing training and guidance. Overcoming these power dynamics was a constant challenge.

Reflections and conclusions

These challenges bring into question what we mean by 'peer' research and critique the notion that simply identifying members of communities affected by a particular health issue is sufficient (Devotta et al. 2016). Our project demonstrates that the value of peer involvement stems in part from involving community members affected by an issue in identifying the structural inequalities that contribute to the issue as well as potential solutions for addressing it both within and outside of communities. Particular health issues do not necessarily affect all members of a community in the same way. Care must be taken to include those who are closest to the problem at hand. A project about violence against women as a problem identified by women in the communities would ideally have involved women as peer researchers. This would have established a closer link between the structural inequalities the project hoped to address and the lived experiences of the peer researchers.

However, this would have had other trade-offs in terms of power relations in the community that should also be taken into consideration. Women in these highly patriarchal settings may have faced more resistance in undertaking project activities than the male peer researchers did. To a certain extent, this was evident in many of the struggles faced by the one female peer researcher, who faced enormous challenges in addressing issues of violence in her community over the course of the project in comparison to the men. The struggles women as peer researchers face in addressing gendered inequalities that drive health issues from violence to HIV have been well-recognised by others (Campbell 2003), and it would be naïve to think that, if done differently, this project would have been an exception.

Our experience engaging peer researchers contributes to other examples of how participatory engagements with communities and community members have helped to produce high-quality data that reflects the problems, identities, norms and dynamics of communities (Wang et al. 2000; Lushey and Munro 2015). As an ideal, peer research approaches stand to make an important contribution to involving individuals in addressing the issues that affect their lives, disrupting the imbalance of power that exists in many (or most) research practices. However, as recognised by others (Guta et al. 2013; Devotta et al. 2016; Strike et al. 2016), the realities of producing good peer research face a number of challenges in terms of pre-existing power dynamics that have the power to undermine many of its benefits.

Preventing gender-based violence against women as an issue brings these power dynamics to the fore in a way that is often not as apparent with other health and social issues. The patriarchal nature of communities with high levels of violence can easily undermine what we mean by peer research. For instance, patriarchal social structures undermine less powerful voices within communities in ways that compromise any research commitment to ensuring community perspectives are valued as part of the research process. With the GAP project this included silencing the voices of those individuals that had originally identified the issue of violence as a community issue (women) and bringing more powerful community actors (men) into the position of peer researchers because of the status this position helped them achieve. If not carefully managed, peer research can act as a 'governing' practice, whereby the process of participation acts to reproduce institutionalised power dynamics and relationships (Guta et al. 2013).

The power dynamics uncovered through our project reinforce the value of taking a feminist approach to participatory action research which promotes inclusion of marginalised voices, values diversity and complexity of lived experiences, and draws attention to the process of knowledge production (Maguire 1996). The issue of gender-based violence is also a product of its own history and alignment with feminist movements of the Global North. In many ways, this makes the involvement of women peer researchers as those most affected by the issue even more important in making the case for addressing violence within communities. Without calls for action from women who have experienced gender-based violence within a community to address gender-based violence, ideas such as gender inequality run the risk of being framed as Western ideologies out-of-sync with local priorities (Tamale 2006).

It is important to recognise that by engaging peer researchers we may be involved in reproducing the same hierarchy of knowledge that has defined research relationships in Indigenous and other local communities for centuries. Peer researchers may be motivated to join research projects because of the status it brings to them in their relationship with their communities, in addition to the genuine pursuit of local knowledge and solutions to local health problems. This creates the challenge of simply replicating the power dynamic between researcher and research participant that is found in more traditional approaches to research. It does not address the underlying issues of epistemic privilege that comes with the relationship between community-based ways of knowing and academic epistemologies. Participation in research can help to highlight these power dynamics. However, addressing them will require more than the use of peer research approaches alone. It will require a reconsideration of the epistemological basis on which we conduct research with communities and a shift away from involving peers to helping them conduct their own research about their lives.

References

Abramsky, T., et al., 2016a. Ecological pathways to prevention: How does the SASA! Community mobilisation model work to prevent physical intimate partner violence against women? *BMC Public Health*, 16, 339. doi:10.1186/s12889-016-3018-9.

Abramsky, T., et al., 2016b. The impact of SASA!, a community mobilisation intervention, on women's experiences of intimate partner violence: Secondary findings from a cluster randomised trial in Kampala, Uganda. *Journal of Epidemiology and Community Health*, 70, 818–825. doi:10.1136/jech-2015-206665.

Anyaegbunam, C., Mefalopulos, P., and Moetsabi, T., 2004. *Participatory Rural Communication Appraisal. Starting with the People*. Rome: FAO.

Arendt, H., 1963. *On Revolution*. New York, NY: Penguin Books.

Bergold, J. and Thomas, S., 2012. Participatory research methods: A methodological approach in motion. *Forum Qualitative Sozialforschung/Forum: Qualitative Social Research*, 13 (1). doi:10.17169/fqs-13.1.1801.

Bollinger, A., 2010. *Monitoring and Evaluating Stepping Stones Using the Outcome Mapping Tool*. Honduras: Plan International.

Campbell, C., 2003. *Letting Them Die: Why HIV/AIDS Prevention Programmes Fail*. Bloomington, IN: Indiana University Press.

Campbell, C. and Mannell, J., 2016. Conceptualising the agency of highly marginalised women: Intimate partner violence in extreme settings. *Global Public Health*, 11 (1–2), 1–16. doi:10.1080/17441692.2015.1109694.

Chacaltana, E., 2013. El 79% de mujeres en Mazán (Iquitos) han sufrido violencia sexual. *Spacio Libre – Web de Noticias. Spacio Libre*. Available from: http://www.spaciolibre.pe/el-79-de-mujeres-en-mazan-iquitos-han-sufrido-violencia-sexual/ [Accessed 1 October 2017].

Cornwall, A. and Jewkes, R., 1995. What is participatory research? *Social Science & Medicine*, 41 (12), 1667–1676. doi:10.1016/0277-9536(95)00127-S.

Devotta, K., et al., 2016. Enriching qualitative research by engaging peer interviewers: A case study. *Qualitative Research*, 16 (6), 661–680. doi:10.1177/1468794115626244.

Devries, K.M., et al., 2013. The global prevalence of intimate partner violence against women. *Science*, 340 (6140), 1527–1528.

Ellsberg, M., et al., 2015. Prevention of violence against women and girls: What does the evidence say? *The Lancet*, 385 (9977), 1555–1566. doi:10.1016/S0140-6736(14)61703-7.

Ferreyra, C., 2006. Practicality, positionality, and emancipation: Reflections on participatory action research with a watershed partnership. *Systemic Practice and Action Research*, 19 (6), 577–598.

Flake, D.F., 2005. Individual, family, and community risk markers for domestic violence in Peru. *Violence Against Women*, 11 (3), 353–373. doi:10.1177/1077801204272129.

Freire, P., 2000. *Pedagogy of the Oppressed: 30th Anniversary Edition*. London: Bloomsbury.

Goeckermann, C.R., Hamberger, L.K., and Barber, K., 1994. Issues of domestic violence unique to rural areas. *Wisconsin Medical Journal*, 93 (9), 473–479.

Guta, A., Flicker, S., and Roche, B., 2013. Governing through community allegiance: A qualitative examination of peer research in community-based participatory research. *Critical Public Health*, 23 (4), 432–451. doi:10.1080/09581596.2012.761675.

Harvey, N. and Holmes, C.A., 2012. Nominal group technique: An effective method for obtaining group consensus. *International Journal of Nursing Practice*, 18 (2), 188–194. doi:10.1111/j.1440-172X.2012.02017.x.

Heise, L.L., 1998. Violence against women: An integrated, ecological framework. *Violence Against Women*, 4 (3), 262–290.

Hult, M. and Lennung, S.-Å., 1980. Towards a definition of action research: A note and bibliography. *Journal of Management Studies*, 17 (2), 241–250. doi:10.1111/j.1467-6486.1980.tb00087.x.

Instituto Nacional de Estadística e Informática, 2011. *Encuesta Demográfica y de Salud Familiar – ENDES 2009*. Lima: Instituto Nacional de Estadística e Informática.

Instituto Promundo, 2012. *Engaging Men to Prevent Gender-Based Violence: A Multi-Country Intervention and Impact Evaluation Study* [Report for the UN Trust Fund]. Available from: http://menengage.org/resources/engaging-men-to-prevent-gender-based-violence-a-multi-country-intervention-and-impact-evaluation-study/ [Accessed 1 March 2018].

Jewkes, R., 2002. Intimate partner violence: Causes and prevention. *The Lancet*, 359 (9315), 1423–1429. doi:10.1016/S0140-6736(02)08357-5.

Jewkes, R., et al., 2008. Impact of stepping stones on incidence of HIV and HSV-2 and sexual behaviour in rural South Africa: Cluster randomised controlled trial. *British Medical Journal*, 337 (7666), 391–395. doi:10.1136/bmj.a506.

Kovach, M., 2015. Emerging from the margins: Indigenous methodologies. In: L. Brown and S. Strega, eds. *Research as Resistance: Revisiting Critical, Indigenous, and Anti-Oppressive Approaches*. Toronto: Canadian Scholars' Press, 99–36.

Lewin, K., 1946. Action research and minority problems. *Journal of Social Issues*, 2 (4), 34–46. doi:10.1111/j.1540-4560.1946.tb02295.x.

Lushey, C.J. and Munro, E.R., 2015. Participatory peer research methodology: An effective method for obtaining young people's perspectives on transitions from care to adulthood? *Qualitative Social Work*, 14 (4), 522–537. doi:10.1177/1473325014559282.

Maguire, P., 1996. Considering more feminist participatory research: What's congruency got to do with it? *Qualitative Inquiry*, 2 (1), 106–118. doi:10.1177/107780049600200115.

Olshansky, E., et al., 2005. Participatory action research to understand and reduce health disparities. *Nursing Outlook*, 53 (3), 121–126. doi:10.1016/j.outlook.2005.03.002.

Orellana, E.R., et al., 2013. Structural factors that increase HIV/STI vulnerability among indigenous people in the Peruvian amazon. *Qualitative Health Research*, 23 (9), 1240–1250. doi:10.1177/1049732313502129.

Peek-Asa, C., et al., 2011. Rural disparity in domestic violence prevalence and access to resources. *Journal of Women's Health*, 20 (11), 1743–1749. doi:10.1089/jwh.2011.2891.

Smith, L.T., 1999. *Decolonizing Methodologies: Research and Indigenous Peoples*. New York, NY: Zed Books.

Strike, C., et al., 2016. Opportunities, challenges and ethical issues associated with conducting community-based participatory research in a hospital setting. *Research Ethics*, 12(3), 149–157. doi:10.1177/1747016115626496.

Tamale, S., 2006. African Feminism: How should we change? *Development*, 49 (1), 38–41. doi:10.1057/palgrave.development.1100205.

Wang, C.C., Cash, J.L., and Powers, L.S., 2000. Who knows the streets as well as the homeless? Promoting personal and community action through photovoice. *Health Promotion Practice*, 1 (1), 81–89. doi:10.1177/152483990000100113.

Section III
Understanding diverse issues

9 Participatory visual research exploring gender and water in Cameroon

A workshop model

Jennifer A. Thompson

Introduction

Participatory research seeks and values voices, knowledges and experiences that have been marginalised, overlooked or excluded from mainstream research. Different participatory approaches invite community engagement to increase the accessibility and meaningfulness of research, to facilitate public dialogue about community issues, and to provoke opportunities for action, including in developing better and more responsive policies and programmes and in supporting social change. Participatory research attempts to address ethical questions about social justice and the difference that research can make to the lives of research participants, challenging historic and ongoing research biases that privilege dominant and normative perspectives. Yet given the potentially tokenistic, exploitative and appropriating uses of participation (Cooke and Kothari 2001), foregrounding questions of power in participatory processes remains ever critical. This chapter considers the methodological implications of two different participatory research traditions: 'peer research' and 'participatory visual methodologies'.

Peer research involves members of a particular group, network or community conducting research with other people similar to themselves. Peer researchers have included people living with HIV (Greene et al. 2009; Logie et al. 2012), people who use drugs (Damon et al. 2017) and children and youth (Burns and Schubotz 2009; Lushey and Munro 2015). Peer researchers often receive research training from researchers and participate as employees, advisors or partners to contribute to research design, data collection and analysis, and dissemination (Roche et al. 2010). Peer research can help to incorporate insider knowledge within research processes, connect with more difficult to reach populations, and support community-based approaches to research (Roche et al. 2010).

In contrast, participatory visual methodologies – including photovoice, drawing, collage, digital storytelling and participatory video – invite research participants to work individually or in groups to produce photographs, videos and other forms of creative media to identify, represent and analyse critical issues in their lives (Mitchell 2011; Mitchell et al. 2017). Working with visual methods offers ways to decentre written text as a primary mode of knowledge production (Gubrium and Harper 2013) and produce alternative texts that represent issues through the eyes of participants. In particular, participant-produced media can speak back to or disrupt dominant or voyeuristic narratives and representations of participants' lived experiences and concerns (Kindon 2003; Mitchell and de Lange 2013).

While participatory visual and peer approaches to research are not necessarily mutually exclusive, they can operationalise participation quite differently and rarely overlap in the literature, perhaps due to their different origins, methods and contexts. Drawing on findings from a collaborative study with a local civil society organisation, this chapter considers these approaches together in the context of doctoral research about gender and water governance with women in four communities in Cameroon's Southwest Region (Thompson 2017). I did not work intentionally with a peer research approach. The project emerged from a participatory visual research as social change framework (Mitchell 2011; Mitchell et al. 2017) and feminist questions about the emancipatory claims of participatory research that fail to acknowledge gender inequalities (Maguire 2006). In elaborating the structure and methodological implications of this study, this chapter seeks to nuance the relationship between peer and visual approaches to participatory research with a particular focus on the diverse experiences, subjectivities and agencies of women.

A workshop model for participatory visual research design

Participatory visual research often brings researchers and participants together in workshop settings. Workshops provide a critical method and space for facilitating interactive group enquiry that enhance the collaborative and peer, participant and community-driven aspects of participatory processes. Participatory visual workshops typically follow a series of media production steps that support the co-creation of engaging, accessible images, dialogue and knowledge for social change. This is a highly facilitated process (Switzer 2018). The behind-the-scenes planning, adapting and decision making that happens before, during and in between workshops significantly shapes how the research unfolds, the types of knowledges that emerge, and the extent to which participants feel ownership or control over the process.

Workshop design can vary in length from a series of relatively short-term sequential events in which projects have a distinct beginning and end, to a longer-term process that may extend across several years or decades (Mitchell 2011). This chapter focuses on shorter-term participatory visual studies conducted over semester-long or multi-month field visits that align with the limited time frames of student research, some funding cycles and study visits.

When participatory visual methodologies are led or instigated by researchers who are outsiders within the research context, workshops are often initiated and conducted collaboratively with a local organisation such as a school or civil society organisation. Working closely with organisations that maintain longer-term relationships with the communities, the research activities contribute to cycles of enquiry and practice at the organisational level, as well as in the communities they support. Collaborative teams involving researchers and practitioners invite community members to workshop settings to facilitate image production and interpretation about particular issues. In studies that involve many participants or multiple participant cohorts from different communities, it may not be feasible or sustainable for every person to be involved at every step of decision making about the research process. Participants may want to participate in media production but not necessarily in planning the wider project or depending on their financial relationship with the project (employed, honorarium, volunteer). Therefore, researchers often work with local organisations and community leaders to co-develop a suitable workshop design.

With this model, workshop facilitators actively design and lead the research activities to support creative group processes and different types of participation at different moments. Working with visual methods that are often new to participants, facilitators make strategic process decisions, including the sequencing and focus of activities as well as what can be realistically accomplished within a given time frame. The workshops are structured loosely ahead of time with 'steps' that provide space for participants to brainstorm the research topic, learn new photography or video-making skills, and discuss their experiences and concerns. This structure enables community participants to lead in identifying, representing and co-analysing the issues affecting their lives. This model can enable a systematic approach across multiple groups and communities, while also allowing for flexible adaptation that responds to the needs of particular groups.

In seeking participants' ways of seeing and thinking about a topic or phenomenon, this workshop model differs from other visual methods in which researchers work with, produce and interpret images from their own perspectives (Rose 2012) or when researchers work with participants individually. While limiting participant ownership to a certain extent, the workshop design facilitates a group process that facilitates collaboration and interaction where participants co-lead data collection and interpretation through making and analysing visual productions. This chapter explicitly investigates how such a workshop format can influence participation, power and knowledge production within approaches to research that aim to position community members at the centre of the research.

Women and water *wahala*: the study

Gender and water in Cameroon

In the areas around Mount Cameroon, fresh water flows abundantly through dense networks of springs and streams. Yet water access and delivery problems persist due to a range of social, political, economic and technical factors. Recent decades have seen policy shifts from public to partially privatised and back to public models of water service provision in urban and semi-urban areas. Community-managed water schemes punctuate rural areas, sometimes coexisting with municipal systems in cities (Folifac and Gaskin 2011; Sally et al. 2014). To study and address these complex and multifaceted aspects of water governance, an interdisciplinary collective involving Canadian and Cameroonian research-ers and civil society organisations explored different platforms for stakeholder engagement in water dialogue in Cameroon's Southwest Region (Thompson et al. 2011; Folifac 2012). Critically, women and girls bear the primary responsi-bility for managing household water and are therefore disproportionately affected by water access challenges. Yet water projects and policies that do not account for these gender roles reinscribe or exacerbate gender inequalities. Drawing on gender and water research about how gender relations shape and are shaped by water use, access and control (Coles and Wallace 2005; Lahiri-Dutt 2011), this research described here sought to work with women and girls to explore the gen-dered nature of water with participatory visual methodologies.

Collaborative design

Concerned about how my positionality as a White researcher from Canada work-ing in Cameroon risks replicating colonial and neocolonial relations, I strove to work *with* communities, local organisations and participants in a way that was culturally appropriate, relevant and meaningful, and that integrated possi-bilities for reciprocity and sustainability (Vanner 2015). During fieldwork, I col-laborated closely with a small, local women-led civil society organisation, called *Changing Mentalities and Empowering Groups* (CHAMEG), that supports a net-work of women from various grassroots associations to promote gender equality, women's empowerment and the active participation of women and girls in local governance.

CHAMEG's director and several Cameroonian academics – all members of the research collective and leaders in their local communities – acted as an advisory committee for the study. While the research proposal had been developed and funding secured prior to travelling to Cameroon, the study design was adjusted in collaboration with the advisory committee before submitting the project to a Canadian university research ethics board. Communities were not consulted directly at this stage, but reliance on the committee's experience ensured feasibil-ity with the local context, cultural protocols and likely participant availabilities. We proposed working in four communities – the urban communities of Buea and Kumba and the villages of Bwitingi and Mudeka – to extend our focus beyond the city of Buea (which had been researched more intensively by University of Buea academics) as well as to support CHAMEG's ongoing work mobilising networks of local women's groups in the Southwest Region.

In preparation for working with either photovoice (Wang and Burris 1997) or participatory video (Milne et al. 2012), I had brought point-and-shoot digital cameras with photograph and video capabilities and a portable photo printer. CHAMEG felt that many participants would have little photography or video-making experience, wanted to learn these skills and would enjoy exploring digital technologies in new ways. Despite the potential redundancy, we opted to use both methods in each community and developed a replicable two-day workshop model.

Facilitator training, pilot study and recruitment

To launch the study, we facilitated participatory visual methodology training attended by fieldworkers – who were local staff working on issues in their own communities – from CHAMEG and from other local civil society organisations, as well as by recent undergraduates from the University of Buea (youth from other regions of Cameroon who were interested in gaining field research experience). This two-day training workshop provided an opportunity to pilot the method and research 'prompt' (Mitchell 2011). Typically distinct from a research question, prompts are carefully designed to facilitate enquiry and focus image production in a way that is specific enough to be clear and accessible, and general enough to include diverse perspectives and experiences (Thompson 2017). We used the same prompt for both photovoice and participatory video activities: *What are some challenges you face with water and what are some solutions?* The training participants became so engaged in the topic and methods that they wanted the photos and videos that they produced during the training to be included as a fifth data set, in addition to the data collected from each of the four communities.

From the group of training participants, we hired ten local facilitators (nine women and one man) to co-facilitate the community-based workshops with me, working with employment contracts typical of those used by CHAMEG with duties and amount of pay in line with local expectations and economy. We prioritised hiring women in order to work with and support experienced and novice women as facilitators, co-researchers and community mobilisers, as part of CHAMEG's wider advocacy work in bolstering women's leadership. These facilitators could be considered peer researchers connected to the communities by at least one social factor (Logie et al. 2012). All Cameroonian – with lived experience of local cultural and community protocols, gender dynamics and water challenges – the facilitators had important insider knowledge about the research topic and within the research communities. They also brought a range of experience and social positions. For instance, the civil society organisation fieldworkers had direct community engagement experience in the region, although not necessarily in the four study sites. The university graduates had academic research methods training but little community engagement experience. None of the facilitators had any previous experience with participatory visual methodologies.

Together, CHAMEG, the facilitators and I fine-tuned the community workshop procedures. For example, while I had initially proposed working with women and girls, CHAMEG and the facilitators disagreed. They felt that the study should prioritise women's experiences, and that some men should be present to hear women's perspectives and to participate in media production. However, the team stipulated that men should not dominate. Therefore, we strategically recruited 'mostly women and some men'.

The facilitators worked in teams of two to four co-facilitators. In each community, the facilitators met with the traditional leaders and other authorities with an introductory letter and customary gift to ask permission to conduct the research and to secure workshop venues. Working with a script approved by both the

Cameroon advisory group and the Canadian university ethics committee, each facilitator team took responsibility for recruiting between 23 and 36 participants per workshop through their personal and professional networks – an example of peer recruitment strategies (Roche et al. 2010). In Kumba, participants constituted higher status individuals who were connected to civil society organisations and government institutions. In Buea, participants were predominantly young women and men attending college, university or secondary school. The Bwitingi facilitators recruited women only: older women, university students and vocational students. Mudeka's village council selected 50% women and 50% men based on community members' interest and availability. In total, we recruited 130 participants: 96 women and 34 men.

Photovoice and participatory video workshops in community

The co-facilitators and I co-organised and co-facilitated the community workshops. While the procedures varied slightly from workshop to workshop, we consistently worked with photovoice on the first day and participatory video on the second day. Each workshop began with individual informed consent, a conversation that we revisited frequently through the two-day workshops.

We began photovoice with a facilitated discussion that involved looking at and thinking about photographs, including visual ethics and the importance of asking for permission before photographing or videoing. Participants then worked in small groups (three to seven people) to brainstorm their answers to the prompt. With the exception of occasional support by facilitators, these small groups were entirely participant-led. Some groups organised themselves according to gender and age (women, men, youths, elders), which provided opportunities for examining shared experiences from particular social groups, and for creating space for the voices of women and youth who are often marginalised in decision-making circles that tend to privilege the perspectives of elder men. Other groups were mixed, which created opportunities for participants to meet and work with people across social hierarchies. Each group left the workshop space independently and travelled into their community to take photographs. In some workshops, groups self-coordinated to ensure representation across community water sources. In other workshops, groups preferred to work independently and wanted to surprise the other participants with their productions. Upon return, each group selected and printed up to 10 photos on the portable printer, arranged photographs on a poster narrative, and added writing to describe, punctuate or supplement their photos. This produced a total of 233 photographs on 28 posters. These analytical procedures were entirely participant-driven. Representatives from each group then presented their photos and analysis, which was also participant-led. We concluded the day with a group discussion facilitated by the facilitators and I about the issues raised in the work, and about ethical considerations relating to anonymity and possible audiences.

We conducted participatory video using a 'No-Editing Required' approach – which avoids the need for editing software and equipment (Mitchell et al. 2017)

– in order to plan, make and screen videos in one day. We began by screening an example *one-shot video* (where the video is filmed in one single take) and facilitating discussion of strategies for no-editing video work. Participants worked, again in small participant-led groups supported by facilitators, to develop a storyboard to explore issues raised the previous day more closely, or to address new topics that might have been missing. Each group then left the workshop and chose the location where they wanted to film, to produce 27 short (two- to six-minute) videos over a two- to three-hour period. Upon return, we screened each video and facilitated group discussion to elicit participant responses to the issues represented in the videos (although often, this particular discussion was rushed because of the time constraints of video production). After media production each day, groups signed Media Release Forms to specify how they wanted their productions to be used for research purposes, shown publicly, published in print or on the Internet.

Participatory analysis workshop

Community participants were involved in identifying and representing issues, as well as analysing the photos and videos produced in their communities. However, because there were different facilitator teams in each community, I was the only person in a position to make sense of the data as a whole. Bringing this concern to the advisory committee, we developed an additional analysis workshop to involve community participants in the interpretation of the entire data set. Whereas traditional member checking verifies preliminary results with participants *after* analysis has been completed, the analysis workshop enabled us to *begin* formulating results together with participants. While it was not feasible to re-convene all 130 participants, CHAMEG and I jointly designed an analysis workshop attended by representatives and a facilitator from each community (11 women and three men) – a group small enough to support interaction and adequate time for reflection. In this workshop, CHAMEG and the facilitators became engrossed as participants in the analysis and I led the facilitation.

To work collaboratively with 233 photographs and 27 videos, we used accessible analysis methods that structured opportunities for us to move back and forth between the larger data set and individual images, allowed time for participant-led discussion, and that were feasible to accomplish in two days. Before the workshop, each participant received a data DVD and notebook along with instructions to pre-screen the entire visual data set and to reflect on a series of writing prompts. During the workshop, we conducted inductive thematic analysis to identify community-specific and general themes that were in the data. Each attendee also selected one or two images that they considered particularly powerful or poignant, and engaged in a close reading and interrogation of these single images using Moletsane and Mitchell's (2007) analytical approach, 'working with a single photograph', in order to identify and interpret the complexity of social issues and relationships encompassed within that image. As a group, we reached consensus over the selection of 27 images (17 photographs and 10 videos) to represent the study and identified community leaders that participants thought should see them.

Outreach and dissemination

At public exhibitions in each community, we displayed the photograph posters and screened each video from that community. We also hosted a 'Decision Maker Dialogue Forum' in Buea to disseminate the study findings and spur wider policy dialogue with people in formal positions of power. This forum was attended by 40 leaders in elected, appointed and inherited positions (including traditional leaders, municipal councillors, ministry representatives) as well as civil society organisations and the media, and participant representatives and facilitators from each of the communities. At the forum, we presented the 27 images and facilitated a 90-minute discussion about women's concerns, which included gender inequalities and water governance in the region.

Findings

The work generated rich provocative descriptions and participant and audience engagement about everyday implicit routines and norms related to gender and water, as well as collective analysis of the similarities and differences across sites. While each community had the infrastructure for piped water supply, access to safe water was unreliable. Different governance factors shaped the *reasons* for water access challenges across municipal and community-managed water systems. However, the resulting impacts on women's daily lives were remarkably similar across the communities. We found that women travelled long journeys to collect household water, sometimes over difficult terrain or to wait at crowded taps, which took time away from other work and education. Not necessarily knowing when or where water would be flowing created uncertainty and daily stress within households. Women described instances of domestic violence and marital troubles related to water at home, and concerns that girls faced sexual harassment while collecting water at busy or secluded taps in the community. Discussion of how households navigated water quality, transportation, billing and storage coincided with contested questions about how to improve water access and gender equality. Significantly, many participants had never thought about the gendered implications of water challenges. Several participants emphasised the importance of bringing communities together and creating space to think and talk about water in a way that valued and legitimised diverse perspectives among local leaders – itself a critical conversation. The fieldwork also led to some concrete outcomes, including Mudeka village's decision to reclaim an abandoned spring.

Among these celebratory narratives, there were also opportunities to reflect critically on participation and power within the workshops. The field activities spanned six months, involving diverse groups and numbers of people at different junctures. This shifting process blurred the nature of participation and relationships between the different actors. Facilitators and community leaders joined media production workshops as participants. Researchers and civil society organisations who we initially considered as potential collaborators became decision makers because of their roles in the water and gender sectors. Each of these sets of relations involve social hierarchies, in which the complexities of power influenced group dynamics.

Reflecting on participation and power

Peer recruitment can help reach those community members who are harder to reach (Roche et al. 2010). In this study, we reached diverse groups of women, many of whom had never participated in research. The participants, aged between 18 and 70, represented diverse social groups, positions and occupations, including teachers, farmers, journalists, business women, university students, labourers, mothers, civil society organisation employees, vocational students, nurses, municipal council officers and elders. This diversity created phenomenal opportunities for intergenerational and intersectoral discussion across social differences and in ways that created important space for new voices and perspectives to be valued and heard. Seeking diverse women's perspectives transgressed traditional hierarchies of whose voice counts in formal fora such as research and community decision making. Exploring gender issues, asking for women's input and expertise, and positioning women's knowledge as important unsettled technocratic and top-down approaches to water governance.

Yet despite our efforts to do so, recruiting participants through the facilitators' existing social networks also excluded lower status community members. Girls and domestic workers were not involved in the study, despite our intention to include them, and their critical role and experiences in daily water management was missed. Given the public nature of the workshops, working with these more vulnerable groups would have required a different study design, access and recruitment strategies, and higher levels of anonymity than could be assured with this study (Thompson 2020). While participatory visual and peer research often target marginalised groups, some participants had relatively privileged age and class status within the research context.

The term 'peer' assumes some sort of sameness, often in relation to age, culture, social position and perhaps (dis)ability. An intersectional perspective raises questions about insider status because of how gender, class, ethnicity and race intersect (Logie et al. 2012) and the effect of difference in position and power. One facilitator who ran a vocational school in her village recruited her students, who were young women who had left secondary school for various reasons. She also recruited her daughter and her daughter's friends who were enrolled as graduate students at the university nearby. A young woman recruited her landlord, who she relied on for affordable housing. Another facilitator recruited her cousins, who she lived with. While peers may share some similarities within a particular community, communities are diverse and heterogeneous such that assumed sameness cannot overlook social hierarchies and the complexities of power in these research relationships.

Women facilitating peer research processes

It was important to have women co-leading and co-facilitating a multi-site study involving 130 community participants. Yet emphasising women's perspectives remained a challenge, despite there being a majority of women in the workshops. Groups often selected the men to speak on behalf of their group, as either a sign of respect or because women felt shy to speak in the workshop. The men and influential women tended to dominate the discussions. Younger women often spoke less than elder women, and those with higher levels of formal education (such as the university students) spoke more frequently. It is difficult, if not impossible, to escape power hierarchies that are embedded and normalised in everyday interactions.

To encourage the expression of more diverse viewpoints, the facilitators and I restructured the workshops. We convened mini-focus group discussions with participants gathered informally around their photographs before presenting to the larger group. We shortened larger group discussion and implemented a 'go around' to create more space for individual voices. Seeking each person's perspective was more significant for some younger women than I had anticipated. In one workshop, a young mother who brought her infant to the workshops was shy at first to speak in front of the group. Prompted by one of the facilitators (her cousin), she reluctantly said a few words. The facilitator later shared with us about how this woman went home and told her family that speaking in the workshop marked an important transition for her, from being a girl to becoming a woman.

Creating opportunities to shift the dynamics of who can traditionally speak can be transformative, even if at small, individual and quite structured scale. Critically, women led the data collection process and orchestrated media production in particular ways. Many women asked men or other community members to hold their group's camera, because the women wanted to *be in the picture*. Women acted and directed simultaneously, disrupting traditional assumptions about power in image production, where the person holding the camera objectifies the photo subject. Many videos show the camera person struggled to keep up, oftentimes quite literally running alongside the act or jostling around crowds to capture the action from a better angle.

Women facilitating together

The facilitators and I worked as peers co-facilitating the workshops. We co-mentored each other to navigate the complexity of processes that involved multiple and simultaneous group dynamics, media productions and technological considerations. We discussed strategies, challenges and activity design, sought advice and guidance from each other at different junctures, and held extensive debriefing meetings after each workshop. Recognising our different ages, skills and social positions, we harnessed our diversity to strengthen our facilitation teams. Some fieldworkers had seasoned experience negotiating community expectations and younger facilitators could troubleshoot digital technologies with ease. My experience working with visual methods helped us adapt media production as required.

We facilitated all of the community-based workshops in Pidgin, a widely spoken *lingua franca* that bridges Cameroon's hundreds of Indigenous languages. Most participants worked together, explained their photos and acted their films in Pidgin, even renaming the study using the Pidgin term, *Wahala*, meaning problems. Working in Pidgin helped to ground our exploration of gender–water relations in local expressions of culture, identity and sociality, and countered how Pidgin is discouraged despite its widespread use (Neba et al. 2006). Conducting research in Pidgin also helped me – as an outsider – to connect in meaningful ways (Thompson 2020). The university student facilitators from Francophone regions of Cameroon struggled with Pidgin, creating the paradoxical situation in which I – the only White and non-Cameroonian facilitator – was the most proficient at speaking the language spoken most frequently in communities, based on my previous experience in West Africa. Doing research in Pidgin offered a critical yet contested cross-linguistic space for seeking more inclusive forms of research about water in the Cameroonian context and challenging dominant social hierarchies.

Our intergenerational mentorship system drew on our individual expertise and introduced opportunities for methodological training and experiential practice – useful skills within the non-profit and research sectors. Co-facilitators supported each other through difficult facilitation moments when alternate framing or explanation was required. Each co-facilitator offered a unique insight, cultural framing and historical and contemporary context. Our age, social status and language differences created more accessible communication pathways for the wide range of community participants.

Women studying up

Laura Nader (1999 [1972]) has advocated for the *studying up* – of powerful as opposed to marginalised groups – to gain insight into bureaucratic power, the attitudes of those who control institutions, and possible avenues for affecting social and political change. As Nader noted, accessing these structures can be challenging – powerful people are busy and difficult to reach, often geographically spread out across different locations. In Cameroon, working across four communities meant navigating six municipal and village councils across three administrative districts. Additionally, our focus on gender and water cut across work in different government and community sectors. The participants, facilitators and I were sometimes uncertain which leaders might take up the research through official leadership roles and positions. We also needed insider knowledge into the subtleties of political influence of different types of leaders, such as salaried civil servants, elected politicians and traditional leaders, within the relatively small urban elite networks composed primarily of men. In addition, many leaders were busy, others did not want to be studied, and it can be dangerous to look too closely given the levels of secrecy and confidentiality required for the control of information and power (Nader 1999 [1972]).

Outreach across multiple bureaucracies took enormous work, waiting and persistence, which took away from our work with communities. Yet, disseminating the research across regional and administrative boundaries generated more far-reaching impact. It also raised questions about who can and cannot access power. CHAMEG, the advisory committee and I had privileged access to leaders, which we leveraged in order to share the study findings. Through us, participants and facilitators had opportunities to voice their concerns up these bureaucratic structures. We also bridged sectoral silos by convening leaders – such as chiefs, government ministry representatives and water organisation leaders – who had not previously met. While participatory research sometimes raises concerns about validity and quality, this study elicited the opposite response. Many leaders valued how the breadth and magnitude of community engagement strengthened the significance, credibility and representativeness of the findings that were grounded in community experience and interpretation.

Conclusion

This chapter presents a workshop model for participatory visual research design and explored the peer research aspects of this model. In reflecting on these participatory traditions together, the chapter offers a methodological reflection about the complex and dynamic nature of participation and collaboration in workshop settings. Focusing in particular on the critical and often overlooked importance of gender relations in participatory and community-based research, the chapter also highlights the complexities of gendered power relations in relation to peer recruitment, supporting women as peer researchers, workshop co-facilitation, and studying up structures of power.

References

Burns, S. and Schubotz, D., 2009. Demonstrating the merits of the peer research process: A Northern Ireland case study. *Field Methods*, 21 (3), 309–326. doi:10.1177/1525822X09333514.

Coles, A. and Wallace, T., eds., 2005. *Gender, Water, and Development*. New York, NY: Berg.

Cooke, B. and Kothari, U., eds., 2001. *Participation: The New Tyranny?* London, and New York, NY: Zed Books.

Damon, W., et al., 2017. Community-based participatory research in a heavily researched inner city neighbourhood: Perspectives of people who use drugs on their experiences as peer researchers. *Social Science & Medicine*, 176, 85–92. doi:10.1016/j.socscimed.2017.01.027.

Folifac, F., 2012. *Towards Improving Knowledge Management and Collaborative Action in Potable Water Delivery at the Local Level: Case of Buea, Cameroon*. Thesis (Doctor of Philosophy), McGill University, Montreal. Available from: http://digitool.Library.McGill.CA:80/R/-?func=dbin-jump-full&object_id=116982&silo_library=GEN01.

Folifac, F. and Gaskin, S., 2011. Joint water supply projects in rural Cameroon: Partnership of profiteering? Lessons from the Mautu-Cameroon Development Corporation (CDC) project. *Water Science & Technology: Water Supply*, 11 (4), 409–417. doi:10.2166/ws.2011.061.

Greene, S., et al., 2009. Between skepticism and empowerment: The experiences of peer research assistants in HIV/AIDS, housing and homelessness community-based research. *International Journal of Social Research Methodology*, 12 (4), 361–373. doi:10.1080/13645570802553780.

Gubrium, A. and Harper, K., 2013. *Participatory Visual and Digital Methods*. Walnut Creek, CA: Left Coast Press.

Kindon, S., 2003. Participatory video in geographic research: A feminist practice of looking? *Area*, 35 (2), 142–153. doi:10.1111/1475-4762.00236.

Lahiri-Dutt, K., ed., 2011. *Fluid Bonds: Views on Gender and Water*, 2nd ed. Kolkata: STREE.

Logie, C., et al., 2012. Opportunities, ethical challenges and lessons learned from working with peer research assistants in a multi-method HIV community-based research study in Ontario, Canada. *Journal of Empirical Research on Human Research Ethics: An International Journal*, 7 (4), 10–19.

Lushey, C.J. and Munro, E.R., 2015. Participatory peer research methodology: An effective method for obtaining young people's perspectives on transitions from care to adulthood? *Qualitative Social Work*, 14 (4), 522–537. doi:10.1177/1473325014559282.

Maguire, P., 2006. Uneven ground: Feminisms and action research. In: P. Reason and H. Bradbury, eds. *Handbook of Action Research: Concise Paperback Edition*. London, Thousand Oaks, CA, and New Delhi: SAGE Publications, 60–70.

Milne, E.J., Mitchell, C., and de Lange, N., eds., 2012. *The Handbook of Participatory Video*. Plymouth: AltaMira Press.

Mitchell, C., 2011. *Doing Visual Research*. New York, NY, and London, UK: SAGE Publications.

Mitchell, C. and de Lange, N., 2013. What can a teacher do with a cellphone? Using participatory visual research to speak back in addressing HIV & AIDS. *South African Journal of Education*, 33 (4), 1–13.

Mitchell, C., de Lange, N., and Moletsane, R., 2017. *Participatory Visual Methodologies: Social Change, Community and Policy*. Los Angeles, CA: SAGE Publications.

Moletsane, R. and Mitchell, C., 2007. On working with a single photograph. In: N. de Lange, C. Mitchell, and J. Stuart, eds. *Putting People in the Picture: Visual Methodologies for Social Change*. Rotterdam, Netherlands: Sense, 131–140.

Nader, L., 1999 [1972]. Up the anthropologist: Perspectives gained from studying up. In: D. Hymes, ed. *Reinventing Anthropology*. Ann Arbor, MI: University of Michigan Press, 284–311.

Neba, A.N., Chibaka, E.F., and Atindogbe, G.G., 2006. Cameroon Pidgin English (CPE) as a tool for empowerment and national development. *African Study Monographs*, 27 (2), 39–61. doi:10.14989/68249.

Roche, B., Guta, A., and Flicker, S., 2010. *Peer Research in Action I: Models of Practice*. Community Based Research Working Paper Series. Toronto: Wellesley Institute.

Rose, G., 2012. *Visual Methodologies: An Introduction to Researching with Visual Materials*, 3rd ed. London, Thousand Oaks, CA, New Delhi, and Singapore: SAGE Publications.

Sally, Z., et al., 2014. The effect of urbanization on community-managed water supply: Case study of Buea, Cameroon. *Community Development Journal*, 49 (4), 524–540. doi:10.1093/cdj/bst054.

Switzer, S., 2018. What's in an image? Towards a critical and interdisciplinary reading of participatory visual methods. In: M. Capous-Desyllas and K. Morgaine, eds. *Creating Social Change Through Creativity: Anti-Oppressive Arts-Based Research Methodologies.* Cham: Palgrave Macmillan, 189–207.

Thompson, J.A., 2017. *Women and Water Wahala: Picturing Gendered Waterscapes in Southwest Cameroon.* Doctoral thesis, McGill University, Montreal.

Thompson, J.A., 2020. Yu Ai Tron! Gender, language and ethics in Cameroon. In: R. Moletsane et al., eds. *Ethical Practice in Participatory Visual Research with Girls and Young Women: A Focus on Rurality, Indigeneity and Transnationality.* New York, NY, and Oxford: Berghahn.

Thompson, J., Folifac, F., and Gaskin, S., 2011. Fetching water in the unholy hours of the night: The impacts of a water crisis on girls' health and sexualities in semi-urban Cameroon. *Girlhood Studies*, 4 (2), 111–129. doi:10.3167/ghs.2011.040208.

Vanner, C., 2015. Positionality at the center: Constructing an epistemological and methodological approach for a Western feminist doctoral candidate conducting research in the postcolonial. *International Journal of Qualitative Methods*, 14 (4), 1–12. doi:10.1177/1609406915618094.

Wang, C. and Burris, M., 1997. Photovoice: Concept, methodology, and use for participatory needs assessment. *Health Education & Behavior*, 24 (3), 369–387. doi:10.1177/109019819702400309.

10 'I am the bridge'

Peer research with women with disabilities in the Philippines and Australia

Liz Gill-Atkinson, Georgia Katsikis, Rowena B Rivera and Cathy Vaughan

Introduction

Across the world, there is a long history of research being done *on* people with disabilities, rather than *with* people with disabilities. This research has often been experienced as irrelevant and intrusive and has led to an incomplete and inaccurate understanding of the lives, health and priorities of people with disabilities. For decades, disability activists and researchers with disabilities have pushed researchers without disabilities to adopt more inclusive approaches to research, and to build on the capacities and expertise of people with disabilities in the way in which research is conducted. Peer research is one strategy increasingly used to engage people with disabilities in research that aims to increase knowledge about the health and social problems they may face, and contribute to positive social change (Burke et al. 2018; Vaughan et al. 2019).

Despite the increasing interest in using peer research approaches in disability research, there is limited critical reflection available from the perspective of people with disabilities themselves about the use of peer research. To address this knowledge gap, in this chapter we draw on our experiences of working together as university-based researchers and as peer researchers on projects with women with disabilities in Australia and the Philippines. Georgia is a psychologist, a woman with a disability, and coordinator of a co-research programme for people with disabilities, who has previously worked as a peer researcher. Rowena (known as Weng) is a Filipina Deaf woman and a well-known advocate for the Deaf community in the Philippines with extensive peer research experience. Liz and Cathy are formally trained researchers based at the University of Melbourne, who do not have lived experience of disability. Liz and Cathy have worked with Weng and Georgia on different peer research projects to increase understanding of the sexual and reproductive health of women with disability in Australia and the Philippines. Considering the historical exploitation of people with disabilities by formally trained researchers without disabilities, we believe that acknowledging our social locations is critical for understanding how our backgrounds and experiences inform our ideas about peer research with women with disabilities.

In this chapter, we explore three issues that have emerged as priorities in our shared experience of peer research – the emotional labour undertaken by peer researchers with disabilities and the consequences of this; what researchers without disability can and should do to support peer researchers during and after their involvement in peer research projects; and the potential of peer research to more effectively contribute to social change than research undertaken without the involvement of communities with the most at stake in the issue being studied. In discussing these themes, we refer to 'university-based researchers' and 'peer researchers' as two different groups, for the purposes of illustration. However, we realise these groups are not mutually exclusive, and that not all formally trained, professional researchers are based in universities. We are also somewhat ambivalent about the label 'peer researcher', noting that the very process of labelling research team members' roles is rarely done collectively, and can act to devalue the contributions of some team members compared to those of others. However, we also recognise that research team members bring to a research project different access to power and resources, different training and experience, and different forms of expertise. We are labelling these two different positions as such, to make clear differences in the power and resources that university-based researchers and peer researchers usually bring to a research project, and the different responsibilities that arise in their research roles.

Background

One in five women worldwide has a disability (WHO and World Bank 2011). Despite being such a significant proportion of women globally, women with disabilities continue to experience disadvantage because of both gender inequality and disability discrimination (CBM Australia 2018). Women with disabilities have greater unmet health needs and reduced access to health information, screening, prevention and care services including minimal access to sexual and reproductive health information and services (McLachlan and Schwartz 2009; WHO and UNFPA 2009). Women with disabilities also experience high levels of violence and are more likely to experience sexual and intimate partner violence than women without disabilities or men with disabilities in their communities (Hughes et al. 2012; Krnjacki et al. 2016). While women with disabilities experience disproportionately poor health and violence-related outcomes, they have traditionally been excluded from active involvement in research about these issues. Despite the established benefits of participatory and peer research approaches, and the longstanding efforts of disability activists, documentation of the active engagement of women with disabilities in the co-creation of knowledge and action to address their health and social priorities is still relatively uncommon in the literature (Chappell et al. 2014; Vaughan et al. 2016, 2019; Burke et al. 2018). In addition, there is little empirical evidence about how women with disabilities themselves experience being a peer researcher. This is particularly the case in relation to research on sensitive topics such as sexual and reproductive health or violence (van der Heijden et al. 2019).

There is growing recognition across the wider literature on peer research approaches that peer researchers may experience emotionally and ethically difficult encounters while collecting data from and with their peers. This is due to the increased likelihood that, because of common aspects of their background or identity, peer researchers may have personally experienced the same issues and experiences that are shared by research participants during data collection, and that this can be unsettling or troubling (Mosavel and Sanders 2014; Vaughan et al. 2019). In discussing their work with South African women with disabilities, van der Heijden and colleagues (2019) note the many advantages of disability-inclusive gender-based violence research and its emancipatory potential, but observe that this requires safeguards and reasonable accommodation. They also highlight the need for university-based researchers to not be patronising of peer researchers, recognising the capacities of women with disabilities and their agency, while also being mindful of the particular risks and costs that may be borne by peer researchers.

One approach to considering how the risks and costs of peer research are distributed is to draw on the notions of reflexivity and solidarity. Reflexivity has been defined as

> the ability to reflect inward toward oneself as an enquirer; outward to the cultural, historical, linguistic, political and other forces that shape everything about the enquiry; and in between researcher and participant to the social interaction they share.
>
> (Sandelowski and Barroso 2002, p. 216)

Reflexivity in peer research requires university-based and peer researchers to identify the power relations in which they are embedded, and for those holding privilege and opportunity to work to address power imbalances. Solidarity has been defined as an enacted commitment to carry financial, social, emotional or other 'costs' to assist others to whom we have a relational duty (Prainsack and Buyx 2017). A framework of reflexive solidarity has been used to examine collaboration between university-based researchers and peer researchers who are women with disabilities to undertake disability inclusive research (Vaughan et al. 2019) and how participatory research approaches can facilitate social action for social change (Davis and Vaughan 2018). In this chapter, notions of reflexivity and solidarity shape our discussion of the emotional labour involved in peer research, what support should be provided to peer researchers, and to reflect upon the contribution of peer research to social change.

Peer researchers' reflections

This chapter draws on Georgia and Weng's experiences working as peer researchers across a range of projects where they experienced varying levels of control over their participation and different degrees of involvement in the research. Peer research occurs across a continuum of engagement, from minimal engagement and input to shared decision making and control (Vaughn et al. 2018). Roche, Guta and Flicker (2010) identify three main models of peer research which are useful for framing the experiences discussed in this chapter. At one end of the continuum is an advisory model, where peer researchers sit on an advisory committee or board and provide guidance and support. In the middle is an employment model, where peer researchers are hired to conduct specific research tasks, such as data collection. At the far end of the continuum is a partner model, where peer researchers are engaged as decision makers and leaders and are actively involved in implementing research activities throughout a research project.

For the drafting of this chapter, Weng and Georgia discussed their experiences working across peer research projects involving employment or partner models with Liz. To address the practical and communication barriers associated with co-authoring a book chapter written in English across time zones, Weng and Georgia filmed their contributions for this chapter. Weng worked with a Filipino Sign Language interpreter who provided a verbal English language translation of Weng's reflections, which was recorded using the video messaging application Marco Polo. Georgia filmed her reflections with Liz. The audio recordings from the videos were then transcribed verbatim and the transcripts were used to develop this chapter.

In her reflections, Weng discusses her first peer research experience in 2009, where she was contracted by a government department to travel to rural areas to interview Deaf women and Deaf men about their livelihoods, and to contribute to the analysis of data. Weng then reflects on her later experience of collecting and analysing data, and designing and implementing peer support groups with other Deaf women and girls for the W-DARE (Women with Disability taking Action on REproductive and sexual health) programme. The W-DARE programme was a three-year (2013–16) mixed method programme of participatory action research in the Philippines that aimed to improve access to sexual and reproductive health and violence response services for women and girls with disabilities (Vaughan et al. 2015). In contributing to this chapter, Georgia reflects on her peer research experiences conducting qualitative interviews and undertaking data analysis in two projects led by the different university-based researchers. The first of these projects examined how people with disabilities in regional Victoria were experiencing the National Disability Insurance Scheme and the impact of the scheme on access to services (Warr et al. 2017). The second project explored factors shaping the sexual and reproductive health of women with disabilities from migrant and refugee backgrounds in Melbourne (Vaughan et al. 2019).

While the projects discussed in this chapter were highly diverse in terms of their stated aims, duration, scope, geographic location, target audience and peer research model, Georgia and Weng reported shared experiences and there were common themes in their reflections, which we discuss below.

Emotional labour and unsettled identities

University-based participatory researchers are increasingly recognising that there may be unintended harms associated with peer research projects, and that these are disproportionately borne by peer researchers and community members. Several accounts of peer research projects, including projects involving women with disabilities as peer researchers, highlight that the very features of peer research approaches that are usually described as its strengths – proximity of peers, knowledge of the community, assumed empathy and rapport because of shared experiences – can be a double-edged sword for peer researchers (Boynton 2002; Warr et al. 2011; Mosavel and Sanders 2014; Vaughan et al. 2019). Peer researchers describe how listening to confronting stories from research participants, that may also reflect their own life experiences, can lead to vicarious trauma and distress (Burke et al. 2018).

Weng reflected that during her experience as a peer researcher it was 'not the women, but their situations [that affected me]. I could feel the sameness with their identity, I could understand what they are going through as a Deaf Filipino woman.' Similarly, Georgia described how she found it 'very difficult to interview the women. Not to speak with them but to hear their experiences and to find a lot of similarities with the experiences that we had as well.' Weng and Georgia's experiences of connection and similarity were often on the basis of shared experiences of disability- and gender-based discrimination, which were present even when many other aspects of their lives were different to those of their research participants.

As peer researchers, Weng and Georgia each reported having had troubling encounters with research participants where they stopped a research interview because they, or the research participant, had become too distressed to continue. For Weng, this occurred during her first experience as a peer researcher on a research project exploring the livelihoods of Deaf people in rural areas of the Philippines in 2009. Weng describes how she had to stop an interview with a young Deaf woman because she became overwhelmed with the severity of the young woman's story, and because of how similar it was to her own life experiences. As Weng described:

> She was able to express herself to me, I think because I was also a Deaf woman and it made me think about my experiences of being a Deaf woman and my own struggles …. I would look at her and I could understand instantly and emphasise with her what she was feeling. She was also a victim [of sexual assault] …. After that she had even more of a mental breakdown, and I could relate to that and it made me cry. I couldn't even complete the research because I got so emotional that I had to stop. And I just felt so completely stressed with anxiety.

When Georgia was a peer researcher on a research project focused on the sexual and reproductive health of women with disabilities from migrant and refugee backgrounds, a young woman shared a particularly confronting story about the sexual violence that she had experienced. Georgia found it challenging in this situation to know how to respond, feeling conflicted between her positions as a psychologist, a researcher and a peer. As she described:

> The most difficult interview was a young lady who I knew of [before the interview] but never met. It was the first meeting I had with her and she had experienced a lot of trauma in her life and I didn't know. My background is in psychology; I used to be a psychologist before my injury and it was very complicated for me and very difficult for me to figure out how I treat this, what do I do. I stopped the interview – that's part of the ethics – you don't want this person to experience anymore trauma than they have already experienced.

In these moments, the distress that Weng and Georgia felt upon hearing about their peers' traumatic experiences was compounded by uncertainty about how to respond, and the conflict they felt between the position of an empathetic peer and the more neutral and objective position that they ascribed to researchers. On these occasions, they found the boundaries between being a peer and being a researcher to be porous, and that this provoked anxiety that was experienced for some time. As Georgia described:

> It was the after. I felt too close to her [the research participant] because we are so similar in other ways. I wanted to help her and it was difficult to do that because as a researcher you can't become involved with the people that you interview. As a psychologist you want to help them as a professional … it was very confusing, and it took me two or three weeks of a lot of soul searching.

Weng described how she managed role conflict when interviewing Deaf women for the W-DARE program, by being 'fluid' in how she presented herself in order to appropriately support the participants through the interviews. As she described:

> The stories and narratives were incredibly sensitive so during the interview I would give them breaks when they needed it, and sometimes other things would come up, so I needed to switch hats and roles – not just being an assessor and doing interviews.

Throughout W-DARE, Weng juggled being a peer, a researcher and an activist.

For all researchers involved in the projects that Weng and Georgia describe, there were challenges in listening to and working with confronting stories of neglect and abuse. However, the emotional labour involved, and the experience of unsettled and conflicted identities, had far more impact on the peer researchers in the team compared to the university-based researchers without disability. During training, peer researchers are often encouraged to 'set boundaries' between themselves and participants. However, in many instances peer researchers are recruited because they can *bridge* boundaries – because their similarities with participants enhances research processes (such as recruitment and data collection). Boundaries cannot easily be turned on and off, and this is work that falls solely on researchers who are also peers. Managing these porous boundaries involves emotional labour for peer researchers and is required even when the research is not about obviously 'sensitive' topics (such as research on livelihoods or the National Disability Insurance Scheme). Researchers who are not peer researchers need to recognise that a peer research approach may give rise to these 'costs' and that it they will not be distributed equally across a research team. In this instance, solidarity from researchers without disability requires anticipation of the potential impact on peer researchers, and ensuring that they have access to adequate training, ongoing mentoring and regular debriefing throughout a research project. It also requires projects to be designed in ways that redistribute resources towards the support and safeguarding of peer researchers.

Support and safety for peer researchers

A range of strategies to support peer researchers to manage the emotional labour involved in their work have been documented. Strategies that have been identified as helpful include peer researchers keeping reflective journals, accessing external psychological support, and having regular debriefing sessions with other peer researchers and formally trained researchers (Chappell et al. 2014; Mosavel and Sanders 2014; Burke et al. 2018; Vaughan et al. 2019). Support for and resourcing of these strategies by university-based researchers is one practical way that they can demonstrate reflexive solidarity with peer researchers (Davis and Vaughan 2018). This includes university-based researchers' willingness and availability to provide emotional support to peer researchers when and where it is needed, and their flexibility and commitment to meeting different peer researchers' needs – what one peer researcher finds helpful may not work for others.

Weng and Georgia's descriptions of what they found helpful after emotionally distressing research encounters highlights the highly varied nature of what individual peer researchers will experience as supportive, and the importance of both formal and informal support being available to peer researchers during and after their involvement in peer research projects.

Georgia found having a list of external psychological support services from whom she could seek support a particularly important support and safeguarding strategy. She explained:

> There should be supports in place before a project begins. They might not need to be used but they should be in place. [As a peer researcher] you need to know who you can speak with … like when we interview someone, and we give them a list of support services if they feel any grief or trauma, then they can call and speak to someone. I think we need to do the same thing for researchers as well.

Georgia also highlighted the importance of being able to debrief with other members of the research team, reporting how much she appreciated the lead researcher on one project reaching out to see how she was after one particularly distressing interview. As she explained, when she [the lead researcher] found out what happened she called me and spoke to me. I think that was a brilliant thing that she did and I said to her that I would be going to speak to my counsellor and to get the confirmation from her that yes, you should go, because usually you are told not to speak to others about it as a researcher – that was comforting.

Georgia emphasised that support should be made available to peer researchers in the weeks and months after a research project ends, because the impacts of distressing research encounters may not be immediately apparent, but may emerge over time. She elaborated, saying that,

there should be ongoing support for peer researchers, and just directing people to where they can get help if they need it. Because trauma is not something that comes up right away, it can come up years later. So just the knowledge of where you can go and seek help. And if they do call you [a university-based researcher] and you are the head of the research, not to hang up but to take five minutes to have a conversation.

In contrast, Weng spoke of how important self-care strategies were for her in managing the immediate and accumulative impacts of being a peer researcher and advocate for other Deaf women in the Philippines. She described how her self-care strategies have evolved over time, from her first distressing peer research experience to her later work as a W-DARE peer researcher examining sensitive issues relating to sexual and reproductive health and experiences of violence:

Over many years I was able to experience W-DARE and compare my experience to how I interviewed women for the first time .... Being a part of W-DARE since 2013 and working with Deaf women in the community has been a really big lesson for me. It hasn't taught me to be perfect, but it has taught me to do a lot of introspective work, looking at myself.

In her reflections upon the experience of interviewing other Deaf women, Weng observed,

it is not easy for me and it is not easy for them. When it is hard I want to say 'ok, are we done?' but once we are done talking I have to go and take care of myself. I have to do my own therapy to process the work that I have done. I do therapy with art and swimming, photography. I find outlets to take myself out of the difficult situations I feel like I am in when I am supporting other Deaf women. It is difficult for me to leave a situation when a Deaf woman has broken down and told me her story .... So I have to find an outlet. If I find that it is affecting me, I take care of myself. I draw pictures, I write and reflect that the world is very different from me.

In reflecting upon the responsibilities of university-based researchers to support and provide appropriate safeguards for peer researchers like Weng and Georgia, we recognise that this in no one-size-fits-all list of appropriate strategies. The resources available to Weng and Georgia in their own communities are very different. However, their experiences do suggest that, at a minimum, researchers leading research teams that include peer researchers who are women with disabilities need to get to know their team members, their personal circumstances, what reasonable accommodations they may require in the workplace, and how they would like to be supported to do what is often difficult work. Their experience also highlights the need to consider how to provide support to peer researchers beyond an initial debriefing during data collection – the impact of holding women's difficult stories, and sitting with peers' trauma, may not emerge until after a project has officially finished. However, acting in solidarity in this instance would require university-based researchers to consider what locally available support can be provided to peer researchers on a long-term basis, particularly if peer researchers continue to engage with research participants and their communities after a project ends in an effort to bring about social change.

Peer research as a strategy towards social change

Participatory approaches to research, including peer research approaches, can contribute to the quality of research endeavours – increasing their rigour, relevance and reach (Balazs and Morello-Frosch 2013). In reflecting upon their experience, Weng and Georgia argue that ensuring that research with people with disabilities is high quality and is relevant to their needs, is key to both the reach of research outcomes and the likelihood that the work will bring about change. Weng felt responsible, as a Deaf woman collecting data from other Deaf women, for making 'sure that that data, which shows that there are many, many more Deaf women who have much less access to everything than differently abled and others in the disability community' is shared widely, increases recognition in the wider disability sector of the specific needs of Deaf women, and contributes to change in the lives of Deaf women. Similarly, Georgia observed that 'you enable change when your research is valid' and that this validity is achieved when peer researchers who have shared lived experiences with the target community of the research are also involved. She described how 'I think you can't have [only formally trained researchers] without [peer researchers] you need to have both. It is the best way of doing research. You come together you bring all the knowledge together.'

While there has been documentation of the contribution of peer research approaches to social change, whether and how individual peer researchers themselves take action to address the needs facing their communities (and why and at what cost), is less well understood. This is an important area for further research, as it is clear that many peer researchers feel compelled to act, beyond what the formal parameters of any particular research project, to improve the conditions facing their communities (Boynton 2002). These actions may involve support-ing individual participants with particular issues identified during the research project. For example, Georgia talked about her support of individual research participants beyond the duration of the research project:

> I think that there should be more flexibility in these cases, that it really should be up to the individual peer researcher to decide how they want to leave it. It should be ok for them to continue a friendly relationship or to support someone they met on the project.

Weng described being moved to find other funding to run follow-up activities for participants in a peer support group she facilitated through W-DARE. She recalled how at the end of the final session,

> all of the participants came up to me, they surrounded me and they all said 'Please run these sessions again, please have them again, please don't forget about us!' They took photos with me, they said they wanted to text me and to stay in touch with me and it is not easy for me to see how many of these women need support.

Beyond supporting change in the lives of individual participants or small local-ised groups, peer research approaches can contribute to broader social change efforts. Georgia described an event where she and other peer researchers and university-based researchers co-presented their research findings to policymakers. This experience highlighted the benefits of putting peer researchers in the same room as policymakers, with Georgia describing how,

> policymakers are used to having academics in the room, who are not usu-ally people with disabilities, so we all went in there and this was a bunch of people with different types of disabilities. We presented this research to [the policymakers] and they really listened and they wouldn't have listened otherwise without our group in the room. I think they become detached when it is just on paper, but when they hear from the people experiencing the problems it becomes real.

This experience illustrates how the act of co-presenting can not only be a dem-onstration of solidarity, but also a more effective strategy for research translation.

Peer researchers are often motivated to become involved in research in the first place to contribute to social change, and can become quite galvanised to do so in response to what they learn about the difficult situations facing their peers. For some peer researchers this is a way of turning the distress that they may have experienced as a result of research into something positive. While peer research-ers can be powerful actors in contributing to social change, it is important to recognise the major structural barriers that may undermine them doing so. Weng discussed how, prior to the passing of the Filipino Sign Language (FSL) Law in

2018, her ability to contribute to advocacy and social change efforts were undermined by the fact that access to sign language interpreters was seen as a luxury rather than a right. As she described,

> now that FSL law is in existence, what a relief .... If there was no FSL law, we wouldn't be able to ask for financing .... If you took away that law, Deaf people would not be able to pay interpreters, so that law is important for all of us.

While the FSL Law is seen as a huge win for the Deaf community, Weng also highlighted that the limited pool of Deaf people with advocacy experience, and the limited availability of resources to fund advocacy for the Deaf community, means that individuals like Weng are overworked, feel supported, and risk mental and emotional burnout. After the closure of the only centre in Manila dedicated to supporting Deaf women, despite her advocacy efforts, Weng described how 'it was devastating .... I wanted to take a step back, and not stop supporting Deaf women, I will always support Deaf women, but I can't solve everyone's issues and problems as much as I want to.' Weng reflects that, over time, she has been worn down by continual exposure to the trauma and distress experienced by other Deaf women in the Philippines: 'Being a long-time advocate for about 15 years has not been easy for me. It doesn't make me want to give up necessarily, but it does make me frustrated.'

As Weng's and Georgia's experiences demonstrate, peer researchers' desire to contribute to social change in their communities doesn't stop when their involvement in a research project ends. In many cases, peer researchers' original motivations are strengthened by what they learn during research projects. However, given the substantial structural barriers to peer researchers' social change efforts, it is imperative that university-based researchers also commit to contributing to social change in solidarity with the wider team. This has implications for researchers' time and material resources, and this must be planned for out the outset of projects.

Conclusion

Peer research approaches can increase the rigour and relevance (Balazs and Morello-Frosch 2013) of research projects, facilitating the generation of rich data and production of analyses based on insider perspectives. Peer researchers themselves enable this by connecting university-based researchers to new communities, new perspectives and new expertise. As Weng describes it, 'I am the bridge – there is the hearing world on one side and the Deaf world on the other side and I am the bridge between two worlds.' However, being a bridge involves risks and costs. It is important that university-based researchers take a reflexive approach in working with peer researchers to jointly analyse what these risks and costs might be, and who is likely to be more affected by them. We suggest that solidarity between university-based researchers and peer researchers requires the management and redistribution of costs. However, we also recognise that this redistribution is unlikely to be sufficient to completely mitigate the structural barriers and discrimination that peer researchers with disabilities may face in contributing to research projects. In addition, university-based researchers can provide practical support to peer researchers working their way through the emotional labour involved in their role – but this does not take this labour away.

University-based researchers working with women with disabilities as peer researchers need to recognise that managing the dual role of peer and researcher can weigh heavily on their colleagues. Solidarity with peer researchers requires a genuine commitment to bearing costs. In our experience, this means university-based researchers ensuring that there are external psychological supports available; that debriefing and other supports are provided when and how they are needed; that reasonable accommodations such as accessible spaces, accessible transport, sign language interpreters, sharing of all information in plain and easy language formats, and so on are prioritised and that this is reflected in the project budget; and that there is also support for sustaining social action after a project has finished. Bridges can only hold if they rest on firm foundations.

References

Balazs, C. and Morello-Frosch, R., 2013. The three Rs: How community-based participatory research strengthens the rigor, relevance, and reach of science. *Environmental Justice*, 6 (1), 9–16.

Boynton, P., 2002. Life on the streets: The experiences of community researchers in a study of prostitution. *Journal of Community & Applied Social Psychology*, 12 (1), 1–12.

Burke, E., le May, A., and Kebe, F., 2018. Experiences of being, and working with, young people with disabilities as peer researchers in Senegal: The impact on data quality, analysis and well-being. *Qualitative Social Work*, 18 (4), 583–600.

CBM Australia, 2018. *Leave No One Behind: Gender Equality, Disability Inclusion and Leadership for Sustainable Development*. Available from: https://www.cbm.org.au/wp-content/uploads/2019/02/CBM-Leave-No-One-Behind-Gender-Equility.pdf [Accessed 13 July 2020].

Chappell, P., et al., 2014. Troubling power dynamics: Youth with disabilities as co-researchers in sexuality research in South Africa. *Childhood*, 21 (3), 385–399.

Davis, E. and Vaughan, C., 2018. Social action for social change. In: S. Banks and M. Brydon-Miller, eds. *Ethics in Participatory Research for Health and Social Well-Being: Cases and Commentaries*. Abingdon: Routledge, 181–206.

Hughes, K., et al., 2012. Prevalence and risk of violence against adults with disabilities: A systematic review and meta-analysis of observational studies. *Lancet*, 379 (9826), 1621–1629.

Krnjacki, L., et al., 2016. Prevalence and risk of violence against people with and without disabilities: Findings from an Australian population-based study. *Australian and New Zealand Journal of Public Health*, 40 (1), 16–21.

McLachlan, M. and Schwartz, L., 2009. *Disability and International Development: Towards Inclusive Global Health*. New York, NY: Springer.

Mosavel, M. and Sanders, K., 2014. Community-engaged research: Cancer survivors as community researchers. *Journal of Empirical Research on Human Research Ethics*, 9 (3), 74–78.

Prainsack, B. and Buyx, A., 2017. What is solidarity? In: B. Prainsack and A. Buyx, eds. *Solidarity in Biomedicine and Beyond.* Cambridge: Cambridge University Press, 43–72.

Roche, B., Guta, A., and Flicker, S., 2010. *Peer Research in Action I: Models of Practice. Community based Research Working Paper Series.* Toronto: Wellesley Institute.

Sandelowski, M. and Barroso, J., 2002. Finding the findings in qualitative studies. *Journal of Nursing Scholarship*, 34 (3), 213–219.

van der Heijden, I., Harries, J., and Abrahams, N., 2019. Ethical considerations for disability-inclusive gender-based violence research: Reflections from a South African qualitative case study. *Global Public Health*, 14 (5), 737–749.

Vaughan, C., et al., 2015. W-DARE: A three-year program of participatory action research to improve the sexual and reproductive health of women with disabilities in the Philippines. *BMC Public Health*, 15, 984. doi:10.1186/s12889-015-2308-y.

Vaughan, C., et al., 2016. Increasing disability inclusion in responses to violence against women in the Philippines: Lessons from W-DARE. *Gender and Development*, 24 (2), 245–260.

Vaughan, C., et al., 2019. 'It is like being put through a blender': Inclusive research in practice in an Australian university. *Disability & Society*, 34 (7–8), 1224–1240.

Vaughn, L., et al., 2018. Partnering with insiders: A review of peer models across community-engaged research, education and social care. *Health and Social Care in the Community*, 26, 769–786.

Warr, D., Mann, R., and Tacticos, T., 2011. Using peer-interviewing methods to explore place-based disadvantage: Dissolving the distance between suits and civilians. *International Journal of Social Research Methodology*, 14 (5), 337–352.

Warr, D., et al., 2017. *Choice, Control and the NDIS.* Melbourne: University of Melbourne.

WHO and UNFPA, 2009. *Promoting Sexual and Reproductive Health for Persons with Disabilities: WHO/UNFPA Guidance Note.* Geneva: WHO.

WHO and the World Bank, 2011. *World Report on Disability.* Geneva: WHO.

11 Reflecting on the role of peer researchers in collaborative Indigenous food security research in the Inuvialuit Settlement Region, Canada

Tiff-Annie Kenny, Sonia D. Wesche and Jullian MacLean

Introduction

Many Indigenous Peoples in Canada are faced with inadequate access to nutritious, culturally preferred foods, such that rates of food insecurity are significantly higher than for the non-Indigenous population. This is particularly true for Inuit, one of three constitutionally recognised Indigenous groups in Canada, the majority of whom live in the sparsely populated Arctic region, where food insecurity is a serious public health issue exacerbated by ongoing changes in social–ecological systems (Council of Canadian Academies 2014). While wild-harvested 'country food' remains fundamental to health and well-being across the Arctic, market foods make up the majority of most contemporary diets. Small, remote Arctic communities are generally serviced by one or two food retailers, providing limited choice to consumers. The high cost of market foods combined with low average incomes in most Arctic communities restricts the affordability of nutritious market foods.

In recognition of such challenges in the Inuvialuit Settlement Region in Arctic Canada, we worked collaboratively with the regional Inuit governance organisation and five peer researchers to conduct a participatory food costing project. The aim was to understand the affordability of healthy diets. The participatory, peer research process was designed to include people with experiential knowledge and contextual understanding of food security, address knowledge gaps that matter to them, and give voice to those impacted by food insecurity, with the aim of influencing regional decision making.

Written from the perspectives of the university-based researchers (Tiff-Annie and Sonia) and a representative of the regional Inuit governance organisation (Jullian), the purpose of this chapter is to describe the evolution of multi-level research relationships among these research partners and community-based peer researchers. This chapter presents learnings and findings from our process of engaging Inuit peer researchers in collaborative food security research in a remote community context.

Background

Inuit food systems

As with Indigenous Peoples globally, Inuit food systems are multifaceted and dynamic, directly linked to and informed by place and culture (Kuhnlein et al. 2009; Harder and Wenzel 2012). While the impacts of colonialism and globalisation have precipitated a dietary transition towards increased reliance on market (i.e. store-bought) food (Kenny et al. 2018b), country food (i.e. locally harvested aquatic, terrestrial and avian wildlife and plants) contributes in numerous ways to Inuit health and well-being, and is central to Inuit identity (Condon et al. 1995).

The majority of Inuit in Canada live in 53 communities spanning four Arctic regions, which collectively make up Inuit Nunangat, the Inuit homeland. Each region is co-managed by Inuit and federal, provincial or territorial governments, resulting from constitutionally recognised land claim agreements. These agreements affirm and delineate extensive rights, such that Inuit hold significant decision-making roles and responsibilities related to their homelands. Advances towards devolutionary Indigenous self-government models are also being made in the Arctic, to bring decision making and the delivery of programs and services closer to Inuit values and priorities.

Most Inuit communities are small and remote, the majority being only accessible by sea during the summer season and year-round by air. Retailers operating in these remote environments experience numerous logistical challenges in transporting and storing market foods and other essential items (e.g. heating fuel, construction material). As a result, market food prices in Arctic Canada are significantly higher than elsewhere in the country. Yet household incomes among Inuit in Inuit Nunangat are dramatically lower than for non-Indigenous households in the region (approximately CAD $70,000/year disparity) (ITK 2018a). This renders access to nutritious market foods challenging for many and is particularly problematic among those who lack access to country foods.

High food prices persist in the Arctic despite the existence of a federally administered food subsidy programme, Nutrition North Canada – a market-based mechanism intended to offset high food transportation costs for remote northern communities. Limited independent research exists regarding the effectiveness, administration and acceptability of the programme. More fundamentally, the active and meaningful participation of Inuit in the design and implementation of the subsidy has been limited (de Schutter 2012). The Inuit-Specific Approach for the Canadian Food Policy (ITK 2017) underscores the fact that current federal funding structures that are purported to support food security often act conversely to remove power from Inuit. It also highlights the importance of Inuit self-determination by ensuring that relevant research and decision making flows through and from Inuit governance structures.

Community leadership and control of research with Inuit

Food insecurity, like other social and health inequities among Inuit, derives from colonisation, systemic disempowerment, institutionalised discrimination and other enduring disparities in power, voice and participation in socio-economic, environmental, political and governance systems in Canada (Adelson 2005). Research involving Inuit communities is steeped in the historical and enduring context of abuse, misrepresentation and exploitation, whereby researchers benefit disproportionately from research partnerships (Brunger and Wall 2016). Supporting food security and food sovereignty for Inuit requires multifaceted approaches that address the multiple dimensions of the food system, while affirming Inuit self-determination and governance in research, and supporting community research capacity (ITK 2018b). As outlined in the *National Inuit Strategy on Research* (ITK 2018b), research in Inuit Nunangat must respect Inuit self-determination in collecting, verifying, analysing and disseminating Inuit-specific data and information. Thus, researchers must work to develop meaningful collaboration through careful, enduring relationship-building and reflection that affirms Inuit governance, partnership and participation in all aspects of the research (Brunger and Wall 2016).

Inuvialuit food security research program

This research is set in the Inuvialuit Settlement Region, the westernmost Inuit land claim settlement area in the Canadian Arctic. The region is governed by the Inuvialuit Regional Corporation (IRC), established at the signing of the Inuvialuit Final Agreement in 1984. The IRC has a governance mandate to improve the economic, social and cultural well-being of Inuvialuit beneficiaries. The region is geographically remote and sparsely populated. Sixty percent of the total population (5,335) reside in the town of Inuvik, the administrative centre for the western Arctic; the rest live in five smaller, predominantly Inuvialuit communities (Statistics Canada 2016a, b). Almost half (46%) of Inuvialuit households in the region experience either moderate or severe food insecurity (Egeland 2010).

Our research programme was initiated in response to the results of a comprehensive cross-sectional study on the health and living conditions of Inuit adults across the Canadian North, emphasising concerns related to diet quality, food security, chronic disease and exposure to environmental contaminants in the Inuvialuit Settlement Region (Egeland 2010). An initial collaborative research process involving the IRC aimed to enhance evidence-based, community-directed decision making around the allocation of resources and programming at regional and local levels (Fillion et al. 2014). From this evolved a number of research projects focused on diverse aspects of food security in the region, involving primary collection of data and analyses of epidemiological data from the Inuit Health Survey. Research activities have acted to reinforce existing relationships between Jullian (who at the time of the research was the Regional

Dietitian, Inuvialuit Settlement Region) at the IRC, and local peer researchers in five remote communities, which led to the initiation of a participatory food costing project.

A participatory food costing project – working with Inuvialuit peer researchers

To address locally identified concerns about retail food pricing, we initiated a participatory food costing project in the five remote Inuvialuit communities (with data collected by Jullian and other local researchers in Inuvik, the sixth community of the region); data was collected each season for a 14-month period between late 2014 and early 2016. Grounded in principles of participatory action research, participatory food costing includes the involvement of those directly affected by issues of food access and food insecurity in research design and collection of food price data (Williams et al. 2012). This comprises hiring, training and supporting peer researchers in communities to engage in research, knowledge translation and other capacity development activities. The participatory methodology was favoured given the potential to enhance research skills of community members and, over the long term, foster capacity for communities to initiate and implement their own food security research. Ethical approval for this research was granted by the University of Ottawa, and a Research License was obtained from the Aurora Research Institute.

Who were the peer researchers?

One Inuvialuit community member was recruited from each of the five remote communities. Two peer researchers were unable to complete the project due to competing demands for time (e.g. family, education, employment); in each case, an alternate peer researcher was identified. Peer researcher recruitment was led by Jullian at the IRC. Headquartered in Inuvik, the regional administrative center, Jullian regularly travelled to the five remote communities, and was able to provide support and oversee research activities both in-person and remotely. Jullian initially contacted each individual by telephone to discuss the food costing project, gauge their interest in participating and establish work agreements. Peer researchers were recruited on contracts and paid for completing food costing activities. This hiring model was key to project feasibility as the selected individuals were already contractually employed by the IRC in a nutrition-related role in their respective communities, thus facilitating logistics and labour relationships (i.e. contracts, timely payment and other financial logistics). Nevertheless, it is important to note that this targeted recruitment process may have excluded some of the more marginalised individuals affected by food insecurity in the community, such as those with no formal wage-based employment experience.

Peer researchers required a functional level of food literacy (e.g. ability to read food labels, understand measurement units) and basic mathematics (e.g. ability to compare food costs).

All the peer researchers had pre-existing training and experience as casual contract-based nutrition workers in their home communities. In their role as community nutrition workers, they were involved in leading regular community cooking circles and food demonstrations to promote healthy eating using affordable country and market foods – activities funded through federal support and administered through the IRC. Although sex and gender were not considered in the recruitment and hiring process, all peer researchers involved in this project were women. Women play important food-related roles in remote Inuit communities, from harvesting, gathering and purchasing, to food preparation and sharing. They are also key caregivers for children, elderly relatives and other extended family members. They are often the primary food shopper in their household and have a keen sense of key aspects of the food system and impacts on community health. Peer researchers were never asked to disclose their experiences of food access. Nevertheless, they often informally shared challenges that they and other community members faced in accessing food in their community. Furthermore, as formal emergency food support programmes (e.g. food banks and soup kitchens) are limited in remote Arctic communities where strong networks of food sharing have traditionally supported community food access, the nutrition education activities they led, which also provisioned food, were likely attended by individuals most in need (Kenny et al. 2018a). Their existing positions meant that they were already connected and aware of services and programmes that supported improved dietary quality and food security in the region. At the same time, involvement in the food costing research project likely enhanced their other community roles and responsibilities.

What training did the peer researchers participate in?

Training was conducted by Tiff-Annie and Jullian in face-to-face community visits at the onset of the project. Peer researchers participated in training sessions (lasting 2–3 days) involving presentations, discussion and hands-on data collection experience. Training materials were co-developed by Tiff-Annie and Jullian and were intended to provide peer researchers with the necessary background, resources and confidence to undertake future data collection independently, and adapt the research methodology to accommodate local issues.

Training involved discussing the goals and expectations of the project, and familiarising peer researchers with the core concepts underscoring the research project, including definitions, principles and tools for appraising food security and the affordability of healthy diets (e.g. 24-hour dietary recall, standardised food basket approaches). Training materials and vocabulary were intended to be adapted to local contexts and levels of education and knowledge. The peer researchers were encouraged to ask questions and engage in open discussion during the training session. These discussions emphasised unique dimensions of the local contexts and underscored the limitations of conventional conceptualisations and approaches to food costing in remote Inuit communities. Peer researchers also participated in an in-depth review and discussion of regional dietary, food security and health results from the Inuit Health Survey, which was designed to provide comprehensive baseline data about Inuit health and living conditions in support of Inuit-specific policies (Saudny et al. 2012). Peer researchers also received training in a participatory food costing methodology, which was adapted and refined iteratively with their input (described below) from standardised training material developed for general/southern community contexts (Williams et al. 2012).

Related to their function as community nutrition workers, the peer researchers continued to participate in various individual and group capacity building and training activities (e.g. food safety certification) led by Jullian. This included periodic (annual or semi-annual) regional group network meetings, lasting approximately three days. These gatherings, held in the regional administrative centre (Inuvik), were also attended by Tiff-Annie and provided a platform to present and discuss project updates/results and solicit feedback on data interpretation with the peer researchers.

How were peer researchers involved in the project?

In addition to independently leading data collection during the study and participating in the interpretation of study results, the peer researchers were involved in the study design from the outset. The peer researchers played a particularly important role in developing the adapted food costing methodology and survey tool from standardised training materials prepared for southern community contexts (Williams et al. 2012). Their involvement was wide-reaching and ensured incorporation of the local socio-economic context of the food system into the methodology, thus helping overcome some of the limitations of conventional assessment measures predicated upon Western economic frameworks (Harder and Wenzel 2012). Through a series of teleconference calls to discuss iterations of the survey instrument, peer researchers provided important input and feedback on the scope of the study and the methods. Their feedback favoured, for instance, the inclusion of items that were actually eaten in the communities and reflected changes in food availability and community dietary habits since the most recent relevant data was collected 10 years previously. Furthermore, as costs can vary between seasons due to local environmental and circumstantial factors – such as the availability of winter roads and barge shipments – the peer researchers dictated the timing of costing activities in their respective communities. As no standardised approach exists for assessing the cost of country food, they also identified the need to include key harvesting equipment (e.g. shotgun shells, heating fuel, gasoline) in the food costing list (Kenny et al. 2018b). The survey instrument was only finalised once they agreed that it was comprehensive and reflective of purchase and consumption patterns of individuals and households at the community scale.

Reflecting on working with peer researchers

Research that explicitly involves community members and community-based organisations is essential to fostering mutually beneficial academic–community partnerships that help to support food security and advance health equity (Wallerstein and Duran 2016). This project benefited from peer researcher involvement in several ways: the development of locally informed approaches to study design; the periodic collection of robust independent data in five remote communities over a significant time period; and mutual learning and capacity development opportunities among academic researchers, the regional Inuit governance organisation and the peer researchers. As study results were predicated upon research processes that affirmed community and regional leadership and built on existing local strengths, knowledge and contexts, they are more likely to be deemed credible and used to inform regional policy. Ultimately, these factors, supported by the structure of our ongoing food security research projects, enhanced the potential for study findings to contribute to local and regional action on food security.

While we affirm the importance of understanding peer researcher experiences and perspectives (Guta et al. 2011), we were unable to involve the peer researchers as co-authors in this chapter due to a complex and lengthy approval process. We also did not appraise peer researcher outcomes and experiences in the project. As with many community-based participatory research studies reported in the literature (Roche et al. 2011), this project did not formalise an explicit peer research model from the onset of the project. Many projects have designed their peer research approach using instinct and experience, but without the benefit of guidance from academic and grey literature on the strengths, challenges and standards of good practice when involving community members in research (Roche et al. 2011). Much collaborative research with Indigenous communities in Canada is founded in the concepts of 'community-based/directed/engaged' and 'participatory' research; rigorous, critical engagement with peer research paradigms is rare. Reflecting on and establishing a peer research approach from the start can strengthen the potential benefits of using these approaches to recalibrate power dynamics in research projects towards more equitable structures of power and status (Roche et al. 2011).

In other settings, involvement in participatory food costing studies has yielded significant personal and professional development benefits for community researchers (e.g. self-esteem, personal growth, leadership and other skills) to help them engage more equitably and effectively in research and action to support local food security (Monteith et al. 2020). In the future, we will aim to embed process evaluation of peer research within our research projects to ensure that peer researchers develop the knowledge, tools and resources needed to successfully undertake, and ultimately lead, future food security research in their communities.

Building community relationships and capacity in remote settings

Peer research models require significant time and sustained investment to develop and maintain. This is particularly challenging in remote Indigenous communities, removed from academic centres, and where elevated research costs can be limiting (e.g. in the Canadian Arctic). Such challenges echo the importance of building human resource capacity in Inuit regions and communities to facilitate Inuit-led research and establish an Inuit Nunangat university, as highlighted in national policy (ITK 2018b).

In this project, Jullian and peer researchers in the remote communities were engaged in research design and data collection, consistent with both advisory (i.e. peers play an advisory role) and employment (i.e. peers act as research employees) models of peer research (Roche et al. 2011). We also strived to support peers as partners and leaders in other aspects of the research over time (i.e. the partner model) (Roche et al. 2011). As the project evolved, peer researcher roles in this study extended beyond data collection to include advocacy in the community (Roche et al. 2011). For example, we have used newly acquired funding for community-driven action on food security to hire one of the peer researchers as a part-time food security coordinator for the region, while she and another peer researcher will develop and implement on-the-ground food security activities.

Constructs of peer researcher and community capacity development are contingent on the social and cultural context of those involved (Labonte and Laverack 2010). Opportunities to support capacity development within research projects – which often emphasise academic journal publications, conference presentations and other academic 'currencies' – may be less meaningful than other forms of training and skill development to peer researchers in remote Indigenous communities. We explored options for involving the peer researchers in such activities (e.g. conferences, workshops) outside of their home community, but most were limited in their ability to travel and participate by family and community responsibilities. It is thus important that training and capacity building opportunities for peer researchers in Indigenous communities be enhanced to recognise the cultural context and emotional impacts of capacity development among peer researchers (Kanuha 2000).

Labour relationships (e.g. recruitment, hiring processes, contracts, wages, training, support and supervision) are important for fostering equitable research relationships in peer research projects (Guta et al. 2011). Critical to this research project was the direct partnership with the IRC, and more specifically Jullian, who also benefited reciprocally from the relationship structure (e.g. through enhanced research capacity and experience). Working closely with the IRC ensured effective and ongoing communication, support and supervision of the peer researchers, building on existing, periodic face-to-face network meetings. It also facilitated communication among academics, peer researchers and other supporting local organisations, such as the Community Corporations, which played an important role in facilitating research logistics (e.g. payment for services, Internet and office access) and the retail store managers. Jullian played a key role in negotiating community labour relationships. In turn, the project may have enhanced organisational ownership over food security research. Partnership with the IRC also ensured the prioritisation of community and regional priorities in the research process, and provided a direct conduit to policy influence.

Our project experiences highlighted the importance of partnership with local health professionals, such as Jullian, who was the regional dietitian at IRC. Public health professionals including nutritionists and dietitians were called upon to extend their focus beyond individual behavioural change to include structural socio-environmental factors, and thus more effectively mitigate the burden of chronic disease and promote health equity (Schubert et al. 2012). Nutrition professionals working to improve the food supply in remote Indigenous communities face unique challenges (Colles et al. 2016). They are often recently qualified, called to engage with a range of community stakeholder groups (e.g. community workers, as well as retail and transportation sector representatives) and expected to perform numerous functions ranging from clinical practice to research and advocacy (Colles et al. 2016; Wilson et al. 2017; Palermo et al. 2019). They may feel that they lack the training and tools to adequately address nutrition-related issues – that stem from multiple interrelated socio-ecological determinants and involve diverse sectors – while ensuring the use of culturally competent, culturally safe approaches (Colles et al. 2016; Palermo et al. 2019). Enhancing their capacity to be more effective in their roles (e.g. through communication and relationship-building skills, cultural adeptness, advocacy) is an important priority for health promotion and health equity in these contexts (Wilson et al. 2017). Working alongside local peer researchers as partners and reciprocal mentors can build the collective capacity of nutrition professionals and peer researchers (Colles et al. 2016).

Peer researcher identities

There are definitional issues regarding 'peers' in such processes, and prospective peer researchers are often asked to self-identify as peers within the community of interest to the research (Roche et al. 2011). In the present context, peer researchers were not asked to disclose their experience with food security and food access. However, food insecurity affects a high percentage of households in the region and the experience of food insecurity in Inuit and other small, remote Indigenous community settings often differs from more populous and non-Indigenous contexts. In these contexts, health is holistically defined, transcending notions of the individual to include the importance of family and kinship ties, relationships to the land, culture, interpersonal and intergenerational issues, and impacts of colonialism (Kral et al. 2011). As such, it is likely that each peer researcher involved in this project had either direct or indirect experience with challenges or concerns related to food insecurity and food access. They drew on this depth of knowledge gleaned through intergenerational lived experience to inform the development of the survey and research methodology, which were critical to project success. This would not have been possible without peer researcher involvement. The application of the peer research paradigm to Indigenous food security-related research indicates the need, however, for an expanded definition of 'peer researcher' beyond those who are most vulnerable and directly involved in the issue at hand. Food security is a social determinant of health, and Inuit health in remote communities is conceived not only at the individual level, but also at the collective, societal level. Thus, issues of food insecurity are experienced as a collective health issue – particularly as many of its determinants derive from enduring legacies of colonisation. As such, any number of community members could act as a prospective peer researcher, bringing their own experience of food-related issues to the role.

While recognising the importance of including a diversity of lived experience in peer researcher processes, the involvement of women in such positions was entirely appropriate in the context of this food costing project. Women play a central role in food production, procurement and preparation within their families and communities. Inuit women, in particular, play a key role in accessing, transforming and sharing market foods (Quintal-Marineau 2019). Interventions that build capacity among women to address structural forces that impact their lives (such as high food costs) have been identified as a priority area for research (Monteith et al. 2020). Among Inuit, food insecurity is experienced differentially by gender, with women (particularly female lone-parent families) experiencing the greatest disparities (Huet et al. 2012). In the current project, the peer researchers were selected based on existing work experience as community nutrition workers, where one of the main activities was leading community cooking circles. This type of activity may tend to predominantly (if not exclusively) draw female applicants. Likewise, due to the centrality of their role in food processes at both household and community levels, the peer researchers were well positioned to report on issues of community food security.

In remote Indigenous communities, local peer researchers can act as local knowledge experts who translate scientific and health-related information into accessible formats, as local champions for healthy eating (Colles et al. 2016). Here, peer researchers brought critical personal and significant professional experience to the project. This includes, among others, professional experience as community nutrition workers, personal experience as residents of remote Indigenous communities and, in some cases, experience as former employees at a local grocery store. Informal discussions and dialogue among the peer researchers, service providers and academic researchers often revolved around subjects such as budgeting skills, community food programme use, and challenges related to employment and familial responsibilities. As described above, these issues will inform ongoing and future community-directed food security research with Inuvialuit communities.

Supporting Indigenous-led food security research and action

For many Indigenous Peoples, control of the research agenda within their territory is a recent movement considered essential to Indigenous governance, self-determination and identity. Enabling community voice and power in informing food security policy is essential. Inuit, supported by scholars and national and international actors (de Schutter 2012) have called for immediate action to support food security in Northern Canada. A key driver of this research project was to address the lack of community 'voice' in publications and public discussion around food cost in the North, something that has been repeatedly highlighted in our interactions with Inuvialuit community members. The participatory food costing approach enabled peer researchers to generate locally relevant independent data that is trusted by community and regional organisations.

Stores in remote community contexts, their management and the quality of the food they provide are critical to the effort to improve the health of Indigenous people living remotely. In the Inuvialuit context, the remote communities have only one or two stores from which to procure food. Moreover, the challenging logistics and supply chain in such contexts makes the food supply (availability, prices and quality) more vulnerable to disruptions and interruptions. As this project demonstrated, multisectoral collaborations between the retail sector, Indigenous organisations and academic researchers have led to the generation and documentation of important knowledge and perspectives about how such dynamics impact the food supply with the goal of supporting healthy food environments and food security in remote community contexts.

Participatory food costing may be helpful in addressing public discontent about food prices in the Inuvialuit Settlement Region by eliciting independent, internally generated (community level) food price data, and empowering community members to contribute to addressing an important community issue. As elsewhere, we are continuing to work with regional-level organisations to use this research to advocate for health equity and policy changes (Williams et al. 2012). At the same time, several peer researchers indicated that their sense of empowerment and enhanced engagement in their communities, which were generated during this project, has added to the success of existing food initiatives. For example, one peer researcher described how involvement in the project heightened her awareness of food cost and availability issues in her community, and expressed a desire to use this knowledge to advocate for change.

In recognition of Inuit self-determination and leadership in decision making, discourse on food security has shifted to recognise important links to *food sovereignty* (QIA 2019). While this participatory food costing project focused largely on market foods, which comprise a major share of contemporary Inuvialuit diets (Kenny et al. 2018b), country foods remain strongly culturally preferred and integral to Inuvialuit food security and food sovereignty (Wenzel et al. 2016). Thus, the retail sector must be addressed as part of a multitude of strategies to improve the health and nutritional intake of remote Indigenous communities (Colles et al. 2016). Due to the complexity of factors that lead to food insecurity, addressing food affordability in isolation from a more comprehensive plan to reduce Inuit food insecurity is insufficient to effect change (ITK 2017). The peer researchers helped adapt survey tools to incorporate the cost of country food harvesting and to interpret research results in the context of Inuit household structures. Ongoing research is being designed to build on these strengths and further engage the peer researchers in analyses that more explicitly reflect these issues and dynamics.

Meanwhile, evidence is lacking concerning the actual processes that might be undertaken to achieve and sustain multifaceted and coordinated approaches in which Indigenous people are central to decision making about their food system (Brimblecombe et al. 2017). Traditional definitions of food security, and consequent assessment measures and tools, tend to emphasise financial and income-related barriers to food access, often overlooking the less tangible social determinants. Peer research structures offer one approach to support the development of research methods and survey instruments that better capture the complex experience of food security in Inuit communities. More specifically, engaging the voice, knowledge and lived experience of peer researchers will ensure the inclusion of food security dimensions that are not typically captured in academic-led approaches.

Moving forward

The study described here was founded on local and regional expertise, while also strengthening research capacity in Inuvialuit communities. Inuit women clearly have important knowledge and experiences that should not be overlooked in designing, undertaking and reporting on food security research. Operationally, it is imperative that peer researchers access and benefit from opportunities to enhance their personal and professional development in ways that are feasible and culturally relevant to them. This goes beyond normative conceptions of capacity building in academic or professional sectors. Capacity building interests should be discussed with peer researchers both early on and periodically throughout a project, and adapted as necessary; to deal meaningfully with these commitments in remote settings, this must be supported by dedicated additional funds, time and resources (Guta et al. 2011).

Peer learning, trust, knowledge sharing and knowledge creation among community members, Indigenous and community-based organisations, and health professionals may help infuse locally relevant priorities, perspectives, and values into food security research projects and support action based on research findings. Mutual capacity building among university-based researchers, peer researchers, service providers and Indigenous organisations sets a strong foundation for future food security research and policy in Canada's northern regions.

While the benefits of peer research are clear, they rely on relationships of respect, reciprocity, and trust, which take time and the right context to develop. Such research paradigms are gaining traction in academia. However, challenges remain with respect to maintaining lines of communication among research teams (including peer researchers) over time, ensuring sufficient time and resources for effective knowledge translation, reconciling community and academic timescales, and actively shifting funding structures to ensure greater continuity, among others. Increased attention and diverse discourse on this topic will only help to illuminate and address many of these challenges.

References

Adelson, N., 2005. The embodiment of inequity: Health disparities in aboriginal Canada. *Canadian Journal of Public Health*, 96 (Suppl. 2), S45–S61.

Brimblecombe, J.K., et al., 2017. Feasibility of a novel participatory multi-sector continuous improvement approach to enhance food security in remote indigenous Australian communities. *SSM – Population Health*, 3, 566–576.

Brunger, F. and Wall, D., 2016. 'What do they really mean by partnerships?' Questioning the unquestionable good in ethics guidelines promoting community engagement in indigenous health research. *Qualitative Health Research*, 26 (13), 1862–1877.

Colles, S.L., Belton, S., and Brimblecombe, J.K., 2016. Insights into nutritionists' practices and experiences in remote Australian aboriginal communities. *Australian and New Zealand Journal of Public Health*, 40 (S1), S7–S13.

Condon, R.G., Collings, P., and Wenzel, G., 1995. The best part of life: Subsistence hunting, ethnicity, and economic adaptation among young adult Inuit males. *Arctic*, 48 (1), 31–46.

Council of Canadian Academies, 2014. *Aboriginal Food Security in Northern Canada: An Assessment of the State of Knowledge*. Ottawa: Council of Canadian Academies.

de Schutter, O., 2012. *Report of the Special Rapporteur on the Right to Food on His Mission to Canada (6 to 16 May 2012)*. United Nations General Assembly. Available from: http://www.srfood.org/images/stories/pdf/officialreports/20121224_canadafinal_en.pdf [Accessed 17 February 2020].

Egeland, G.M., 2010. *Inuit Health Survey 2007–2008: Inuvialuit Settlement Region*. Montreal, QC: Centre for Indigenous Peoples' Nutrition and Environment.

Fillion, M., et al., 2014. Development of a strategic plan for food security and safety in the Inuvialuit Settlement Region, Canada. *International Journal of Circumpolar Health*, 73 (1), 25091.

Guta, A., Roche, B., and Flicker, S., 2011. *Peer Research in Action II: Management, Support and Supervision*. Toronto: Wellesley Institute.

Harder, M.T. and Wenzel, G.W., 2012. Inuit subsistence, social economy and food security in Clyde River, Nunavut. *Arctic*, 65 (3), 305–318.

Huet, C., Rosol, R., and Egeland, G.M., 2012. The prevalence of food insecurity is high and the diet quality poor in Inuit communities. *Journal of Nutrition*, 142 (3), 541–547.

ITK, 2017. *An Inuit-Specific Approach for the Canadian Food Policy*. Ottawa: Inuit Tapiriit Kanatami.

ITK, 2018a. *Inuit Statistical Profile 2018*. Ottawa: Inuit Tapiriit Kanatami.

ITK, 2018b. *National Inuit Strategy on Research*. Ottawa: Inuit Tapiriit Kanatami.

Kanuha, V., 2000. 'Being' native versus 'going native': Conducting social work research as an insider. *Social Work*, 45 (5), 439–447.

Kenny, T.A., et al., 2018a. Supporting Inuit food security: A synthesis of initiatives in the Inuvialuit Settlement Region, Northwest Territories. *Canadian Food Studies*, 5 (2), 73–110.

Kenny, T.A., et al., 2018b. Dietary sources of energy and nutrients in the contemporary diet of Inuit adults: Results from the 2007–08 Inuit Health Survey. *Public Health Nutrition*, 21 (7), 1319–1331.

Kral, M.J., et al., 2011. Unikkaartuit: Meanings of well-being, unhappiness, health, and community change among Inuit in Nunavut, Canada. *American Journal of Community Psychology*, 48 (3–4), 426–438.

Kuhnlein, H.V., Erasmus, B., and Spigelski, D., 2009. *Indigenous Peoples' Food Systems: The Many Dimensions of Culture, Diversity and Environment for Nutrition and Health*. Rome: FAO.

Labonte, R. and Laverack, G., 2010. Capacity building in health promotion, part 1: For whom? And for what purpose? *Critical Public Health*, 11 (2), 111–127.

Monteith, H., Anderson, B., and Williams, P., 2020. Capacity building and personal empowerment: Participatory food costing in Nova Scotia, Canada. *Health Promotion International*, 35 (2), 321–330.

Palermo, C., et al., 2019. Using unfolding case studies to better prepare the public health nutrition workforce to address the social determinants of health. *Public Health Nutrition*, 22 (1), 180–183.

QIA, 2019. *Food Sovereignty and Harvesting*. Iqaluit: Qikiqtani Inuit Association.

Quintal-Marineau, M., 2019. Feeding our families: That's what we have been doing for centuries'. *Hunter Gatherer Research*, 3 (4), 583–599.

Roche, B., Guta, A., and Flicker, S., 2011. *Peer Research in Action I: Models of Practice*. Toronto: Wellesley Institute.

Saudny, H., Leggee, D., and Egeland, G.M., 2012. Design and methods of the Adult Inuit Health Survey 2007–2008. *International Journal of Circumpolar Health*, 71 (1), 19752.

Schubert, L., et al., 2012. Re-imagining the "social" in the nutrition sciences. *Public Health Nutrition*, 15 (2), 352–359.

Statistics Canada, 2016a. *Aboriginal Population Profile, 2016 Census – Inuvialuit Region [Inuit Region], Northwest Territories*. Ottawa: Statistics Canada.

Statistics Canada, 2016b. *Aboriginal Population Profile, 2016 Census – Inuvik [Population Centre], Northwest Territories and Saskatchewan [Province]*. Ottawa: Statistics Canada.

Wallerstein, N.B. and Duran, B., 2016. Using community-based participatory research to address health disparities: *Health Promotion Practice*, 7 (3), 312–323.

Wenzel, G., Dolan, J., and Brown, C., 2016. Wild resources, harvest data and food security in Nunavut's Qikiqtaaluk region: A diachronic analysis. *Arctic*, 69 (2), 147–159.

Williams, P., et al., 2012. A participatory food costing model: In Nova Scotia. *Canadian Journal of Dietetic Practice and Research*, 73 (4), 181–188.

Wilson, A.M., Delbridge, R., and Palermo, C., 2017. Supporting dietitians to work in aboriginal health: Qualitative evaluation of a community of practice mentoring circle. *Nutrition & Dietetics*, 74 (5), 488–494.

Section IV

Ethical considerations

12 Socio-ethical considerations in peer research with newly arrived migrant and refugee young people in Denmark

Reflections from a peer researcher

Nina Langer Primdahl, Alaa Nached and Morten Skovdal

Introduction

In 2015, a number of European countries experienced a rapid influx in migrants and refugees, resulting in a large number of asylum seekers. Arguably due to public concern about the so-called 'refugee crisis', research interest and resources were channelled into the study of opportunities and challenges faced by newly arrived migrants and refugees in their adjustment to a new host country, as well as the health and social challenges they faced as a result of past and present experiences as 'people on the move'. We secured funds from the European Commission, together with colleagues in five other European countries, to test and contextualise a selection of school-based mental health promoting interventions for newly arrived migrant and refugee young people, aged 12–21. In Denmark, the project involved schools from 24 municipalities, spread across the country. In this chapter, we reflect on the experience of embedding elements of peer research into the project.

Working with migrant and refugee peer researchers

Every year, around 6,000 young people arrive from other countries to gain residence in Denmark (Danmarks Statistik 2019). Reasons for migrating vary from labour migration from one European country to another, to fleeing war or political persecution. Some come with family members, others come alone. The challenges that young people experience when moving to Denmark are as multifaceted as the reasons for migrating, and include loneliness (Leth et al. 2014; Rich Madsen et al. 2016); stress related to past experiences of trauma, interrupted schooling and family separation (Center for Udsatte Flygtninge 2016); and issues pertaining to the migration and asylum system (Montgomery and Foldspang 2007; Larsen 2011; Goosen et al. 2014; Barghadouch et al. 2016). In addition, discursive actors such as policymakers, municipal authorities, news media and researchers continue to construct newly arrived refugee and migrant young people as 'problems' (Moldenhawer 2017). For young migrants and refugees, the upheaval of moving from one country to another is compounded by liminality associated with being in between countries, languages and life stages. Research has shown that arriving to a new country in the last school years decreases the chances of young people finishing their exams and continuing secondary education compared to arriving earlier (Kristjansdottir and Pérez 2016; Bakunzi 2018). Providing space for newly arrived adolescents to learn Danish, gain sociocultural competence and develop a social network upon arrival is important.

Since the 1970s, preparatory classes have been used as a gateway for newly arrived children and young people into the Danish society, language and educational system (Kristjansdottir and Pérez 2016). Preparatory classes are smaller than usual, typically located in mainstream schools, and facilitate a gradual transfer into mainstream classes, depending on young people's Danish language skills. The classes often consist of refugees, asylum seekers and Non-European and European migrants with completely different life histories, migration experiences, cultural backgrounds and levels of schooling.

We sought to embed peer research into the project, because this approach is increasingly considered 'good practice' in migration and refugee research (Mackenzie et al. 2007; Marlowe et al. 2015). Peer research has been described as a strategy to reduce power imbalances and create more trust between the researchers and research participants (Castleden et al. 2008). Although an exact definition of peer research has not been agreed on, mutual lived experiences between the peer researcher and research participant are usually pivotal (Logie et al. 2012). Migrant and refugee peer researchers have been involved in research in different ways across diverse settings (Marlowe et al. 2015; O'Reilly-de Brún et al. 2016; Bakunzi 2018) and methodologies (Phillimore et al. 2015; Brigham et al. 2018). Such peer researchers have been referred to as 'insiders', 'group members', and 'bilingual' or 'bicultural workers', who are engaged in a research process because they can also be viewed as part of the target group (Lee et al. 2014; Marlowe et al. 2015).

Inviting newly arrived migrants or refugees as insiders, group representatives or peers to participate in the research process is justified by claims that doing so can reduce historical power imbalances within research and knowledge production; create fuller and more representative knowledge about specific groups; and work as an emancipating and empowering practice for the peer researcher (Seal 2018). Peer research is therefore both a methodological strategy and an ethical project. While all research is influenced by power relations informed by class, gender and race, refugee and migrant research is often complicated by inequalities of language, living situation and residency, together with anti-Muslim discourses created by and influencing the political climate. Peer research enables a partial deflection of these power imbalances, as important structural positions are shared between researcher and participants (Mackenzie et al. 2007).

At a more practical level, peer research minimises the use of translators and eases the flow of conversation when recruiting and interviewing participants. In our research, identifying a peer researcher who could seamlessly communicate with study participants was a key consideration. In cross-cultural research, communication is about language, implied cultural knowledge and interpretation (Liamputtong 2008), and is central to recruitment processes and asking 'questions in a culturally relevant and explicit manner' (Dunbar et al. 2002, p. 294). For instance, we suspected that many study participants would still be in the process of asylum-seeking, making them susceptible to linking the immigration process with our study, perhaps thinking that participation might either aid or inhibit their application for asylum. Carling et al. (2013) have previously noted how those researching newly arrived migrants and refugees may be perceived as representatives of the state and their research may contribute to policy changes which will make the situation for refugees and migrants more vulnerable. Complex relational and cross-cultural research encounters like these can influence the trust and corporation between researcher and participants, affecting the quality of data generated and eventually the knowledge that is produced (Israel et al. 1998). By involving a peer researcher, we hoped to minimise misunderstandings, foster trust, and get closer to emic (insider, participant) perspectives on salient issues.

As an ethical project, refugee, migrant, diasporic and racialised groups have historically been excluded from the production of knowledge about their lives and experiences (Pottie and Gabriel 2014). Research practices and knowledge production are still largely based on Western epistemologies, while non-Western subjectivities, philosophies and thought systems are seen as interpretations rather than the 'objective knowledge' some academic research strives to produce. This inequality in knowledge production has been described as 'epistemic injustice' (Fricker 2007), existing partly based on inequalities in how credible and trustworthy we perceive people to be when sharing their stories. By inviting peer researchers to lead the collection and interpretation of data with racialised population groups, peer research approaches can overcome such injustices by getting closer to research participants' lived experiences associated with being a refugee, migrant or other identity. In turn, data generated during peer research can help re-frame future policymaking and programming to fit with their diverse lived experiences, rather than the version of these experiences produced by others (Collumbien et al. 2009).

Much has been written about the methodological difficulties (Jacobsen and Landau 2003; Block et al. 2012) and socio-ethical dilemmas (Birman 2006; Doná 2007; Mackenzie et al. 2007; Thorstensson Dávila 2014) involved in conducting migrant and refugee research. However, little has been done to identify and reflect on the socio-ethical opportunities and challenges experienced by peer researchers (Ganga and Scott 2006). Against this background, and in the interest of identifying implications for peer migrant and refugee research, we describe the socio-ethical opportunities and challenges experienced by Alaa Nached – one of the authors of this chapter – who was employed as a peer researcher on the RefugeesWellSchool project.

The RefugeesWellSchool project

The RefugeesWellSchool project is an intervention study (2018–22) testing the effectiveness of school-based interventions in improving the psychosocial and mental well-being of refugee and migrant young people in diverse European settings. The project is funded by the European Union's Horizon 2020 programme and involves partner universities in Belgium, Denmark, Finland, Norway, Sweden and the UK. The interventions are implemented in different school settings and evaluated using data from self-reported questionnaires and focus groups with young people, teachers and parents.

In Denmark, we tested two interventions in preparatory classes for newly arrived young refugees and migrants. These were designed to establish classroom cultures of sharing, connection and belonging, so that students could collaboratively, and in conditions of trust and mutual support, engage with and seek to transform conditions of adversity. The first intervention involved drama therapists who visited seven preparatory classes in public schools located on Zealand, eastern Denmark, on a weekly basis over a nine-week period to run drama, dance and storytelling exercises in drama workshops. The second intervention, called Welcome to School, consisted of a 14-session curriculum designed for teachers of preparatory classes to facilitate dialogue around topics such as friendship, health and home.

The interventions were evaluated with baseline and follow-up surveys in both control and intervention schools, capturing assessments of young migrants' and refugees' mental health, well-being and resilience, among other things. Evaluation data collection was completed in July 2020 and analyses of the evaluative data will run until 2022. Drawing on realist evaluation (Maxwell 2012) and implementation science principles (Brownson et al. 2017), qualitative research at baseline and endpoints of the study sought to understand people's experiences of the interventions and unpack the range of contextual factors that may shape intervention successes or failures.

In Denmark, the research took place in 34 preparatory classes located in 29 schools spread across 24 urban and rural municipalities. The participants were a mix of young migrants and refugees aged 12–21, representing 44 nationalities. Recruitment of study participants was a major challenge. Once a school and its teachers agreed to participate in the study, it was necessary to describe the study to potential participants and recruit young migrants and refugees, and parents, into the study. We required parental consent for some of the younger participants. Given the recent arrival of refugees from the Middle East, and Syria in particular, Arabic-speaking adolescents made up a significant proportion of our study participants. The largest nationality group was from Syria, accounting for around 35% of participants. For these reasons, we employed a Syrian peer researcher who would lead communication with Arabic-speaking participants and families.

Working with Alaa, a Syrian peer researcher living in Copenhagen

Alaa Nached – a Syrian and Arabic speaker with personal experience of migration – joined the project in October 2018 as a research assistant to improve engagement with study participants in qualitative and quantitative research processes. She was responsible for recruiting Arabic-speaking participants, providing potential participants with initial information about the project in Arabic in a way that was sensitive to their circumstances. At baseline stage, Alaa translated a self-reported questionnaire, which was sent to around 500 newly arrived parents and 1,200 students in all six countries. The questionnaire consisted of a range of measurement scales and scores, some of which have been validated in Arabic. Parts of the questionnaire were therefore already translated. However, Alaa was not satisfied with the quality of the validated Arabic translations as the language did not flow naturally and appeared strange to a native speaker. She played a critical role in instigating discussion on the validity of the self-reported question-naire, and her inputs were incorporated into the questionnaire. Alaa also led the collection of qualitative data through three in-depth focus group discussions with Arabic-speaking students and parents; other (non-peer) researchers were respon-sible for focus groups with participants of other nationalities. She transcribed the recorded focus groups into English but was then offered a full-time position in another institution and left the project. For this reason, Alaa did not participate further in the analytical part of the work.

Alaa was originally from Aleppo in Syria, and her mother tongue is the Syrian dialect of Arabic. Alaa emigrated from Syria nearly a decade ago, first to Lebanon and later to Denmark where her husband, who had migrated before her, had received refugee status. She now lives in Copenhagen with her family. She has a background in business administration and before the war in Syria broke out, worked in student support at a private language school. Prior to her recruitment in the study, she worked at an international pharmaceutical company and com-pleted an internship in risk management with UNICEF.

With regard to being a 'peer', Alaa shared many aspects of her identity with informants.

This included her Syrian nationality and her Syrian dialect of Arabic, which was a central commonality between her and the research participants. Alaa's migration status was shared with all the participants. Being Muslim, clearly shown by wearing a hijab, she also worked as an identity marker, signalling affiliation between Alaa and Muslim participants, especially those who themselves wore hijabs. Supported by these shared identities, Alaa's position as a peer should be viewed as a configura-tion of lived experiences, cultural norms and belief systems, which made it possible for her to connect and communicate closely with participants.

In line with the elasticity of identity, other parts of Alaa's identity and experi-ences – including her age, gender, educational background and socio-economic status and parts of her migration experience – were not necessarily shared with informants. For instance, Alaa had left Syria several years before the participants and had therefore not experienced the same war as many of them. This meant that although her experience of leaving behind her country to move to another country to start a new life was shared with participants, first-hand experiences of long-lasting civil war, as well as the human and economic consequences of this war, was not.

Training is vital in peer research processes, especially if peer researchers have no formal education or research experience. Given Alaa's professional background, we opted for an informal, 'learning on the job' approach. Alaa was fully briefed on project aims and methods and had an in-depth conversation with one of the experienced researchers about what a focus group discussion is and how best to facilitate it. She then co-facilitated a focus group with another researcher, getting some initial experience. Following a de-debrief, she felt ready to facilitate her own focus group discussion. Similarly, her first experience of recruiting participants was undertaken together with a seasoned researcher before doing it independently. Alaa proactively asked questions and sought support when uncertainties arose and approached the activities confidently. This informal approach seemed appropriate given Alaa's background, confidence and continuous contact with the research team.

Socio-ethical considerations in peer research with migrant and refugee young people

In this section, I – Alaa – write about my experiences of conducting research with Syrian peers in which I was simultaneously a peer, a sister, a role model and a researcher. I occupied what Dwyer and Buckle (2009, p. 60) call a 'space in between', alluding to the multiple relationships and shifting positions of power that I had to negotiate. These introduced socio-ethical research opportunities and dilemmas that I will reflect on.

Being a peer researcher was a rewarding experience

My experience as a peer researcher in the project proved overwhelmingly to be a positive experience. Drawing on writing on participatory research with refugees by Doná (2007), I link my experiences to three forms of representation – descriptive, instrumental, personalist – that peer researchers use to connect with peers. Descriptive representation refers to us looking and being alike. Being and looking Syrian, speaking the Syrian dialect of Arabic and sharing the same culture as young people and their parents, I, in many ways, was similar to them. Our connection became clear through common dialect and cultural reference points, or when sharing memories from specific places in Syria.

This shared identity and sense of connection with many participants contributed to pleasant and relatable interactions. These relations with research participants also put me in a unique position within the broader research team, as I knew that I was able to encourage participants to talk in a way other research team members could not. In the first focus group discussion, which I conducted with a Danish colleague, one of the Syrian boys told a story about his school in Syria and how the teachers there would be violent towards students. The other boys agreed with him in a mix of Danish and Arabic, interrupting each other. Where my Danish colleague was confused about the story and slightly shocked by the violence of the teacher, I was able to relate and immediately comprehend the story by connecting it to my own experiences of Syrian schools. I could then retell her what they had said and confirm what the boys meant.

Instrumental representation is defined as 'acting on behalf of' (Doná 2007, p. 220) the research participants, which I was able to do with participants by passing along their stories as research data. Meeting and speaking with fellow Syrians and being able to give them a voice in relation to the struggles and experiences related to starting a new life in Denmark was a tremendously gratifying experience. I was given the power to make their voices heard by the research community and hopefully reach policymakers in Denmark and Europe. Being a migrant myself and knowing to some extent the hopelessness that comes with being newly arrived in a host country, it was important for me to help them convey their experiences and stories. When I spoke to newly arrived parents, worries about raising a young adult in exile while balancing their heritage and culture with integrating into Danish society were dominant. One parent explained how his young son was shy and how this made it more difficult to make new friends in school. He explained how this shyness was increased by the fact that the son's classmates in the Danish school, girls in particular, dressed differently than his classmates in Syria. His father said this made him even more shy around these girls, and he would avoid looking too much at them. Sensitive stories like these, thick with nuance, were shared quickly and casually with me, since the parents seemed to trust that I would understand. The father was not critical nor judgemental of the girls' dress style but wanted to explain how his son was feeling. He trusted me to represent him in passing on his story about his son with its nuances and depth, instead of the possible oversimplification that could have been feared in a Danish researcher's perception and portrayal of Muslim immigrants' view on western clothing.

Personalist representation concerns the values and orientations projected to participants. I believe many of the participants saw me as a role model, both by being someone who they could trust to make sure their story was heard in right way, but also by being a Syrian woman now working at a university in Denmark. The young people would ask me how I got my job, express how impressed they were by my job, and realise that this career choice might also be possible for them. One parent, who himself was a graduate of higher education in Syria, asked me for advice on how to get a job like mine. My position as a Syrian researcher in Denmark not only gave them a glimmer of hope, but also made me feel a sense of achievement.

Establishing rapport because 'we speak the same language'

This project was my first time facilitating focus group discussions. I quickly learned that my Syrian background, the Syrian dialect I spoke, my religion and my migrant background were shared characteristics that helped me establish rapport between me and the participants. On some occasions, additional identity markers or lived experiences were shared. Speaking with women and girls, our gender worked as a common marker, enabling conversations about gender inequalities or job opportunities for women. Speaking with fellow parents, being a mother also worked as a shared identity marker, enabling deep conversations about parenting in exile, parental relationships with schools and religious parenting. With young people I was able to share schooling experiences as we were all acquainted with educational systems in Syria, Denmark or both, eliciting conversation about spatial and material differences between the school systems as well as teacher–student relationships and forms of discipline. Each of these shared markers and experiences came with practical, methodological and socio-ethical benefits and implications.

There were practical benefits of having a shared language. For instance, participants were defined as 'newly arrived', which meant having arrived in Denmark within the past six years. My ability to speak directly and naturally with participants most probably saved the project time during recruitment. Although some young people were capable of participating in focus group discussions in Danish or English, interpreters would have been necessary for focus groups with parents. Using interpreters, though useful in situations where it is the only alternative, brings high costs to the project, and creates methodological challenges associated with ensuring the quality of interpretations and negotiating the role of the interpreter. The difficulties of interpreters, who are active, influential agents in research processes, are often ignored in methodological reflections (Temple 2002; Squires 2009). Being linguistically fluent in Syrian Arabic enabled me to facilitate conversations free of translation-related interruption from interpreters in the room. My role as a reflexive part of the research team was not ignored. Being able to push the translation of interviews until after the interview created a space that, to me, felt safer for participants. This allowed me to enter sometimes quick debates, such as a heated discussion between a group of Syrian refugee girls about whether or not they would have the same career opportunities in Syria as in Denmark, without pausing to translate and ruining the dynamic of the discussion.

Having a shared language and lived experience is pivotal for generating meaningful data, which in the case of our project meant honest, emic insights into what it is like to be new to a country and a school system. It became apparent to me how a shared language relates closely to cultural understanding and closeness in a research setting, which support building of rapport and trust so that participants were willing to confide in me with their layered stories. For instance, one parent spoke about how a school decided to meet the needs of Muslim refugees by giving them money to buy modest swimsuits so the daughters could participate more comfortably in swimming lessons. The father used this example to acknowledge the school's helpfulness. However, the compromises associated with enabling Muslim girls to participate in swimming classes is a controversial topic in Denmark. This made it risky for Muslim participants to speak about, especially where language barriers can lead to potential misunderstanding. In this case, the father knew that he was able to express his opinion to a fellow Muslim, who in addition spoke his dialect, allowing him to express himself clearly.

The difficulty of being in 'a space in between': Being a 'sister' and a 'researcher'

In refugee and migration research, there is a tendency to position peer researchers as insiders or group members based on ethno-nationality (Collet 2008; Carling et al. 2013; Dwyer and Buckle 2009). Focusing only on ethno-national origin creates a simplistic insider–outsider divide (Carling et al. 2013), which reproduces an essentialist view of migrants and refugees, which reduces them to being *only* that, which is never the case. I am not just a Syrian migrant, but represent an intersection of dynamic identities and positions, according to my gender, age, class, educational background, migration status and religious beliefs. These affected my role as a peer researcher in different and complex ways. I gained trust and connected with some research participants through shared identities and experiences, but struggled to connect with others precisely because specific identities or experiences as refugees in Denmark were different. The hierarchical imbalance between researcher and participant is not removed by common language, nationality or lived experience. Thus, I, like other researchers, was working in a space of entering and exiting communities, shifting between being an insider or outsider. The subjective experience and ethical dilemmas of 'the space in between' (Dwyer and Buckle 2009, p. 60) for peer researchers is rarely documented in the context of refugee and migration research.

In most situations I had many identity markers in common with participants, which led young people to often refer to me as 'sister'. This label emphasised the closeness I felt I had gained with them. It also suggested that our relationship was 'more' than a professional one and that we had a familiarity that extended further than the research project. This is confirmed today, when I meet participants by coincidence and am greeted with the warmth and interest of a relative. By being their sister, I paved the way for useful and honest data.

However, I was not only a sister. I was also someone who had managed to secure a role at a respectable university as a researcher. This role became especially apparent in research situations where participants discussed and criticised the societal and cultural conditions for refugees in Denmark. Even though I invited participants to speak openly and freely, the fact that I as a researcher was not only representing them but also the Danish state came into play. On occasions, parents forgot that I was a researcher during interviews, and communicated with me retrospectively that some of the things I had just been told should not go into the study. In one conversation we talked about the difficulties of raising our children Muslim in Danish society, which led us into a discussion about differences in values. The discussion quickly turned casual between two parents. However, all of a sudden, a parent paused, as if he was re-registering that the dialogue took place in a research setting and had to moderate himself.

There were also moments where – when discussing differences between Syria and Denmark – I was told not to translate something into English, as participants did not want my co-researchers to hear what they just said. On multiple occasions, participants asked to tell me something off the record or to not use some information for the research project. At other times, I found it challenging to understand whether discussion was on or off the record. Participants seemed very conscious about not being portrayed as negative, ungrateful refugees, being a burden to the Danish state – a common portrayal, especially amongst the far-right parties in parliament, that they were afraid of reproducing. They wanted to project a good image of Syrians in Denmark in front of the authority that the research project represented. Similar challenges in other peer research studies have been described elsewhere (Marlowe et al. 2015).

This constant balance between respecting study participants' wish to be repre-sented in a particular way, my role as a researcher respecting scientific rigour and transparency, and my personal motivation to give voice to my peers was difficult. Not knowing how to exercise my power in this 'in between space' constituted a major dilemma, which became more apparent during transcription where I had to make decisions on how to translate and phrase the sentences. My research colleagues had told me to transcribe the focus groups verbatim, except for the parts where participants had made explicit requests not to be quoted. This was fairly straightforward. In more sensitive sections of the focus groups, where criti-cism of Denmark was made, I struggled to transcribe verbatim because I knew the participants would not appreciate being quoted for saying what they said, and how they said it. Because participants were so careful about how they represented themselves, I felt a responsibility to moderate any slips of this control. While I know this goes against some perceptions of scientific rigour, I felt it was right for me to do the transcription and make decisions around how to paraphrase the participants, given the relationship I had with them.

Final thoughts

In this chapter, we have described how we used a peer research approach to gather quantitative and qualitative data from Syrian migrants and refugees. Alaa's experi-ential testimonies and reflections as a peer researcher show how peer research can strengthen knowledge production by facilitating improved communication and trust between researchers and research participants, creating richer data. However, Alaa also had to navigate difficult dilemmas that arose and were amplified by her many roles – as researcher, sister, role model and translator – when acting as a node between her allegiance to the study participants or the 'rigour' of the study. Alaa's experiences have taught us the importance of ongoing ethical discussions and prep-arations for peer researchers working in migrant and refugee research. Often, access to, communicating with and the development of trust and rapport with research participants does not always extend beyond the peer researcher. This poses specific challenges pertaining to the translation and analytic work required to disseminate findings in academic and policy spaces. Peer research should be facilitated by trans-parent procedures relating to the dilemmas faced by the peer researcher in their brokerage between different roles, and social support from research colleagues who understand, respect and create safe social spaces for dialogue about these dilemmas. By so doing, it is possible to embrace and act upon the ethical complexities that peer research approaches inevitably introduce.

Acknowledgements

We thank participants for their time and insights. We also thank colleagues within the research consortium for input and support. The RefugeesWellSchool project (2018–22) is funded by Horizon 2020 (EU) (https://cordis.europa.eu/project/rcn/212677_en.html).

References

Bakunzi, W., 2018. Working with peer researchers in refugee communities. *Forced Migration Review*, 59, 58–59.

Barghadouch, A., et al., 2016. Refugee children have fewer contacts to psychiatric healthcare services: An analysis of a subset of refugee children compared to Danish-born peers. *Social Psychiatry and Psychiatric Epidemiology*, 51 (8), 1125–1136.

Birman, D., 2006. Ethical issues in research with immigrants and refugees. In: J.E. Trimble and C.B. Fisher, eds. *The Handbook of Ethical Research with Ethnocultural Populations & Communities*. London: SAGE Publications, 156–177.

Block, K., et al., 2012. Addressing ethical and methodological challenges in research with refugee-background young people: Reflections from the field. *Journal of Refugee Studies*, 26 (1), 69–87.

Brigham, S.M., Abidi, C.B., and Zhang, Y., 2018. What participatory photography can tell us about immigrant and refugee women's learning in atlantic Canada. *International Journal of Lifelong Education*, 37 (2), 234–254.

Brownson, R.C., Colditz, G.A., and Proctor, E.K., eds., 2017. *Dissemination and Implementation Research in Health: Translating Science to Practice*, 2nd ed. New York, NY: Oxford University Press.

Carling, J., Erdal, M.B., and Ezzati, R., 2013. Beyond the insider–outsider divide in migration research. *Migration Studies*, 2 (1) 36–54.

Castleden, H., Garvin, T., and Huu-ay-aht First Nation, 2008. Modifying Photovoice for community-based participatory indigenous research. *Social Science & Medicine*, 66 (6), 1393–1405.

Center for Udsatte Flygtninge, 2016. *Flygtningebørn i folkeskolen: En guide til modtagelsen af flygtningebørn og deres familier*. Copenhagen: Center for Udsatte Flygtninge.

Collet, B., 2008. Confronting the insider-outsider polemic in conducting research with diasporic communities: Towards a community-based approach. *Refuge: Canada's Journal on Refugees*, 25 (1), 77–83.

Collumbien, M., et al., 2009. Understanding the context of male and transgender sex work using peer ethnography. *Sexually Transmitted Infections*, 85 (Suppl. 2), 3–7.

Danmarks Statistik, 2019. Opholdstilladelser (år) efter opholdstilladelsestype, statsborgerskab, køn og alder. Available from: https://www.statistikbanken.dk/10024 [Accessed 30 July 2020].

Doná, G., 2007. The microphysics of participation in refugee research. *Journal of Refugee Studies*, 20 (2), 210–229. doi:10.1093/jrs/fem013.

Dunbar, C., Rodriguez, D., and Parker, L., 2002. Race, subjectivity, and the interview process. In: J.F. Gubrium and J.A. Holstein, eds. *Handbook of Interview Research: Context and Method*. Thousand Oaks, CA: SAGE Publications, 279–298.

Dwyer, S.C. and Buckle, J.L., 2009. The space between: On being an insider-outsider in qualitative research. *International Journal of Qualitative Methods*, 8 (1), 54–63.

Fricker, M., 2007. *Epistemic Injustice: Power and the Ethics of Knowing*. Oxford: Oxford University Press.

Ganga, D. and Scott, S., 2006. 'Cultural insiders' and the issue of positionality in qualitative migration research: Moving 'across' and moving 'along' researcher-participant divides.

Forum Qualitative Sozialforschung/Forum: Qualitative Social Research, 7 (3). doi:10.17169/fqs-7.3.134.

Goosen, S., Stronks, K., and Kunst, A.E., 2014. Frequent relocations between asylum-seeker centres are associated with mental distress in asylum-seeking children: A longitudinal medical record study. *International Journal of Epidemiology*, 43 (1), 94–104.

Israel, B.A., et al., 1998. Review of community-based research: Assessing partnership approaches to improve public health. *Annual Review of Public Health*, 19 (1), 173–202.

Jacobsen, K. and Landau, L., 2003. The dual imperative in refugee research: Some methodological and ethical considerations in social science research on forced migration. *Disasters*, 27, 185–206.

Kristjansdottir, B. and Pérez, S.J., 2016. Nyankomne børn og unge i det danske uddannelsessystem: Lovgrundlag og organisering. *Norand*, 11 (2), 35–63.

Larsen, B.R., 2011. Becoming part of welfare scandinavia: Integration through the spatial dispersal of newly arrived refugees in Denmark. *Journal of Ethnic and Migration Studies: 'Integration': Migrants and Refugees between Scandinavian Welfare Societies and Family Relations*, 37 (2), 333–350.

Lee, S.K., Sulaiman-Hill, C.R., and Thompson, S.C., 2014. Overcoming language barriers in community-based research with refugee and migrant populations: Options for using bilingual workers. *BMC International Health and Human Rights*, 14 (1), 11.

Leth, I., et al., 2014. Psychological difficulties among children and adolescents with ethnic danish, immigrant, and refugee backgrounds. *Scandinavian Journal of Child and Adolescent Psychiatry and Psychology*, 2 (1), 29–37.

Liamputtong, P., ed., 2008. *Doing Cross-Cultural Research: Ethical and Methodological Perspectives*. Social Indicators Research Series, vol. 34. Dordrecht: Springer.

Logie, C., et al., 2012. Opportunities, ethical challenges, and lessons learned from working with peer research assistants in a multi-method HIV community-based research Study in Ontario, Canada. *Journal of Empirical Research on Human Research Ethics*, 7 (4), 10–19.

Mackenzie, C., McDowell, C., and Pittaway, E., 2007. Beyond 'do no harm': The challenge of constructing ethical relationships in refugee research. *Journal of Refugee Studies*, 20 (2), 299–319.

Marlowe, J.M., et al., 2015. Conducting post-disaster research with refugee background peer researchers and their communities. *Qualitative Social Work*, 14 (3), 383–398.

Maxwell, J.A., 2012. *A Realist Approach for Qualitative Research*. Thousand Oaks, CA: SAGE Publications.

Moldenhawer, B., 2017. «Vi prøver at gøre det så godt for dem som muligt, mens de er her». *Tidsskrift for velferdsforskning*, 20 (4), 302–316.

Montgomery, E. and Foldspang, A., 2007. Discrimination, mental problems and social adaptation in young refugees. *European Journal of Public Health*, 18 (2), 156–161.

O'Reilly-de Brún, M., et al., 2016. Using participatory learning & action research to access and engage with 'hard to reach' migrants in primary healthcare research. *BMC Health Services Research*, 16 (1), 25.

Phillimore, J., et al., 2015. Understanding healthcare practices in superdiverse neighbourhoods and developing the concept of welfare bricolage: Protocol of a cross-national mixed-methods study. *BMC International Health and Human Rights*, 15 (1), 16.

Pottie, K. and Gabriel, P., 2014. Ethical issues across the spectrum of migration and health research. In: M.B. Schenker, X. Castañeda, and A. Rodriguez-Lainz, eds. *Migration and Health: A Research Methods Handbook*. Berkeley: University of California Press, 345–360.

Rich Madsen, K., et al., 2016. Loneliness, immigration background and self-identified ethnicity: A nationally representative study of adolescents in Denmark. *Journal of Ethnic and Migration Studies*, 42 (12), 1977–1995.

Seal, M., 2018. Peer research: Epistemological symbolism, proxy trust, conscious partiality and the near-peer. In: M. Seal, ed. *Participatory Pedagogic Impact Research*. London: Routledge, 60–74.

Squires, A., 2009. Methodological challenges in cross-language qualitative research: A research review. *International Journal of Nursing Studies*, 46 (2), 277–287.

Temple, B., 2002. Crossed wires: Interpreters, translators, and bilingual workers in cross-language research. *Qualitative Health Research*, 12 (6), 844–854.

Thorstensson Dávila, L., 2014. Representing refugee youth in qualitative research: Questions of ethics, language and authenticity. *Diaspora, Indigenous, and Minority Education*, 8 (1), 21–31.

13 The ethical dilemmas of working safely with community researchers

Lessons from community-based research with lesbian, gay, bisexual, transgender and queer communities

Ashley Lacombe-Duncan and Carmen H. Logie

Introduction

The ongoing stigmatisation of lesbian, gay, bisexual, transgender and queer (LGBTQ) people internationally contributes to significant health disparities, which may be better understood through community-based research in which LGBTQ people are engaged as community researchers. However, stigmatising social and political contexts create challenges for working safely and effectively with members of these populations. Drawing on reflections of multi-method community-based research studies with LGBTQ populations in Canada, Jamaica, Swaziland and Lesotho, this chapter discusses some of the ethical challenges experienced working with and by community researchers from LGBTQ communities internationally. Particular challenges include exploitation and tokenism; the navigation of conflicting identities; stigma associated with being a community researcher investigating 'taboo' issues to do with sexuality, gender and race, particularly in socially conservative settings; and the physical and mental tolls of community research, including burnout. Critical attention to power and privilege is fundamental to promoting safe work with LGBTQ populations in international contexts. We end with some practical suggestions to promote community researcher safety in the context of conducting research with marginalised populations.

Background

Internationally, there have been increased human rights protections for LGBTQ and other sexual and gender minority persons, evidenced through new instances of decriminalisation of same-sex practices and marriage equality. Yet ongoing stigma, violence and legally sanctioned persecution of these communities remain in many places (Mendos 2019). Within these contexts of stigma, health disparities among LGBTQ people become entrenched. Stigma can lead to social and institutional discrimination against LGBTQ people including acts of violence (Logie 2012). These acts, in turn, are associated with poor mental and physical health, such as depression and HIV, among other outcomes, for LGBTQ people. Stigma and discrimination based on sexual orientation and gender identity/expression also limit LGBTQ peoples' access to key social determinants of health, including income, employment, housing and healthcare (Fredriksen-Goldsen et al. 2013).

Understanding these disparities – in addition to translating this understanding into real-world solutions and social justice-oriented change – has been the focus of our work as academic researchers. We use community-based research methods that draw on meaningful engagement with communities in order to understand their needs and produce research with greater potential impact (Israel et al.1998). Community-based research approaches often involve the hiring of peer researchers. While definition of what is meant by the term 'peer researcher' changes across time and context, the term tends to refer to researchers who share key aspects of individual experience (e.g. poverty, homelessness) and/or specific identities (e.g. gender, sexual orientation) with study participants (Greene 2013). However, the term 'peer researcher' can overestimate commonalities between peer researcher and study participants when, in fact, communities are complex, diverse and heterogeneous. Importantly, an individual peer researcher's lived experiences cannot be representative of the myriad experiences across members of a community. In this chapter, we use the term 'community researchers' more broadly to encompass those researchers working outside academic settings who share some commonalities across experiences or identities with study participants, just as we do as queer-identified academic researchers.

In the research we do, community researchers are perceived and positioned as equals to academic researchers, bringing distinctive knowledge, experience and expertise to the research process (Greene et al. 2009). Community researchers may benefit from acquiring new skills, conducting meaningful work, and making personal and professional connections with their communities, researchers and organisations (Logie et al. 2012). Yet studies have also highlighted some of the ethical challenges to working with, and experienced by, community researchers, including issues of defining and engaging in capacity building; conflicting perspectives on payment, career advancement and professional obligations; navigating multiple relationships; balancing personal and professional responsibilities; and emotional and physical tolls (Greene et al. 2009; Logie et al. 2012; Guta et al. 2013).

Methods

In order to do this, we draw on reflections from three multi-method research studies with LGBTQ populations in four settings.

Study 1: Understanding access to HIV-related and gender-affirming healthcare for trans women with HIV in Canada – a mixed methods study

The first study – doctoral research conducted in 2016 by the first author with mentoring support from the second author – focused on understanding barriers and facilitators to accessing medical care for trans women living with HIV, and was designed in partnership with a recognised leader in the trans community. It used baseline survey data from the Canadian HIV Women's Sexual and Reproductive Health Cohort Study (CHIWOS), in which women living with HIV were included from study inception, from shaping the study, to developing the survey, recruiting participants, collecting data and disseminating findings (Loutfy et al. 2016).

CHIWOS baseline data were collected between 2013 and 2015 in Ontario, British Columbia and Quebec, Canada. The full sample included 1,422 women living with HIV (including 54 trans women) aged 16 or older who were recruited by community researchers, who in this case were women living with HIV who were hired and trained to conduct research (Loutfy et al. 2016). A subset of trans women living with HIV (n = 11) who completed the baseline CHIWOS survey also participated in individual interviews. For this qualitative arm of the mixed methods study, community researchers were involved in participant recruitment and qualitative data collection. Community researchers also participated in study oversight, through participation in the CHIWOS Trans Community Advisory Board and in conference presentations and publications.

Support for CHIWOS community researchers included in-person training over the course of several days (Loutfy et al. 2016). During this training, researchers discussed the project, provided practical training around recruitment, informed consent and administering the online survey, and reviewed self-care support. An online version of the training was also created for refreshers or newly hired community researchers. Follow-up training was held at waves two and three of longitudinal data collection. Monthly teleconferences or in-person meetings were held to provide ongoing updates and support. Training on qualitative data collection (interviewing) was also provided and recordings of community researchers' first interviews were reviewed to provide tailored feedback as data was collected.

Study 2: Towards an understanding of structural drivers of HIV/STIs and protective factors among sexual and gender minority youth in Kingston, Jamaica

The second study comes from a multi-method community-based research project that examined the HIV prevention needs of LGBTQ youth in Jamaica, with a focus on stigma. The study was led by the second author and was designed and conducted in partnership with 'Jamaica AIDS Support for Life', a community-based organisation focused on HIV prevention and LGBTQ health in Kingston, Montego Bay and Ocho Rios, Jamaica. The first author became involved in the project during phase two as a doctoral student and research assistant. Six further organisations focused on LGBTQ issues were involved in participant recruitment and key informant interviews as part of the qualitative phase of work.

The first phase of data collection involved 63 individual interviews with young LGBTQ people and key informants from LGBTQ organisations, HIV clinicians and outreach workers in Kingston. Three focus groups also took place. For this phase, the team hired and trained three community researchers aged 18–29 who self-identified as LGBTQ to conduct outreach and interviews with participants. Community researchers were identified by Jamaica AIDS Support for Life due to their perceived leadership in LGBTQ communities, intimate knowledge and connections to the LGBTQ community, and training and/or comfort level discussing HIV issues. Community researchers also pilot tested the qualitative interview guide questions.

In a second phase of work, seven community researchers (two continuing from the first phase, with another five rotating in and out through phase two) were recruited and trained. These community researchers self-identified as LGBTQ or as other sexual and/or gender minorities and were from Kingston, Ocho Rios or Montego Bay and surrounding areas. Drawing on the expertise of these seven community researchers as well as our community partners, we developed and implemented a survey with young LGBTQ people (n = 911).

Community researchers recruited participants from their social networks, and those who worked as HIV outreach workers also shared study information with potential participants during outreach shifts. Community researchers obtained informed consent from all participants and collected survey data and played an active role in data interpretation and reviewing manuscripts for publication. Training was delivered over the course of four days, covering conducting in-depth interviews (16 hours) and implementing computerised (tablet-based) data collection methods (16 hours). Weekly supervision was provided by research coordinators in Kingston and Ocho Rios. Community researchers received further in-person training in booster sessions as well as weekly supervision to discuss data quality issues and data collection procedures.

Study 3: Using performance ethnography as an innovative approach to challenge stigma and promote empowerment among sexual and gender minorities in Swaziland and Lesotho

The third study involved qualitative data collection followed by development and pilot testing of a participatory theatre intervention to reduce the general public's stigma toward LGBTQ people in Swaziland and Lesotho (Logie et al. 2018, 2019). The study was built on pre-existing partnerships between academic researchers (including the second author as principle investigator) and community-based LGBTQ organisations in Swaziland (The Rock of Hope) and Lesotho (Matrix Support Group). The Rock of Hope and Matrix Support Group participated in all phases of study planning and implementation, including developing a series of participatory theatre vignettes, conducting data collection and assisting with data interpretation.

Six community researchers were hired across the two partner organisations. These community researchers identified as LGBTQ and were identified by partner organisations based on their involvement with the LGBTQ community and interest in learning research methods (Logie et al. 2018). Community researchers identified LGBTQ individuals willing to participate in the research, assisting in the development and refinement of the qualitative interview guide for appropriateness to Swaziland and Lesotho contexts, conducting qualitative interviews, analysing qualitative data, and then working with local theatre groups, the academic research team and partner organisations to create three short skits tailored to local contexts (Logie et al. 2019).

Finally, community researchers participated in developing solutions to anti-LGBTQ stigma to be presented during the participatory theatre intervention performances and facilitating post-intervention focus groups. Training was provided in research methods and ethics (two six-hour sessions), and following the qualitative data collection, a two-day workshop took place with a local theatre group. Following skit development, there was further training about participatory theatre planning as well as focus group training (two six-hour sessions). Each participatory theatre event was followed by debriefing with community researchers.

Ethical dilemmas of working safely with community researchers

Preventing exploitation and tokenism

Community-based research is best characterised by authentic partnerships, meaningful community engagement and reciprocal learning among academic and community researchers (Israel et al. 1998). While aspirational, these ideals – authenticity, meaning, reciprocity – are challenging to operationalise. Albeit unintentional, concerns have been raised about exploitative processes through community-based research from the perspective both of academic researchers and community researchers, as well as the experiences of tokenism sometimes described by community researchers (Greene et al. 2009; Greene 2013).

Community researchers may experience exploitation in many ways – being expected to offer free labour, receiving low wages, not being reimbursed for extra time and money spent engaging with participants, and not receiving prompt payment (Logie et al. 2012; Boilevin et al. 2019). Exploitation can also occur when research work results in greater gains for the academic partner than for the community researchers or the participating communities (Guta et al. 2013). Tokenism occurs when involvement of community researchers functions superficially to make a research project 'look good on paper' when, in reality, little power is shared between community and academic researchers (Boilevin et al. 2019). We reflect on how we mitigated (and sometimes failed) to address these dilemmas.

Limited engagement of community researchers in the research process

It was beneficial for study 1 to be embedded within the larger CHIWOS study where processes of meaningful engagement of women living with HIV and shared decision making between academic and community researchers were already well established. For example, existing CHIWOS support mechanisms included a built-in fair compensation mechanism for community researchers assisting with qualitative study recruitment; community researchers who had already received training on participant recruitment and research ethics, necessitating only brief follow up conversations or training sessions in new skills areas; and an established trans community advisory board whose members were committed to the CHIWOS project.

As a researcher who became involved after the initiation of CHIWOS, the first author participated in several CHIWOS initiatives over time (e.g. team celebrations) which helped build trust, commitment and reciprocity between her and the CHIWOS team. This type of ongoing, deep engagement with community researchers helped flatten hierarchies that can inhibit meaningful inclusion and provides opportunities for critical reflection among all members of the research team. For example, the first author reflected on the process of doing a PhD as a self-fulfilling endeavour, recognising that there is almost no way that the community researchers she worked with would benefit as much as she had personally from completing her work. Consequently, she sought to equalise power by supporting community researchers with their work and career development priorities, such as assisting with grant applications to support service provision within the community-based organisation or funding applications to support their attendance and presentations at conferences.

While building strong and reciprocal collaborations with the community-based organisation, the second author often found it hard to build and maintain long-term relationships with community researchers due to high turnover. For instance, during study 2, there was considerable mobility among LGBTQ young people in Jamaica. While two community researchers were involved throughout both phases of the study, some researchers were only partially involved in phase two. Experiences of social exclusion of LGBTQ persons in family, religious, legal, educational and employment systems resulted in many moving between cities, and some migrating to North America or the United Kingdom during the study.

Superficial understanding of research contexts

If academic researchers spend inadequate time engaging meaningfully with community researchers, a superficial understanding of the contexts may affect the research and the lives of community researchers, inadvertently perpetuating marginalisation. For example, at one point the first author learned of trans peoples' historical and ongoing struggle to fight for prioritisation within HIV research due to it being primarily led by cisgender researchers like herself (Namaste 2015). This led to critical conversations with trans researchers about her role as a cisgender queer woman doing this work. As a result, the first author made a more conscious effort to raise awareness of the contributions of trans team members – past and present – throughout the dissertation process. This was done to highlight the historical and contemporary activism led by trans community members and prioritise community voices and perspectives.

Swaziland has same-sex criminalisation laws (that have been enforced), which made it challenging to find a local academic partner. The LGBTQ organisation identified a senior female researcher who was employed at a religious academic institution and who played a supportive role throughout the two-year project. At the end of this project, a news reporter attended a community forum where the study team were sharing their research findings. The reporter critiqued this researcher's involvement in a research project with LGBTQ people, a criminalised and religiously unacceptable population, and the researcher then experienced negative feedback from her institution due to be being involved in the study.

While the study may have created positive change for participants, the larger stigmatising sociocultural and political contexts remained intact. The reporter's actions may dissuade other academic researchers (particularly more junior scholars) from focusing on LGBTQ issues. It also caused the research team to wonder whether the results should have been shared in a private rather than public forum. However, the team questioned whether stigmatising *community-level* norms can be transformed without employing a community-based approach to sharing study findings on the impacts of stigma. This example highlights the importance of fully understanding the context influencing the research process, and how sharing research findings can create potential ramifications for study team members.

Adequate preparation of community researchers in research skills

Adequate training of community researchers in research skills is key to avoiding the tokenistic involvement of community members in research processes. In the Jamaica study, the second author found that roles such as focus group co-facilitation can be difficult for community researchers who may lack these specific research skills or the confidence to manage research in such complex group settings. Moreover, it was difficult for focus group co-facilitators to challenge stigmatising language used in the focus groups by participants that could offend other participants. At one point, a participant in the gay and bisexual men's focus group started complaining about 'flamboyant' men being a problem for the gay or bisexual men's community. The second author had to step in to reaffirm the acceptability of all gender presentations and remind participants about the need to respect diversity within the focus group that was reflective of diversity in the larger LGBTQ community. However, having an academic researcher take a leadership role in focus group facilitation in the presence of a community researcher, as described in this example, may reinforce hierarchies between academic and community researchers.

Acknowledging challenges of navigating multiple roles and relationships

Community researchers can oscillate between the roles of researcher, service provider and community member, or may experience these roles simultaneously throughout a study. We describe some of the ethical dilemmas of promoting community researchers' safe navigation of multiple roles and relationships in terms of a loss of, or changing, relationships and concerns about confidentiality.

Loss of, or changing, relationships

Community researchers may not be prepared for the positive and negative impacts that their research role has on existing social relationships (Guta et al. 2014a). There can be particular challenges of managing new interpersonal dynamics and potential ethical dilemmas associated with holding multiple roles. Some CHIWOS community researchers identified cases of being perceived and treated differently by women in the community due to their new research position (Loutfy et al. 2016). Academic researchers must also listen to community researchers' concerns about participation (e.g. hesitancy about study recruitment of potential participants with whom they engage socially) and respect their boundaries (e.g. assign them to recruitment of other potential participants with whom they engage less socially). In study 1, the first author worked closely with a community researcher who set boundaries around when, how and who she would recruit for the qualitative sub-study. For example, she was comfortable inviting a participant if she encountered them in her everyday life, as long as the participant appeared to be doing well and not exhibiting signs of distress or seeking support from her. Academic researchers need to be aware of the myriad of ways that existing social relationships may impact community researchers' engagement. For example, some community researchers may feel uncomfortable asserting power with known others, particularly if they are service providers and sources of support in their communities (Logie et al. 2012). In the aforementioned example, the community researcher was also a service provider working with trans women of colour. As one of the only service providers working with this group, she was cautious not to let the research take precedence over her clinical work, so as not to impede her client's access to support.

Confidentiality

Community researchers may experience challenges of managing confidentiality when conducting research with people within existing social or community networks (Guta et al. 2014b). In study 1, the first author tried to maintain participant confidentiality when sharing data with the broader research team through the removal of identifiable story elements (e.g. specific acts of violence, specific types of healthcare settings where stigmatisation occurred, specific countries where participants immigrated from). However, even when such identifiable elements are removed, participants may be identifiable to academic and community researchers if they have close, established relationships with the participants. The potential for this breach of confidentiality to occur should be specified in the informed consent process and academic and community researchers should discuss processes for how to proceed if such a breach occurs. Participants' stories (e.g. narratives about violence) may deeply affect community researchers, particularly if they know the person whose story is being shared and if the violence was based on an identity or experience (e.g. gender identity, sexual orientation, HIV status) shared by the community researcher. Community researchers collecting data may experience emotional reactions to interview content in the moment which needs to be managed, but researchers may also feel a responsibility to provide supportive counselling. It takes time to foster skills to differentiate between one's role as researcher, community member and service provider, in these situations. Support should also be in place to enable community researchers to debrief a process difficult emotions arising during the research process.

There is also the risk of loss of confidentiality among community researchers themselves, which can result in negative experiences, particularly in the context of stigma. In the Jamaica, Swaziland and Lesotho contexts, community researchers had to manage the disclosure of their sexual orientation and gender identity to other community members during recruitment and data collection procedures. In Jamaica, the cisgender lesbian, gay and bisexual men and women community researchers tended to be university students and recent graduates who had access to wider range of support systems beyond personal networks to help manage any repercussions from disclosing their sexual orientation in community research settings. In contrast, the trans women community researchers were more marginalised from formal education and employment sectors, and used their personal networks to recruit participants. Not only did this result in a lack of confidentiality about their study involvement, but they also lacked support networks beyond the people who were involved in the study.

Stigmatisation within and beyond the research project

Confidentiality concerns are distinctly associated with fear and experiences of stigma in the research process and in people's daily lives. Seeing research as one element of community researchers' lives – embedded within larger relationships, hopes, fears, struggles – can help academic researchers to broaden the lens from which they understand stigma experienced by community researchers. Identifying as a community researcher is a label that may mark people as belonging to a marginalised group due to the subject matter being researched, which in turn may affect their safety and well-being depending on the context within which the study is taking place. It is important to consider the ethics of having self-disclosure of parts of one's core identity or experience as a prerequisite for employment (Guta et al. 2013). As university researchers, this type of disclosure is not always required – although we may share identities and experiences with participants – because we often have the privilege of other identities associated with our employment or country and culture of residence, choosing when and how parts of our selves are shared with others. Researchers can also consider the socio-emotional impacts of experiencing stigma and witnessing stigma among community researchers. In community-based research, we have a responsibility to ensure that we work with community researchers in ways that reduce the potential stigmatisation experienced throughout the research process, as well as stigmatisation experienced in society more broadly, while balancing our place as outsiders within international contexts.

Stigmatisation experienced throughout the research process

In some contexts, identifying as an 'out', visible representative of one's community can increase experiences of stigma, including social exclusion, or interpersonal verbal and physical violence. In Jamaica, same-sex sexual practices are criminalised, dating back to 1864, during British colonial rule, with the Offences Against the Person Act, Article 76, which states that 'buggery' (anal intercourse) is punishable with up to 10 years' imprisonment with possible hard labour (Jamaican Forum for Lesbians, All-Sexuals, and Gays 2012). Under Article 79, gay, bisexual and other men who have sex with men and trans women who are mislabelled as male can also receive up to two years' imprisonment with possible hard labour if convicted of 'being a male person who is party to the commission of any act of gross indecency with another male person' (Jamaica Forum for Lesbians, All-Sexuals, and Gays 2012, p. 1). Thus, for the work in Jamaica, all study information was shared by word-of-mouth (as opposed to study flyers or posters) to promote the safety of potential participants and community researchers. On one occasion when the second author arrived in Kingston to conduct research training with community researchers, the trans community researcher did not show up. No one from the team could reach her, but later they heard that she had been arrested and imprisoned for walking around doing outreach for her HIV prevention job in the evening. While not directly related to the study in hand, it was clear that community researchers who are well connected and employed in recognised outreach roles are not immune to the effects of criminalisation. The academic team did their best to support the trans community researchers to conduct study activities in times and places that they perceived as safe, and the community collaborators conducted anti-stigma training with the police, but we were limited in our capacity to effect change due to the larger legal context.

During study one, trans women living with HIV experienced increased targeted public violence directly as a result of their visibility related to participation in research studies as well as public stigma-reduction campaigns and advocacy. While Canada is considered a world leader in advancing the rights of LGBQ people, having decriminalised same-sex sexual activities between consenting adults in 1969 (Government of Canada 2017), gender identity and expression have only recently been added as prohibited grounds of discrimination to the Canadian Human Rights Act in 2017. Moreover, HIV stigma remains pervasive. As such, constant attention had to be paid to how community researchers were introduced in particular spaces (e.g. a dinner with some members of the research team and some non-members, such as other academics, in attendance). This attention was particularly important when community researchers had not explicitly agreed to participate as community members and to refer to them as community researchers would disclose their HIV status to non-members of the team.

Including community researchers on publications and presentations can be a good way of mitigating power differentials and contributing to the personal and professional development of community researchers. However, when a publication says that a community researcher holds a particular identity or experience, their confidentiality may become difficult to protect. This was true for the Jamaica, Swaziland and Lesotho studies where only a few community researchers wanted to be included as co-authors on publications. In Lesotho, same-sex practices between consenting adult men were decriminalised in 2012. However same-sex practices between men are a common-law offence in Swaziland, for which there have been convictions (Carroll and Mendos 2017).

There is also the intersection between a lack of training in research methods, and a lack of training with regards to reducing stigma and challenging it when it occurs in the research process. For instance, when one of the interventions by participants in the community forum in Swaziland elicited a transphobic response, the second author realised that she needed to act as no one else was challenging the transphobia. She pointed out the issue with the language used in a non-judgmental way and invited another community researcher to act out a more supportive response. If there are expectations that community researchers should challenge stigma as it occurs in research processes, information and strategies should be provided about how to do so effectively, particularly in contexts where there may not be many examples or suitable role models to follow.

Stigmatisation experienced in society

As researchers, we also have a responsibility to fight stigma at interpersonal and structural levels against the communities that we are a part of and work with, with the leadership of community researchers. During study one, the first author worked closely with a community researcher to challenge stigma by ensuring that the research findings were shared broadly, most often by the community researcher. This community leadership, however, requires material and emotional support to be sustainable. For example, the first author and community researcher planned a workshop for health and social service providers to share study findings. This workshop required financial support for event logistics (e.g. food, space) as well as the community researcher's time spent organising the event, recruiting attendees and carrying out the event. The team worked closely together to mitigate the stress associated with planning and carrying out a large public event.

Our work in Jamaica involved the production of several publications (e.g. Logie et al. 2016, 2017) with a focus on human rights in order to highlight the systemic violence faced by LGBTQ populations that perpetuate health inequalities. We have done so urgently, given peoples' lived experiences of these issues. The second author was contacted by US lawyers to provide expert testimony for a trans woman asylum seeker from Jamaica in the USA. There is so little research on police harassment and violence targeting trans women, the study findings were used successfully in arguing her case for asylum. It is equally important to try to ensure that research brings about local change. Our findings on trans women's HIV care needs were later used by the community partner in Jamaica to secure funding for trans specific programmes. We also conducted a community forum attended by more than 150 people at which presentations were given by gender diverse sex workers and LGBTQ people about their experiences participating in the study, with recommendations made about how best to challenge stigma.

Promoting mental and physical well-being

The stigmatisation of community researchers can impact physical and mental health, as can participation in community-based research. The emotional labour expended by community researchers can have short-term (e.g. distress) and long-term consequences (e.g. depression) (Greene 2013). Following study 1, trans women living with HIV reflected on the burdens they experienced as a result of participating in activism, including research. They identified reduced HIV health as evidenced by experiencing opportunistic infections and depression as a result of ongoing engagement to the point of exhaustion and exasperation at the slow process of social change resulting from their work. The negative mental and physical health consequences of being a community researcher may be exacerbated by inadequate access to resources for managing stress or burnout, or by the research team's lack of consideration for the ongoing life circumstances of community researchers.

Community researchers may need additional support for mental health and assistance navigating health and social service systems. For instance, in the Jamaica study, community researchers felt emotional after hearing the stories and responses from the surveys. Thus, we worked with Jamaica AIDS Support to hire a psychologist to provide free counselling sessions for community researchers. This cost had not been built into the research grant so was an additional cost for the community organisation to bear. In addition to health issues, community researchers may face similar struggles to those who are researched – including issues such as poverty, social isolation, stigma and housing insecurity (Logie et al. 2012). Studies are rarely set up to help address these larger social and structural concerns.

A major challenge to addressing stress and burnout among community researchers derives from lack of recognition of these issues. In study 1, attempts were made to mitigate these concerns by checking in with community researchers regularly, asking questions about self-care, providing breaks in the research timetable and celebrating vacations. Academic researchers may have access to additional resources not available to community researchers, whereby full-time salaried academic staff can take days off without loss of pay or have access to additional benefits for psychosocial support (e.g. counselling). These privileges are not often afforded to community researchers and should be taken into account in project funding and implementation processes.

Working safely with community researchers

We close with some suggestions for enhancing ethical practice with community researchers. First, to prevent exploitation and tokenism, academic researchers should reflect on their social positions and identities, including the inequitable distribution of access to power and resources between academic and community researchers. Academic researchers should also reflect on their dual relationships with other members of the research team, including both academic and community researchers, as well as with the communities being studied. Regular meetings can provide opportunities to discuss power differences and develop partnership agreements. Taking into account time, travel and the informal work that community researchers engage in during research – such as the work they may need to do to maintain the social networks that are used for recruitment – can increase the likelihood of fair compensation.

Second, researchers can be more transparent about the risks of participating as a community researcher in terms of the shifting ways people may perceive or respond to community researchers, particularly community members that are already known to community researchers prior to study commencement. Action can be taken to reduce such risks. For example, researchers can have frank and detailed conversations about potential safety issues and about what being a community researcher on a project will mean for their safety and well-being. Researchers can explore community researcher preferences for sharing personal information (e.g. by email or face-to-face) with other team members, recruitment strategies (e.g. times, places, materials) and preferences regarding inclusion in publications and conference abstracts. Community researchers can also review the final write up of findings to provide perspectives and interpretation. Furthermore, research training can help community researchers to manage boundaries and relationships. This might involve the inclusion of real-life experiences where community researchers have had to negotiate one's multiple positions with a focus on role play and skill building. Community researchers can practice politely interrupting a participant who discloses an issue they are struggling with during the course of the interview that is not relevant to the overarching research question, redirecting the participant to the focus of the research and offering to talk further about the issue after the interview.

Third, academic researchers can prepare better for local impact by learning more about historical and current sociopolitical situations within countries they are working in, and working to understand partner organisations' and community researchers' social justice and sociopolitical change goals and initiatives. Conversations about community researchers' contextualised needs and agendas should be built into the research development phase, allowing community researchers to play an active role in shaping the research questions that are most relevant to their communities. Community researchers should also be given opportunities to advise on appropriate dissemination strategies (e.g. policy brief) for different target audiences (e.g. policymakers) to ensure local impact, alongside academic dissemination strategies.

Finally, academic researchers can commit to checking in with and express genuine interest in community researchers' physical and mental well-being as part of study protocols and procedures, while respecting that some issues should remain private. During study design and training, there is opportunity to create research environments that systematically support community researchers to be fully engaging in self-care practices.

Ultimately, more research is needed that further explores the ethical dilemmas of working safely with community researchers from diverse backgrounds. Academic researchers can start by reading materials written by community researchers that focus on their ethical treatment and meaningful inclusion (Boilevin et al. 2019). For it is only when community researchers are fully and ethically engaged in a project, that the full social justice potential of community-based research can be realised.

References

Boilevin, L., et al., 2019. *Research 101: A Manifesto for Ethical Research in the Downtown Eastside*. Available from Homeless Hub: https://www.homelesshub.ca/resource/research-101-manifesto-ethical-research-downtown-eastside [Accessed 19 February 2020].

Carroll, A. and Mendos, L.R., 2017. *State Sponsored Homophobia 2017: A World Survey of Sexual Orientation Laws: Criminalisation, Protection and Recognition*. Available from The International Lesbian, Gay, Bisexual, Trans and Intersect Association: https://ilga.org/ilga-state-sponsored-homophobia-report-2017 [Accessed 19 February 2020].

Fredriksen-Goldsen, K.I.P., et al., 2013. The physical and mental health of lesbian, gay male, and bisexual (LGB) older adults: The role of key health indicators and risk and protective factors. *The Gerontologist*, 53 (4), 664–675.

Government of Canada, 2017. *Rights of LGBTI Persons*. Available from: https://www.canada.ca/en/canadian-heritage/services/rights-lgbti-persons.html [Accessed 19 February 2020].

Greene, S., 2013. Peer research assistantships and the ethics of reciprocity in community-based research. *Journal of Empirical Research on Human Research Ethics*, 8 (2), 141–152.

Greene, S., et al., 2009. Between skepticism and empowerment: The experiences of peer research assistants in HIV/AIDS, housing and homelessness community-based research. *International Journal of Social Research Methodology*, 12 (4), 361–373.

Guta, A., Flicker, S., and Roche, B., 2013. Governing through community allegiance: A qualitative examination of peer research in community-based participatory research. *Critical Public Health*, 23 (4), 432–451.

Guta, A., et al., 2014a. *HIV CBR Ethics: Managing Multiple Roles and Boundaries*. Available from: http://www.hivethicscbr.com/documents/HIVCBREthics_FactSheet03.pdf [Accessed 19 February 2020].

Guta, A., et al., 2014b. *HIV CBR Ethics: Confidentiality in Close-Knit Communities*. Available from: http://www.hivethicscbr.com/documents/HIVCBREthics_FactSheet06.pdf [Accessed 19 February 2020].

Israel, B.A., et al., 1998. Review of community-based research: Assessing partnership approaches to improve public health. *Annual Review of Public Health*, 19, 173–202.

Jamaican Forum for Lesbians, All-Sexuals, and Gays (J-Flag), 2012. *Human Rights First: LGBT Issues in Jamaica*. Available from Human Rights First Organization Website: http://www.humanrightsfirst.org/sites/default/files/Jamaica-LGBT-Fact-Sheet.pdf [Accessed 19 February 2020].

Logie, C., 2012. The case for the World Health Organization's commission on the social determinants of health to address sexual orientation. *American Journal of Public Health*, 102 (7), 1243–1246.

Logie, C., et al., 2012. Opportunities, ethical challenges, and lessons learned from working with peer research assistants in a multi-method HIV community-based research study in Ontario, Canada. *Journal of Empirical Research on Human Research Ethics*, 7 (4), 10–19.

Logie, C.H., et al., 2016. Exploring lived experiences of violence and coping among lesbian, gay, bisexual and transgender youth in Kingston, Jamaica. *International Journal of Sexual Health*, 28 (4), 343–353.

Logie, C.H., et al., 2017. Associations between police harassment and HIV vulnerabilities among men who have sex with men and transgender women in Jamaica. *Health and Human Rights*, 19 (2), 147.

Logie, C.H., et al., 2018. Exploring experiences of heterosexism and coping strategies among lesbian, gay, bisexual, and transgender persons in Swaziland. *Gender and Development*, 26 (1), 15–32.

Logie, C.H., et al., 2019. Exploring the potential of participatory theatre to reduce stigma and promote health equity for lesbian, gay, bisexual, and transgender (LGBT) People in Swaziland and Lesotho. *Health Education & Behavior*, 46 (1), 146–156.

Loutfy, M., et al., 2016. Establishing the Canadian HIV women's sexual and reproductive health cohort study (CHIWOS): Operationalizing community-based research in a large national quantitative study. *BMC Medical Research Methodology*, 16 (1), 101.

Mendos, L.R., 2019. *State Sponsored Homophobia 2019*. Available from The International Lesbian, Gay, Bisexual, Trans and Intersect Association: https://ilga.org/state-sponsored-homophobia-report [Accessed 19 February 2020].

Namaste, V., 2015. *Oversight: Critical Reflections on Feminist Research and Politics*. Toronto: Canadian Scholar's Press.

14 Blurred lines

Treading the path between 'research' and 'social intervention' with peer researchers and participants in a study about youth health in South Africa

Rebecca Hodes

Introduction

Recent decades have seen the growing popularity and use of community-based peer research approaches across a swathe of academic disciplines. This chapter describes the ethical challenges of conducting peer research within the largest known longitudinal, community-traced, mixed methods study about medicines-taking and sexual health among HIV-positive young people (aged 11–19). The study, named Mzantsi Wakho (isiXhosa for 'Your South Africa'), began in 2013, and primary research continued for the next half a decade, concluding in 2018. Together with peer researchers and participants, study investigators developed, piloted and implemented an array of research methods to explore aspects of youth health.

The peer-led, participatory methods used in the study, and attending ethical challenges, have been written about elsewhere (Vale et al. 2017; Hodes et al. 2018a; Hodes and Gittings 2019). However, to date no publication has focused at length on the ethical challenges of conducting community-based peer research over the course of this study. This chapter seeks to document and describe the difficulties and imperatives of working with peer researchers to study the intimate health and social experiences of young people living in with HIV. It examines the interplay between formal study protocols, intended to ensure safe and ethical research conduct, and researchers' real-world adaptations when put to the test within study sites, including public healthcare facilities. The chapter explores an instance which dissolved the parameters between 'pure research' and 'social intervention', challenging prohibitions against intervening in the healthcare of people not enrolled in the study, when faced with a medical emergency.

This chapter focuses on the qualitative component of the Mzantsi Wakho study in which I – as the study's co-principal investigator and lead investigator of qualitative research – collaborated with two peer researchers, Mildred Thabeng (19 years old at the start of the study) and Kanya Makabane (21 years old at the start of his work with the study in 2014). Mildred and Kanya are young

South Africans with no formal qualifications in conducting research. From 2013, Mildred worked as a peer researcher on the qualitative component of the study and, from 2014, Kanya joined our team – initially as a 'community guide', and later as a peer researcher. Together, we conducted in-depth, qualitative research on the medicines-taking and sexual health practices of 66 young people living with HIV, as well as the experiences of their families, friends and sexual and romantic partners.

This chapter describes an event in which the qualitative research team (then comprised of Mildred and I), in consultation with a healthcare worker, took the decision to contravene the study protocol (which expressly prohibited intervening in the healthcare of non-study participants) and to help an adult in a medical emergency. It explores the critical role of peer researchers, and indeed study participants (in this case, a senior nurse), in informing a collective decision, and reflects on the – arguably fictitious – divide between 'research' and 'intervention' within studies on young people's health in contexts of poverty and precarity.

The location and relevance of research sites

After the lethal years of AIDS denialism, during which South African President Thabo Mbeki and Health Minister Tshabalala-Msimang questioned the link between HIV and AIDS, and obstructed public access to antiretroviral therapy (ART) (Nattrass 2007), the Government has 'rolled out' ART in clinics across the country. Over four million people in South Africa had been initiated onto ART by 2018, constituting one of the largest health interventions in global history (Simbayi et al. 2019).

ART is now readily available in many healthcare facilities, and South Africa's AIDS mortality rates have at last begun to decline (Johnson et al. 2017), but HIV prevalence and incidence remain high. Young people aged 15–24 in South Africa have the highest HIV incidence than any other age group (Simbayi et al. 2019). Nationally, young people are not benefitting proportionately from ART roll-out, and continue to experience higher rates of virologic failure on ART, and higher rates of AIDS-related mortality, than do other age groups. Both of these health outcomes, of greater morbidity and mortality, are related to non-adherence to ART (Agwu and Fairlie 2013; Maskew et al. 2016).

There are many studies on HIV, led by non-governmental organisations which leverage copious clinical expertise, and which are funded by bilateral agencies, which have gleaned remarkable results about the successes of HIV interventions. In contrast, far fewer research studies investigate the provision of ART at its most ordinary, in places in Eastern and Southern Africa which are home to the global majority of people living with HIV (UNAIDS 2019). In order to investigate the provision of health and social services, and the lived realities of young people with HIV and their families in the era that has come to be designated as 'post-Apartheid', it was essential to locate the study at the fulcrum of democratic development, in areas previously designated as 'bantustans'. This study was based in the Amathole District and the Buffalo City Metropolitan Municipality of South Africa's Eastern Cape province, in rural, peri-urban and urban settings.

Some parts of the province have been the particular focus of state funding in the post-Apartheid era, including through the building of schools and clinics (Gumede 2001; Freund 2019). But the Eastern Cape remains among South Africa's poorest and worst-served provinces, rent by corruption and dysfunctionality within local government (Everatt 2008; Olver 2017), and with soaring rates of unemployment (Statistics South Africa 2018). Working in these locations provides insights into the legacies of Apartheid privation, as well as the successes and failures of South Africa's democratic transition, specifically in relation to public healthcare.

A community-located peer-led research approach

Large longitudinal studies on health behaviours are usually located at healthcare facilities, which provide ready access to a steady stream of prospective research participants. Our research was about adherence to ART and the sexual health practices of young people, including those who were 'non-compliant' to their treatment, so we adopted a peer-led, community-based approach. Because we were interested in real world health practices, most of our primary research – in the form of interviews, focus groups and observations – was conducted with young people and their families within their own homes and neighbourhoods. The focus of the research was on the sensitive, personal and often stigmatised practices of (non-)compliance with medicines. Seeking out participants in their homes might attract the curiosity of neighbours and other community members, potentially compromising their privacy.

In navigating this difficult terrain, it was imperative to be guided by peer researchers who were of a similar age to young participants and who spoke the same vernacular – while also able to switch to more formal disquisition with older relatives – and who were familiar with the neighbourhoods and surrounding areas in which young people lived and mingled. Rather than arriving at a young person's home in a strange car and as an obvious outsider, the peer researchers within the study's qualitative component mostly relied on public transport. Because they looked and dressed like the study participants, they could pass as visiting friends or cousins if questioned by neighbours – a common occurrence during fieldwork visits. Due to the similarities between peer researchers and study participants – concerning age, familiarity with the surroundings and fluency in local languages – the collective hope of all members of the qualitative research team was that participants would be more able to 'be themselves', and to speak more freely about the challenges and meanings of living with HIV. The peer researchers with whom I worked – Mildred and Kanya – belonged to the same 'communities' as young research participants, in the sense that they lived in the same areas, were of similar ages, had endured the death of their parents at a young age (many study participants had lost parents to AIDS while children), and faced the same socio-economic challenges of subsisting in the Eastern Cape.

The racial divisions demarcated with brutal force by five decades of Apartheid continue to define post-Apartheid demography and political economy (Posel 2001), including the distribution of wealth and access to education and employment, particularly among the 'black' working-classes (Seekings and Nattrass 2006; Southall 2016). Racial categories remain primary markers of social identity in contemporary South Africa.[1] As a 'white' South African, my presence in many locations within the study sites was peculiar and notable, arousing attention and suspicion. Under Apartheid's segregation laws, most of the neighbourhoods in the study districts had been previously designated for 'black' or 'coloured' South Africans, while nearby, more affluent cities and suburbs – exceedingly better-served by municipal authorities, and with greater access to healthcare and education – had been reserved for 'whites'. The importance of working with peer researchers who were, in general, the same race as research participants – including in seeking to avoid arousing scrutiny and perhaps compromising confidentiality – felt, at times, like a capitulation to the racial architecture of the Apartheid past, and its continued structural and socio-economic power in the present. Confronting these realities, and considering the difficult subject of this research, it was arguably more important to pursue every possible measure to maintain the trust and privacy of research participants, and to seek their participation in ways that would mitigate against further surveillance and scrutiny by their neighbours, rather than to obfuscate or aim to subvert them.

While most of the qualitative research was conducted in young people's homes, by Mildred and Kanya (young, 'black' peer researchers), I (an older, 'white', South African woman) would occasionally join household visits if it had been established – usually over the course of three or four prior visits to a home – that my presence was welcomed or indeed requested. Families, particularly the adult caregivers of young people, often insisted on meeting other staff members working on the study, perhaps wanting to ascertain the nature of the project's organisation and to further assess the motives or characters of its leads. In these instances, both participants and peer researchers explained, if I aroused the curiosity or suspicion of their neighbours, families might explain my presence as part of their church activities, or as related to a non-governmental organisation or government project (the last of which, due to the study's partnership with South Africa's National Department of Health, was in general correct).

In parallel with primary research conducted in participants' homes, I led another component of the qualitative study, located in healthcare facilities. Here, the presence of 'whites' was more familiar, although again infused with the portents of the racialised power of Apartheid and its aftermath. Medical doctors – of all 'races' – are required by South African law to spend one year of 'community service' working within public health services (Reid et al. 2018). Newly qualified doctors and other healthcare workers (such as dentists and pharmacists) are therefore common figures within public health facilities across South Africa. They often conduct their 'community service' in areas that are vastly different – geographically and demographically – from the places in which they have grown up and received their education. In the careful reading of these trainee healthcare workers by patients and healthcare workers within public facilities, they may instantly be regarded as 'outsiders' to a particular community, but their presence may be more widely accepted as a part of an established, nation-wide, and government-sanctioned initiative, rather than as an imposition, peculiarity or even prospective threat.

Within the qualitative component of the study located at healthcare facilities, I spent over two thousand hours speaking with and observing staff working within antenatal, sexual health, HIV treatment and trauma wards. My age (I was in my early to mid-thirties at this time and thus typical of a young doctor or medical specialist) and race seemed to suggest, both to staff and to patients, that I was a healthcare worker or researcher visiting facilities to learn first-hand about the challenges of public health provision. Moreover, my familiarity with healthcare workers, established over years of observation, suggested that I had procured the requisite permissions and indeed the approvals and trust of healthcare workers to work within their facilities (which was indeed the case). Within this component of the research, the focus was on the ways in which HIV and sexual health treatments were provided. During these clinic visits, for which explicit permissions had been sought and obtained by clinic staff, Mildred and Kanya would mingle with patients in the waiting areas, observing the goings-on of facilities, and perhaps conducting interviews with participants if conditions of confidentiality and consent were met.

At the peak of the Mzantsi Wakho project's primary research, the study employed over 70 people at two offices in the Eastern Cape, with academic and administrative staff based at the Universities of Cape Town and Oxford. University staff dealt with study operations within academic departments and faculties, and within the broader operations of research institutions – working, for example, with contracts offices to ensure compliance with Labour and Intellectual Property laws. But, because the primary research was located in the Eastern Cape – and not within the cities of Cape Town and Oxford where investigators' academic homes were located – most of the project staff in the Eastern Cape offices were local, and living in study sites. Most, but not all of these researchers, were 'black' South Africans who had completed high school, but very few had any tertiary education. They were recruited on the basis of their interest and experience in youth health – many had worked for non-governmental organisations or for government projects in the past – and, simplistically, because they were seeking work and the study offered prospective employment.

Within the cut-throat world of HIV research funding, the smaller the study budget, and the more ambitious its methods and commitments (including to reaching a sample size that ensures statistical significance in logistical regression), the more 'competitive', and likely to receive funding, a research project becomes. The Mzantsi Wakho study was no exception. We aimed to reach 1,500 adolescents, and to study them longitudinally, over at least three waves of data collection. Project staff in the Eastern Cape, who would collect the data, and whose demographic similarities with study participants might strengthen their familiarity and trust, were paid marginally more than the minimum wage, which was all the study could afford.

The labour of students and interns – who were essentially paid in scholarships or the prospects of CV-strengthening, and who gained experience through data collection and analysis, supervision by investigators and other researchers on the study – was also fundamental to its functioning and its financial sustainability. These realities – of the minimum payments for project staff and of the necessity of free labour to the subsistence of HIV studies – are common features of the research domain but are rarely described in reports and publications. Indeed, the ability of research studies to absorb these kinds of challenges, and function or even thrive in spite of them, is a core marker of success in large, longitudinal, survey studies. But, the quality of analysis from the data gathered remains largely dependent on work of peer researchers, and – within qualitative research – on their insights in deciphering themes, co-creating findings, and deciding how research questions should evolve in response.

Over the course of five years, the study enrolled over 1,500 young people, and included patient data gathered from 108 healthcare facilities (Cluver et al. 2018; Dyer et al. 2019). A team of quantitative peer researchers traced participants to their homes and interviewed them three times using a survey that incorporated 32 measures and constructs regarding health and social support. The result was a rich and rigorous longitudinal data set on the health behaviours and needs of HIV-positive adolescents.

In its early phases, investigators sought and secured ethical permissions to conduct the study from the Universities of Cape Town and Oxford, and the Eastern Cape Provincial Departments of Health and Education. The University of Cape Town ethics protocol detailed a number of fieldwork hazards as well as their prospective management. It dealt with both intricate and mundane challenges, including, for instance, how researchers would ensure the confidentiality and protection of HIV-positive minors, as well as what we would do if confronted by aggressive animals.

Publications about the study explore how methods and results may be integrated through combined quantitative and qualitative analysis (Cluver et al. 2015; Toska et al. 2015; Hodes et al. 2018b). But the methodological complexities and the practical challenges of having conducted this research are usually condensed into a single paragraph in these publications. This chapter focuses in greater depth on the practical difficulties of one particular issue – namely, upholding the ethical requirement of 'observation only' in health emergencies. It provides a frank account of the workings of a mixed methods study that relied in large part on the collaboration of peer researchers to collect and analyse data. In doing so, it unpacks some of the baggage that remains sealed from the glare and scrutiny of donor reports, conference presentations and peer-reviewed publications. To protect the anonymity of people and places, pseudonyms are used throughout.

The case of the absent ambulance

Over the course of five years, I conducted qualitative research in a range of state healthcare facilities. I would begin my day's research at clinic opening hours when initial patient screenings were conducted by nurses, witnessing how they triaged care in response to a dizzying array of needs. In interviews with Mzantsi Wakho participants, they often spoke about their experiences at public health facilities, including their impressions of healthcare workers. One nurse in particular, Sister September, was mentioned by a number of participants. She was known as being extremely strict, but with a reputation as an excellent healthcare provider who went beyond the call of duty in caring for her patients.

On an initial visit to Okhoyo Day Hospital where she worked, I consulted with facilities managers and was introduced to Sister September herself, the 'in charge' (i.e. head nurse) of the family planning clinic. We had a discussion about the study, and I asked if she would be willing to participate in both interviews and observations. She readily agreed. Our study had already secured ethical permission from Okhoyo's director and from the Eastern Cape Department of Health. Because of the strong integration of ART, antenatal and family planning services at Okhoyo, I hoped to study the Day Hospital as a potential model of care. Sister September was a charismatic figure, renowned for her midwifery skills. She was often 'deployed' by provincial health authorities to other healthcare facilities to improve the quality of their services. She was also known for her successes in tracing patients who had defaulted on ART, particularly in pregnancy.

My research in healthcare facilities surfaced a range of ethical challenges, some of which were procedural (for instance, learning which steps to follow when referring participants who were being abused by their caregivers for psychosocial intervention and support, while maintaining their trust and avoiding further victimisation). Other challenges had arisen from the difficulty of separating a research project from a social intervention. Often, these challenges coalesced around specific instances, one of which occurred during a visit to Okhoyo Day Hospital in June 2015.

At 12:30 in the afternoon on Tuesday 11 June, an 18 year old patient, and primigravida, presented at the clinic in obstetric emergency. The patient, Cebisa, had booked previously into an antenatal clinic, but had subsequently moved residence. She had presented at the clinic closest to her new residence on the correct date for her next antenatal booking, but was refused an appointment because she had not booked a previous appointment at that clinic. The patient explained to the nurse there that she had experienced recurring pain in her abdomen for the last three days, and that she was struggling to eat and sleep. She was given a return date for an appointment at that facility a week later. Cebisa's pain worsened and, anxious about her health and her pregnancy, she asked a friend to journey with her to Okhoyo Day Hospital which was renowned for its high quality of antenatal care, in part because of Sister September's excellent work there. Beginning at dawn, the women had taken four different taxis to reach the facility, travelling over 200 kilometres.

With perpetually full waiting rooms outside the antenatal and family planning wards, Okhoyo nurses practised forms of triage by scanning the patients, identifying who among them was in need of emergency care, and consulting them first. Cebisa was sitting in the waiting room with her friend, Zinzi. Mildred had gone to sit next to Cebisa and Zinzi, and to speak with Cebisa who was obviously in an advanced stage of pregnancy. Scanning the waiting room between clinic consultations, Sister September saw that Mildred was speaking with a worried-seeming patient, and she approached them. Sister September summoned Cebisa into the consulting room for a medical examination, after which Cebisa returned to the waiting room and rejoined Mildred and Zinzi on a bench. I was standing nearby, in a section of the waiting room separated by a curtain from the patients' benches. Because of space constraints, the nurses in the family planning and antenatal ward had repurposed this part of the waiting room to conduct certain procedures, such as weighing patients, giving contraceptive injections, or inserting subdermal contraceptive implants.

After examining Cebisa, Sister September approached me and explained that Cebisa needed emergency medical attention and should be taken to Aeden Hospital (the largest and best-resourced hospital in the district). The facility ambulance, however, was absent. Lunchtime had just begun, and it would likely be at least another two hours before Cebisa could be transported to the hospital. My hired research car was parked in the clinic lot outside, and the pieces of this ethical puzzle were thus in place: should I drive Cebisa to the hospital for emergency treatment, or should I remain an impartial observer, upholding the strictures of non-interventionism regarded as a fundament of sound qualitative research? And what would Mildred and Sister September advise? Mildred was a peer researcher, with direct and personal experience as a patient within the public health sector, while Sister September was known for her excellence as a nurse, with decades of experience in providing antenatal care.

Both Mildred and I knew that it would be a violation of the study's ethical protocols to transport Cebisa and Zinzi to Aeden Hospital. All researchers had been briefed, copiously, about not giving lifts to study participants or anyone else for that matter. We worried that, should an accident occur, we could be held legally liable for its consequences. Despite meticulous safety precautions, numerous car accidents had indeed occurred over the course of the study, and some project staff had been badly hurt. We were also worried that Cebisa's health might worsen during the drive, which would take about 20 minutes, and that – lacking medical training – we would not know how to help her.

Sister September, Mildred and I knew that the ambulance's timely return to Okhoyo after the lunch hour, and its rapid transport of Cebisa to Aeden Hospital, were doubtful. Corruption within the ambulance service is a commonplace reality in the Eastern Cape (Bateman 2013; MedicalBrief 2020). On 23 July 2016, while travelling between the cities of Port Elizabeth and East London after attending a national rally of the African National Congress (South Africa's ruling political party), I had driven behind an ambulance picking up and dropping passengers who were holding signs offering cash for transport on the highway. The ambulance had been operating as a taxi.

With a project car standing empty in the clinic parking lot, it seemed a moral necessity that we should drive Cebisa to the hospital ourselves. Mildred was vehemently in favour of this course of action, as was Sister September. But I waivered.

Mzantsi Wakho was explicitly an observational research project, stipulated by its ethical protocols. In the case of current or prospective harm, such as the sexual abuse of minors, we were legally bound to act to protect participants, and to ensure their direct linkage with healthcare and social services. But Cebisa was 18, an adult according to South African law. One of the study's ethical axioms, an inversion of the heroics of social and medical interventions, was 'Don't just do something, stand there'. Rather than seeking to direct or to change the actions of participants, we sought to uphold the ideals of observational research: to watch and witness, but not to intervene. With little time to reason this further, I relied on the insights – indeed the compulsions – of Mildred and Sister September. For Mildred in particular, who had been painstakingly trained in techniques for open-ended, 'amoral' research conduct, the arcane features of the study protocol seemed irrelevant in the face of this medical emergency, and whatever negative consequences might accrue were worth the risk.

Sister September, Mildred and I approached Cebisa and Zinzi, who were seated on the clinic benches, to talk over the prospects of me driving them to the hospital. The nurse explained that time of the taxi's return to the clinic was uncertain, and that I could give them a lift to the hospital if they agreed. Wanting to ensure their consent, I asked Cebisa and Zinzi explicitly if that was what they wanted, and they confirmed that it was. I then asked the group if anyone would hold me responsible in the dreaded case of an accident, or if Cebisa's condition should worsen during the journey. All agreed that they would not. As there would be no fee charged for the journey, I had a vague understanding that I could not be held legally liable in the case of an accident, nor could the wider research study. But in reality, I was not thinking about these legalities. Absorbed in the immediacy of the crisis, I failed to consider the wider implications for the research project if an accident or death should occur while driving Cebisa to the hospital.

After this brief conversation, Sister September returned to her other patients, and Mildred, Cebisa, Zinzi and I walked the short distance to the car. We got inside and fastened our seatbelts. The atmosphere was, understandably, extremely tense, and I focused intently on the road. Mildred, whose skills as an interlocuter and whose knack for 'breaking the ice' in even the most awkward and distressing of situations were invaluable in her role as a peer researcher, made light conversation with Zinzi, who held her friend's hand on the backseat while Cebisa stared out of the window. She tried to smile when she got out of the car, before walking resolutely through the doors of the emergency unit. We learned later, from Sister September, that Cebisa had given birth in the emergency ward that day, and that both she and her baby were well.

Conclusion

Within the humanities and social sciences and in the disciplines of public health, there is a presumed distinction between 'observational research' and 'social/health/development interventions'. But, in contexts of poverty and inequality in particular – such as Mzantsi Wakho's sites – all research constituted an intervention of sorts. Not intervening in particular cases (such as health emergencies), in the name of adhering to ethical guidelines that stipulated the research was only 'observational', violated the fundamental commitment to humane research: to do no harm, whether through action or inaction. In cases of obvious, imminent harm through inaction, such as that of Cebisa and the absent ambulance, I believe it is the researchers' ethical duty to disregard the role of a mere 'observer', and to intervene decisively in seeking emergency medical care.

'Emergency' interventions are not without their consequences. Perhaps, by driving Cebisa to the hospital, I absolved the absent ambulance driver of professional negligence. Had Cebisa died at Okhoyo Day Hospital, an investigation might have found other people guilty of negligence, including the nurse who had refused Cebisa antenatal care at the previous clinic in spite of the severity of her symptoms. Perhaps it might have brought to light the crippling combination of corruption, exhaustion and indifference with which many of those working within the health sector are confronted, and in which many are complicit.

But the risks we took in helping Cebisa were potentially severe. If something had gone wrong in the course of the trip to the hospital, formal permissions for the study granted by university committees and government health authorities might have been withdrawn. What was at stake in this decision was, therefore, the work of hundreds of researchers and participants over the course of half a decade, on a subject that was central to public health: how to improve medicines-taking and sexual health among young people. But in conducting this work, together with peer researchers and healthcare workers with direct experiences of the health systems failures, we could not comply with the study protocol at the expense of helping someone whose neglect by the public health system had precipitated exactly the kind of crisis that our study had aspired to document and resolve. In real-world contexts, the lines between 'pure research' and 'social/healthcare and intervention' are often blurred. The mere presence of researchers, and their acts of observation, are embroiled within the dynamics of power and identity already at play within particular contexts, even while these dynamics are in perennial flux in relation to political changes and healthcare advances (as is the case in the treatment of HIV in post-Apartheid South Africa).

Intervening actively in observational studies may damage research projects. It may introduce biases, reifying power differentials between researchers and participants, and recasting studies as 'interventions' rather than exercises in data gathering and observation. It may also undo years of careful work in managing participants' expectations about what research project can give to them, and how this may be sustained once studies are completed. Intervening in the context of a research study may also confuse researchers, whose job it is – though this is difficult – to watch and witness rather than to interfere. And, despite the lengthiest and most detailed of ethical protocols, there will always be unforeseen instances in which researchers are required to make difficult decisions beyond their remit. In these instances, I believe it is up to individual researchers – in collaboration with their colleagues and medical experts if possible – to choose the lesser of two prospective evils, and to intervene to perhaps save a life no matter what the professional consequences.

Acknowledgements

Thanks go to the participants, researchers and funders of the Mzantsi Wakho study (further information available at http://www.mzantsiwakho.org). The ethics committees of the Centre for Social Science Research and the Humanities and Health Sciences Faculties at the University of Cape Town provided crucial guidance on how to mitigate and manage the study's potential risks. This chapter has benefitted immensely from the insights of the editors of this volume.

Note

1 Race is a social construct, reified through Apartheid's system of racial categorisation and segregation. Racial descriptors continue to hold immense power in post-Apartheid South Africa. Racial terms are used in this chapter as commonplace demographic demarcations in contemporary South Africa, but their use must not be read as an acceptance of their biological validity, and must be interpreted with an awareness of the dangers of ascribing race an essential biologism or of accepting and legitimising racial differences and persistent inequalities.

References

Agwu, A.L. and Fairlie, L., 2013. Antiretroviral treatment, management challenges and outcomes in perinatally HIV-infected adolescents. *Journal of the International AIDS Society*, 16 (18579), 1–13.

Bateman, C., 2013. E. Cape's corruption busting DG finally ousted. *South African Medical Journal*, 203 (4), 215–217.

Cluver, L., et al., 2015. 'HIV is like a tsotsi, ARVs are your guns': Associations between HIV disclosure and adherence to antiretroviral treatment among adolescents in South Africa. *AIDS*, 29 (Suppl. 1), S57–S65.

Cluver, L., et al., 2018. Violence exposure and adolescent antiretroviral non-adherence in South Africa. *AIDS*, 32 (8), 975–983.

Dyer, C., et al., 2019. Are youth living with HIV in South Africa reaching the sustainable development goals? CSSR Working Paper No. 434. University of Cape Town.

Everatt, D., 2008. The undeserving poor: Poverty and the politics of service delivery in the poorest nodes of South Africa. *Politikon*, 35 (3), 213–319.

Freund, B., 2019. *Twentieth-Century South Africa: A Developmental History*. Cambridge: Cambridge University Press.

Gumede, W., 2001. Delivering the democratic developmental state in South Africa. In: A. McLennan and B. Munslow, eds. *The Politics of Service Delivery*. Milton Park: Taylor & Francis, Ltd., 43–103.

Hodes, R., et al., 2018a. Yummy or crummy? The multisensory components of medicines-taking among HIV-positive youth. *Global Public Health*, August (2018), 284–299.

Hodes, R., et al., 2018b. Pesky metrics: The challenges of measuring antiretroviral treatment adherence among HIV-positive adolescents in South Africa. *Critical Public Health*, 28 (4), S1–S12.

Hodes, R. and Gittings, G., 2019. Kasi curriculum: What young men learn and teach about sex in a South African township. *Sex Education*, 19 (4), 436–454. doi:10.1080/1 4681811.2019.1606792.

Johnson, L.F., et al., 2017. Estimating the impact of antiretroviral treatment on adult mortality trends in South Africa: A mathematical modelling study. *PLOS Med*, 14 (12). doi:10.1371/journal.pmed.1002468.

Maskew, M., et al., 2016. Insights into adherence among a cohort of adolescents aged 12–20 years in South Africa: Reported barriers to Antiretroviral Treatment. *AIDS Research and Treatment*, 2016, 4161738. doi:10.1155/2016/4161738.

MedicalBrief, 2020. Cape controversy over motorbike ambulances and clinics. *MedicalBrief: Africa's Medical Media Digest*, 15 July. Available from: https://www.medicalbrief.co.za/ archives/ec-controversy-over-motorbike-ambulances-and-clinics/.

Nattrass, N., 2007. *Mortal Combat: AIDS Denialism and the Struggle for Antiretrovirals in South Africa*. Pietermartizburg: University of KwaZulu-Natal Press.

Olver, C., 2017. *How to Steal a City: The Battle for Nelson Mandela Bay, An Inside Account*. Johannesburg: Jonathan Ball.

Posel, D., 2001. What's in a name? Racial categorisations under apartheid and their afterlife. *Transformation*, 47, 50–74.

Reid, S., et al., 2018. Compulsory community service for doctors in South Africa: A 15-year review. *South African Medical Journal*, 108 (9), 741–747.

Seekings, J. and Nattrass, N., 2006. *Class, Race and Inequality in South Africa*. Scottsville, VA: University of KwaZulu-Natal Press.

Simbayi, L.C., et al., 2019. *South African National HIV Prevalence, Incidence, Behaviour and Communication Survey*. Cape Town: HSRC Press.

Southall, R., 2016. *The New Black Middle Class in South Africa*. Johannesburg: Jacana.

Statistics South Africa, 2018. *Quarterly Labour Force Survey, QLFS: Q2: 2018*, 31 July 2018. Available from: http://www.statssa.gov.za/?p=11361 [Accessed 27 September 2020].

Toska, E., et al., 2015. Sex and secrecy: How HIV-status disclosure affects safe sex among HIV-positive adolescents. *AIDS Care*, 27 (1) Supplement 1, 47–58.

UNAIDS, 2019. People living with HIV (all ages) by region. *AIDSinfo*. Available from: http://aidsinfo.unaids.org/ [Accessed 23 October 2019].

Vale, B., et al., 2017. Bureaucracies of blood and belonging: What documents tell us about the relationship between HIV-positive youth and the South African state. *Development and Change*, 48 (6), 1287–1309.

Section V
Influencing policy and practice

15 Farmer-led change

Addressing environmental and health problems caused by widespread pesticide use in Costa Rica, Nicaragua and Honduras

Laura Sims

Introduction

Food security is essential to human survival. There exist major concerns about the environmental sustainability of agricultural production in Central America because of frequent occurrences of pesticide toxicities in rural communities, high incidences of elevated pesticide residues in food sold at local markets, and widespread environmental pollution (Sage 2012; Shiva 2013). Intending to address poverty-reduction strategies in Costa Rica, Nicaragua and Honduras by improving human and environmental health and increasing agricultural productivity, the Canadian International Development Agency's (CIDA) *Community-based pest management in Central American agriculture project* (2006–13) focused on developing mechanisms that could impact local, national and regional methods, programmes and policies regarding the handling, storage and use of pesticides to increase farm income and productivity (Mulock and Herrera 2013).

Within the field of international development, participatory approaches to governance have been promoted as a way to engage communities in decision-making processes to increase the success of interventions, enhance perceptions of legitimacy, and ensure sustainable learning outcomes and capacity building (Rist et al. 2007). Development interventions should address local needs and reflect local priorities as they focus on poverty reduction, human health and/or environmental problems (Green 2010). In the food security and environmental sustainability sector, some international development agencies collaborate with local institutions to encourage agro-ecological practices and capacity building in rural communities (Taylor et al. 2012; Sims 2017). However, initiatives often fail for lack of meaningful public involvement in decision-making processes (Diduck et al. 2012; Guta et al. 2013). Within such contexts, research approaches that engage community members as researchers in their own communities can enable better access to marginalised communities, increase understanding of local realities, contexts and cultural practices, and involve local people in the creation of activities and services that more appropriately respond to community needs (Price and Hawkins 2002).

Community-based participatory research approaches involve a range of partners – including academic researchers, disadvantaged communities and public sector actors – in a research process, recognising their strengths while addressing issues of importance to the community (Logie et al. 2012). Such a 'bottom-up' approach tries to value contributions local people make to the shared development of knowledge, using that knowledge to inform action (Carlisle and Cropper 2009). The benefits of community involvement in research are many, including greater representation of marginalised groups in research, data that are more representative of community needs, and increased opportunities for local capacity building and empowerment (Guta et al. 2013). Peer research approaches – in which members of a target population are trained to participate in research studies as co-researchers – are often central to enabling more meaningful community involvement in research and subsequent action that arises from study findings. A key premise here is that peer researchers act as 'key informants', facilitating relationship building and authentic knowledge sharing between academic and/or professional researchers with the marginalised communities they seek to understand (Price and Hawkins 2002). Porter (2016) describes how peer research is usually part of larger, mixed methods research approaches to understanding particular contexts or communities, often with the aim of providing improved service delivery to them (Coupland et al. 2005; Elmusharaf et al. 2017).

Drawing on CIDA's *Community-based pest management in Central American agriculture project* as a case study, this chapter examines the roles of farmers in collaborative research that aimed to bring about changes in agricultural practices and policies regarding the harmful use of pesticides. With a particular focus on the use of farmer-led demonstration plots and demonstration days, it explores the role of farmers working as peer researchers in data collection and analysis activities, and changes brought about through their sharing of innovative, beneficial agricultural practices with other local farmers.

Community-based pest management project

In this community-based pest management project, universities from four countries collaborated to increase food security with rural communities and stakeholders through improved agricultural practices and to contribute to more effective government programmes and policies concerning pesticides. The participating universities included the Universidad Nacional Agraria (Nicaragua), Universidad de Costa Rica, Universidad Nacional Autónoma de Honduras and University of Manitoba (Canada). Over 2,200 participants from rural communities, academia, government and local organisations were involved. However, participating farmers were instrumental in experimenting with, collecting data and sharing results around beneficial agricultural practices with the broader community.

This community-based pest management project consisted of three complementary components: the community development component involved work with farm families to understand their farming and pest management practices; the technical component involved working with farmers to implement demonstration plots and facilitate educational outreach activities with a focus on safer pesticide storage, handling and use and the provision of alternatives to pesticides;

and the policy component developed indicators to monitor changes in practices over time (Sims 2017). University collaborators from each country jointly developed a common methodological framework where broad guidelines for objectives and activities were established. This allowed for a similar approach to be taken to address a regional problem yet permitted enough flexibility to adapt activities to specific contexts according to local needs and community characteristics. A detailed description of the project and learning results is published elsewhere (Sims 2017).

Research activities were central to each component of the project. For example, during the community development component, baseline surveys and participant observation – conducted by university students living with farm families – were used to understand how and why farm families farm the way they do in local contexts. Information gathered through these methods was fundamental for planning technical outreach activities to address local priority concerns. However, the focus of this chapter is on the role of farmer peer researchers during technical activities – such as workshops, farm-level demonstration plots and demonstration days – which occurred in the three Central American countries.

The data presented below was collected during my involvement in the work as project manager (2008–11), community-development team member (2008–13) and researcher (2008–16). I draw from semi-annual field visits involving participant observation, discussions with participants and project collaborators (2008–11); project reports (Chibi 2011; Mulock and Herrera 2013); and results from a qualitative case study that aimed to understand what participants had learnt through participation in the CIDA project (Sims 2017). This case study involved two rounds of interviews: the first conducted directly following project completion (December 2012 – February 2013) and the second conducted three years later (May 2016). These interviews involved farmer peer researchers who had 'hosted' demonstration plots and members of the technical teams. In this chapter, direct quotations from this case study highlight participant voice, bringing authenticity to the sharing of their experiences. At participants' own request, real names have been used.

Peer research through farmer-led demonstration plots

This project was about developing skills and knowledge around good, culturally appropriate pest-management practices, looking to improve human health and the environment, and provide a better life for producers. Implemented during the second year of the project (2008), farm-level demonstration plots and demonstration days were critical aspects in trying to realise these objectives. Demonstration plots were venues for farmer peer researchers and technical teams to experiment with and learn from various alternative and conventional agricultural approaches. Demonstration days took place on demonstration plots and provided opportunities for farmer peer researchers to highlight strategies they were experimenting with, share their experiences and promote beneficial practices to other farmers in the community. Below I describe the research process and farmers' experiences as peer researchers in Costa Rica and Nicaragua. Obstacles to implementing this work in Honduras are also examined.

Recruiting, training and supporting farmer peer researchers

In Costa Rica, three farmers and their families – Minor, Ricardo and Marvin – were asked to host demonstration plots and act as peer researchers. They were chosen as they represented different communities, located in relatively close proximity from one another near the city of Pacayas in the province of Cartago, and within an hour's drive of the Universidad de Costa Rica. This region has very irregular topography with steep slopes. These farmers also represented differ-ent approaches to farming – Minor used conventional farming practices whereas Ricardo farmed organically, and Marvin had livestock. Each farmer was known to be highly collaborative and open to new ideas, and were considered leaders in their communities.

Costa Rican project teams and participating farmers decided to experi-ment with alternative to conventional chemical-intensive practices along-side approaches considered 'good agricultural practices' (Izquierdo et al. 2007) to address persistent challenges within that farmer's current farming system. The Costa Rican technical team was made up of four academic, agricultural technicians. They made weekly visits to the farmer peer researchers, begin-ning well before the growing season, to identify key issues facing the farmers. They wanted to understand the farmers' intentions in terms of crop production, usual strategies and approaches to deal with pest management, concerns and persistent challenges. The technical team would propose possible alternative approaches to conventional chemical use drawing on other good agricultural practices, and together they discussed potential benefits and limitations of the proposed approaches. The farmer peer researchers then decided whether or not to try the approach. For example, Minor – a conventional potato farmer who generally relied on chemical inputs to grow crops (e.g. to fertilise soil, control pests) – struggled with 'white flies' (i.e. *aleyrodidae*) and soil erosion. The tech-nical team suggested experimenting with pheromones traps to lure flies into sticky traps, and creating drainage rows to help reduce erosion. Then, Minor, in collaboration with the project team, evaluated the efficacy of these approaches (e.g. taking soil samples, counting the moths in the traps). Associated costs were paid by the project. In this process, Minor was a co-researcher on his farm. Based on his observations, results from the tests, and in consultation with the technical team, he was able to make informed farm-level decisions mov-ing forward. Minor (farmer peer researcher, Costa Rica, 2013) described his experience:

> In the field they showed me about soil conservation …. It makes me think about my children, that if we continue with bad practices, things won't change. So, we've changed how we till the soil to protect it …. A month before planting they asked what products I was applying and why. We decided

we could change certain products …. I use these new practices consciously as I'm convinced it's the right thing to do. The plots were marvelous – the harvest was superior, not only because of the amount produced but because we've a clear conscience that we're lowering the chemicals that were making us and consumers sick.

In Nicaragua, the technical team consisted of three academic, agricultural technicians. They held workshops in different collaborating communities in the municipality of Tisma, located in the department of Masaya, to explain the concept of demonstration plots and invited potential volunteers to host demonstration plots on their farms. Tisma's climate is tropical savanna with a generally flat landscape. There were eventually three demonstration plots in this country, including one farm family (Leticia and Ofilio, and their two adult sons) and two small groups of farmers – one composed of a local women's organisation (hosted by Lejía) and one of men (Rafael and Antonio, hosted by Antonio) – who also acted as peer researchers. Similar to Costa Rica, these farmers represented different communities located within relatively close proximity to each other, were within an hour's drive of the Universidad Nacional Agraria, were known as being collaborative, open to new ideas, and reliable, and were considered leaders in their communities.

The Nicaraguan project team decided to experiment with a whole-systems, agro-ecological approach to farming, testing the efficacy of intercropping, vermi-composting and producing naturally occurring insecticides among other approaches. On the demonstration plots (approximately 100 m × 50 m), half the plot was experimental (controlled by the Nicaraguan technical team) and half was farmed by the farmers using their conventional methods. Similar crops were planted, following the lead of what the farmer peer researchers chose to plant. The technical team worked closely with the farmers to identify key issues and try to address them. Together, farmers and university collaborators analysed the progress of the crops and the efficacy of the different practices on a weekly basis (during the growing season). Guided by the technical team, farmers learned how to systematically document their work, identify persistent challenges, diseases and pests, assess whether an intervention was necessary and, if so, decide on appropriate measures to take. Together, they analysed the effectiveness and limitations of the approaches they were testing on their farms. Antonio (farmer peer researcher, Nicaragua, 2013) described his experience:

They came weekly to help, teach us. They developed alternative options with us that produced good results. We're always open to experimenting with other options, other varieties to plant. With this project, we learned to write, save what we do, compare what happened. We learned to be independent of the national market. Now, we know how to classify the plantings, what crops are best for our area …. It was excellent that the university accompanied us for three years, they were there to review, see if the changes were working.

In both Nicaragua and Costa Rica, ongoing technical support combined with experiential field-based training and critical reflective dialogue around what farmers were observing was essential in farmers learning to be researchers on their own land. This hands-on, one-on-one training was accompanied by community-level workshops featuring topics chosen by farmers. As identified in other peer research work (Carlisle and Cropper 2009; Logie et al. 2012), in-depth training and support were essential to success. Technical teams tried to work around farmers' schedules and within their existing constraints. Farm demonstration plots were located on farmers' land, which was beneficial in terms of access and potential benefit if new approaches were successful. But this also involved risks as precious land was being given up for uncertain gain. Farmer peer researchers and technical teams discussed which approaches to try on the demonstration plots, but farmer peer researchers made final decisions as to what they wanted to implement. The only exception to this was on the Nicaraguan technical team's half of the demonstration plot.

Data collection methods varied depending on what was happening on each farm. In the case of Minor in Costa Rica, using pheromones traps and monitoring white flies caught taught farmers about trap efficacy, the extent of infestations and how these changed over time. Soil samples, used to determine nutrient content, composition and other characteristics, were used to evaluate soil quality over time. Doing meticulous pest observations in the demonstration plots – by learning to identify beneficial versus harmful insects and by counting levels of infestations – taught farmer peer researchers the difference between beneficial and toxic pests and how to systematically document their observations in field notes.

Data analysis was an iterative process. Farmer peer researchers analysed the data in collaboration with technical teams who helped them make sense of what they were seeing and make decisions around when, or not, to implement certain approaches. Data were analysed with the aim of understanding how to improve production and the well-being of families and the environment. Over time, and in light of analysis and findings, farmers adopted approaches that they assessed as beneficial. This information was then shared with other regional teams at international meetings to inform next project steps and discuss best practices and potential policy development.

Dissemination of findings through demonstration days, project meetings, final symposium

Demonstration plots served as educational venues for the community, particularly for highlighting innovative, beneficial practices during demonstration days where other farmers would come to learn about what was being done. At demonstration days, participating farmer peer researchers, supported by local university technical teams, would share the results from their experiences experimenting on the demonstration plots. Over the course of the study, for instance, they presented findings on how to vermicompost, create natural insecticles, use cover crops, do crop rotation, use pheromone traps and create drainage rows. Demonstration days provided authentic and culturally appropriate opportunities for farmer peer researchers to share their work with others farming in similar environments. Due to the nature of the demonstation plots, as living experimental labs located in the community, farmer peer researchers ongoing modelling of practices and casual conversations with neighbours also helped disseminate research findings during and beyond the life of the project.

Apart from sharing results from their experiences at farm demonstration days, farmer peer researchers also shared their work with the international project team (meaning all the national project teams together) during team meetings involving project teams from all four countries that took place in their country (e.g., January 2009 in Costa Rica, April 2010 in Nicaragua). On these occasions, transport permitting, either the whole team or simply the technical teams visited the farmer peer researchers to witness and discuss what they were doing on their demonstration plots. Peer researchers from all three countries shared their experiences and findings at an international symposium for the project in Nicaragua (February 2013), where all 69 participants were in attendance (i.e., project team members, farmers, students and other project collaborators).

Changes related to well-being and sustainability

The research undertaken documented changes in farming practices and a sense of responsibility that contributed to food security, poverty reduction, improved environmental and human health, and increased agricultural productivity. As reported elsewhere (Sims 2017), farmer-led demonstration plots and demonstration days facilitated significant learning outcomes for farmer peer researchers and among wider community members around the health and environmental impacts of inappropriate pesticide use. Farm-level sustainability action outcomes included the implementation of alternative farming techniques and use of protective gear when handling and applying pesticides. For the farmer peer researchers, learning about the impacts of pesticides often resulted in a deep feeling of responsibility to show leadership in their communities to protect the environment and human health (Sims 2017).

Antonio (farmer peer researcher, Nicaragua, 2013) explained how learning specific farming practices taught him how to protect his health and the environment and control pests:

> We learned how biodiversity helps improve crops; how to rotate crops to eliminate pest reproduction … using organic matter and diversifying crops to produce healthier products …. This project has transformed me. I'm motivated to open minds, to seek out ways to engage producers, so that they change their practices. We have to care for the earth, to not pollute.
>
> (Sims 2017, p. 547, 549)

In 2016, Antonio shared how he continues to apply his skills and knowledge acquired through being a peer researcher:

> The plots were like our school … there was a whole learning around pest control and using resources from your farm …. On my farm I'm still applying what I learnt, I've innovated too …. I wanted to experiment with a small tomato crop from seed until harvest – with conventional and non-chemical practices …. I applied a certain amount of organic vermi-compost to every five plants – each having a label, application date, what I applied.

This sense of responsibility to show leadership manifested itself in different ways. It included farmer peer researchers implementing and modelling beneficial agro-conservation farming practices on their farms. It also involved promoting these innovative practices in their communities. Ricardo (farmer peer researcher, Costa Rica, 2013) stated:

> I can help the community. I still use the practices because they're good. Before we were technicians but now we're professionals, we've the knowledge to make intelligent decisions. With this project, I learned how to save money using different techniques and products that are less expensive, natural.
>
> (Sims 2017, p. 549)

According to Ricardo, in 2013 his farm was 90% more productive as a result of his involvement as a peer researcher in the project. Minor (farmer peer researcher, Costa Rica, 2013) articulated the relationship between learning, his sense of responsibility, and his change in practice:

> They showed me about soil conservation and the harmful effects of conventional practices …. Consequently, we've changed the way we work the land to protect the soil. I feel more at peace. I don't want to contribute to people getting sick …. We have to be more environmentally responsible, to change in order to leave something good for our children. I have to teach them.
>
> (Sims 2017, p. 550)

This sense of responsibility led to ongoing dissemination of information. Beatriz (technical team, Costa Rica, 2016) explained how farmer peer researchers acted as community-level promoters of beneficial practices and educators, particularly when they continued to model agro-conservation techniques on their farms:

> Minor, for example, has pheromone gallons that everyone can see. Farmers stop. Minor explains what they are, where they should be located, where to get them. They then call me. One strategy is putting them in strategic visible places, having someone who knows how they work. These farmers-as-trainers are important.

Interviews in 2016 revealed that Antonio and Minor were still applying beneficial agro-conservation practices including the incorporation of new practices. Sadly, due to family illness, Ricardo had to find more stable employment. Certainly, for continued implementation, these farmers had to see that what they were doing was beneficial for themselves, others and/or the environment. Having resources accessible on their farm (e.g., manure to feed composting worms) facilitated continued implementation.

For farmer peer researchers, this learning resulted in changes that contributed to their well-being (health, quality of life), food security and livelihood viability through increased agricultural productivity and reduced costs, and environmental sustainability. As their words attest, this learning resulted in changes in agricultural practices and in their perceptions about their roles and responsibilities around human and environmental health in their communities. Importantly, the development of leadership capacity by engaging peer researchers in decision-making processes can contribute to local governance structures (Sims 2017).

Reflections on working with farmer peer researchers

Benefits of participation to the research and to peer researchers themselves

There were undoubted benefits for the research project associated with farmer peer researchers' essential role as intermediaries between technical teams, their communities and policymakers, and researchers in the international community in this study (Logie et al. 2012; Guta et al. 2013). Through their farm demonstration plots, farmer peer researchers were able to experiment and see successes themselves and then share these approaches and address concerns with other farmers in their community in the local vernacular (Porter 2016). Through these exchanges with other community members, they learned about local concerns, which they were able to share with the technical teams during weekly visits, and later at national meetings and international symposium. As such, farmer peer researchers enabled access to marginalised communities and their local understandings and realities (Porter 2016). They also facilitated the exchange of information and knowledge between service providers, policymakers and researchers on one hand, and through existing authentic, trusted relationships, with community members like themselves on the other (Logie et al. 2012; Guta et al. 2013).

Furthermore, demonstration plots – as contexts through and in which peer research occurred – exemplified environmental enquiry, whereby they were highly experiential and opportunities to learn actively from the natural environment where embedded in these sites. A focus and outcome of the project was on responsible environmental stewardship (Sims 2017). Similar to other studies focusing on agro-conservation development initiatives (Sinclair et al. 2009; Taylor et al. 2012), working with farmer peer researchers through these situated experiential activities enabled dialogue and reflection in the identification of new solutions to ongoing environmental challenges.

However, the farmer peer researchers also benefitted from participation. As with other studies (Logie et al. 2012; Porter 2016), they appreciated the relationship building (e.g. with other farmers, local technical teams, and with project members and farmers from other countries), and skills development in terms of learning about alternative farming practices, human and natural environments, and safer pesticide use. In some cases, these benefits were reported as changing 'their perspective about life and their role in society' (Sims 2017, p. 539). For Minor, as evidenced earlier, a change in his approach to soil conservation and pest management as a result of participating in this study led to a transformation in the way he acts, thinks and sees his role as an environmental steward (Sims 2017).

In 2016, former peer researchers – Minor, Antonio, Leticia, and Ofilio in particular – stated how learning through demonstration plots made them more resilient in the face of challenges. As with other peer research approaches (Elmusharaf et al. 2017), capacity building, experimentation, reflection and dialogue helped them understand their realities better and provided them with practical strategies, analytical skills and communal networks to support them moving forward. These farmers continued using methods that they had learned in spite of changing circumstances. For example, as a result of participating as peer researchers in the project, Leticia and her family (farmers in Nicaragua) recognised the need to reflect on food and livelihood security and integrate strategies for resilience at a farm level. They subsequently planted hoquote trees with the technical team's support. Over the years, selling fruit from these trees paid for two modest homes for their sons' families. The trees reduce erosion, provide shade, are a food source, and create income.

Significant in terms of realising project goals, farmer peer researchers continued to disseminate and model beneficial practices in the communities, even after the 'research' project had finished. For instance, in visiting Nicaragua in 2016, Antonio proudly showed me the used pesticide container recycling depot (resembling a small shed) he had built on his land for communal use. Speaking to the power of peer dissemination, Antonio explained that at the final symposium, he learned from 'his Honduran brothers' about how beneficial these depots could be to community well-being and the environment. Inspired to act, he built one on his land. Similarly, Minor in Costa Rica described how he continued to model and share strategies he learnt with his neighbours, both through casual encounters and more strategic attendance at gatherings hosted by the local agrochemical outlet. He continued to collaborate with the university, sharing his model farm with agricultural students and encouraging them to disseminate this information when they become agro-technicians.

Successes and challenges in the peer research process

Several factors enabled the successful integration of farmer peer researchers in this study (see also Logie et al. 2012). First, farmer peer researchers explained that the technical teams' regular visits over three years and six growing seasons in

Costa Rica and Nicaragua provided them with excellent ongoing research training and they felt supported in their decisions. Second, the farmer peer researchers appreciated the warm, respectful relationship with members of the technical teams, which were particularly important given the perceived possible livelihood risks and consequences of failure associated with farming their land in new ways. Such emotional support is documented as important in peer research with other marginalised communities (Price and Hawkins 2002; Coupland et al. 2005; Logie et al. 2012). Third, a participatory, flexible and iterative approach to project management (Sims 2017) permitted us to build project activities based on what farmers were telling us, their needs and circumstances, and what we were observing, as well as according to unpredictable changes within natural systems. Finally, empirical studies (Sims and Sinclair 2008; Sims 2012, 2017; Taylor et al. 2012) confirmed the influence of cultural practices and contexts on the effectiveness of participatory approaches to learning and capacity building. We were collaborating with small-scale farmers who needed to 'see to believe' (Sims 2017), and the experiential nature of the demonstration plots, their location in communities, and opportunities to share findings through demonstration days all contributed to the success of the project.

Yet there were challenges working with peer researchers. One issue was protecting peer researchers from potential hazards and risks (Porter et al. 2010). In this case study, this included potential financial risk if something were to go wrong in the demonstration plots (e.g. crop failure), which could be addressed by ensuring international development projects include comprehensive compensation for contributions of land and time in research costs, especially in terms of study failure. Another risk was the harassment of farmer peer researchers by local 'middlemen' (i.e. *coyotes*) or agro-chemical representatives who perceived changes in farming practices as a direct threat to profit margins. This is more challenging, particularly in contexts where violence is common and life is often precarious (Lakhani 2018). Establishing supportive networks around peer researchers could help mitigate the situation. However, the concern is real and full disclosure of potential risks prior to informed consent when participating in research is essential.

Yet another challenge concerned the ability to provide adequate ongoing training and support throughout the process, which we experienced in the case of the Honduran demonstration plots. Although their intentions were good, the Honduran technical team was unable to provide adequate ongoing technical and logistical support to those responsible for the demonstration plots due to flooding, political unrest, internal university politics, student strikes and one field site being a six-hour drive from the university. In the case of Nicaragua, we started with six demonstration plots, but this proved too ambitious in terms of the ability to provide adequate support due to their regular academic responsibilities.

Working in Central American farming contexts where farming tends to be done by men also created challenges engaging women and men as peer researchers. While farm families were actively involved in many project activities, with demonstration plots, it was predominately men who were peer researchers. There

were two exceptions. In Nicaragua, one demonstration plot involved participation of the whole family (Leticia, Ofilio, two adult sons) as peer researchers.
Another demonstration plot involved a local women's group. However, as with
other peer research studies (Porter et al. 2010), these women had other household and family responsibilities and found it hard to fulfil their roles and responsibilities as peer researchers with the demonstration plot, with the work finally
being left, in the case of the women's organisation, to Lejía who hosted the demonstration plot.

Reflecting on power relationships between team members and farmer peer researchers

Ethical questions have been raised around relations of power between peer
researchers and researchers in established institutions during decision making in
peer research approaches (Guta et al. 2013). Reflecting on observations, demonstration plot visits and discussions with the national teams and farmer peer
researchers during my involvement in the project over six years, I believe that
the farmer peer researchers had substantial decision-making power during demonstration plot activities. Over the years they built trusting relationships with the
national project teams, and made collaborative decisions on their own farms as
to what crops to grow and which strategies to experiment with. At farm demonstration days, peer researchers' knowledge and hands-on experiences were valued
when they shared their work with other community members. Involvement of
peer researchers in community-based research should be a continuous, respectful
negotiation to ensure that research is relevant and responsive to peer researchers
(Logie et al. 2012). This peer research approach was consistent with the larger
participatory approach taken when designing and implementing the project, that
was intentionally meant to mitigate power inequities, to promote learning, and
involve actors in meaningful ways in decision making (Sinclair et al. 2009; Sims
2012, 2017). Despite these aims, much effort is required to limit the possible
influence of power differentials in participatory commuity-based research projects given that primary responsibility for research remains within academic or
professional communities (Carlisle and Cropper 2009), which was the case with
this community-based pest management project.

Concluding comments

The most valuable aspect of having farmers as peer researchers in terms of
improving food security, well-being and environmental sustainability at a farm
and community level was the learning that occurred and how the project benefitted from their contributions. Farm-level demonstration plots were productive
forums for learning for farm families and technical teams and provided authentic venues for sharing experiences with other community members. Through
experiential fieldwork in the plots, technical team members and farmers – acting
as peer researchers – learnt how to identify persistent challenges, diseases and

pests, problem-solve together, observe results, experiment in a systematic way, and innovate. Farmer peer researchers gained confidence, carrying these skills forward beyond the life of the project, continuing to be curious and experiment. Their role as intermediaries allowed for the project to be adapted to suit their needs and, conversely, their participation increased the dissemination of research findings in communities and the promotion of beneficial practices.

References

Carlisle, S. and Cropper, S., 2009. Investing in lay researchers for community-based health action research: Implications for research, policy and practice. *Critical Public Health*, 19 (1), 59–70. doi:10.1080/09581590802225712.

Chibi, A., 2011. *Contributions of University Partnerships in Cooperation and Development (UPCD) Tier 2 Projects to Marginalized Populations*. Ottawa: Association of Universities and Colleges Canada.

Coupland, H., et al., 2005. Clients or colleagues? Reflections on the process of participatory action research with young injection drug users. *International Journal of Drug Policy*, 16, 191–198. doi:10.1016/j.drugpo.2004.12.002.

Diduck, A.P., et al., 2012. Transformative learning theory, public involvement and natural resource and environmental management. *Journal of Environmental Planning and Management*, 55 (10), 1311–1330. doi:10.1080/09640568.2011.645718.

Elmusharaf, K., et al., 2017. Participatory ethnographic evaluation and research: Reflections on the research approach used to understand the complexity of maternal health issues in South Sudan. *Qualitative Health Research*, 27 (9), 1345–1358. doi:10.1177/1049732316673975.

Green, M., 2010. Making development agents: Participation as boundary object in international development. *Journal of Development Studies*, 46 (7), 1240–1263. doi:10.1080/00220388.2010.487099.

Guta, A., Flicker, S., and Roche, B., 2013. Governing through community allegiance: A qualitative examination of peer research in community-based participatory research. *Critical Public Health*, 23 (4), 432–451. doi:10.1080/09581596.2012.761675.

Izquierdo, J., Rodriguez Fazzone, M., and Duran, M., 2007. *Guidelines "Good Agricultural Practices for Family Agriculture"*. Colombia, SC: Food and Agriculture Organization of the United Nations. Available from: http://www.fao.org/3/a-a1193e.pdf.

Lakhani, N., 2018. Justice for Cáceres's killers – But bloodshed continues. *The Guardian Weekly*, 7 December, 24–25.

Logie, C., et al., 2012. Opportunities, ethical challenges, and lessons learned working with peer researcher assistants in a multi-method HIV community-based research study in Ontario, Canada. *Journal of Empirical Research on Human Research Ethics*, 7 (4), 10–19. doi:10.1525/jer.2012.7.4.10.

Mulock, B. and Herrera, J., 2013. *Community-based Pest Management in Central American Agriculture Final Narrative Report*. Ottawa: Association of Universities and Colleges Canada.

Porter, G., 2016. Reflections on co-investigation through peer research with young people and older people in sub-Saharan Africa. *Qualitative Research*, 16 (3), 293–304. doi:10.1177/1468794115619001.

Porter, G., et al., 2010. Children as research collaborators: Issues and reflections from a mobility study in sub-Saharan Africa. *American Journal of Community Psychology*, 46, 215–227. doi:10.1007/s10464-010-9317-x.

Price, N. and Hawkins, K., 2002. Researching sexual reproductive behaviour: A peer ethnographic approach. *Social Science and Medicine*, 55, 1325–1336.

Rist, S., et al., 2007. Moving from sustainable management to sustainable governance of natural resources: The role of social learning processes in rural India, Bolivia, and Mali. *Journal of Rural Studies*, 23, 23–37. doi:10.1016/j.jrurstud.2006.02.006.

Sage, C., 2012. *Environment and Food*. New York, NY: Routledge.

Shiva, V., 2013. *Making Peace with the Earth*. Halifax: Fernwood Publishing.

Sims, L., 2012. Taking a learning approach to community-based strategic environmental assessment: Results from a Costa Rican case study. *Impact Assessment and Project Appraisal*, 30, 242–252. doi:10.1080/14615517.2012.736761.

Sims, L., 2017. Learning for sustainability through CIDA's 'community-based pest management in Central American agriculture project': A deliberative, experiential and iterative process. *Journal of Environmental Planning and Management*, 60 (3), 538–557. doi:10.1080/09640568.2016.1165188.

Sims, L. and Sinclair, A.J., 2008. Learning through participatory programs: Case studies from Costa Rica. *Adult Education Quarterly*, 58 (2), 151–168. doi:10.1177/0741713607309802.

Sinclair, A.J., Sims, L., and Spaling, H., 2009. Community-based approaches to strategic environmental assessment: Lessons from Costa Rica. *Environmental Impact Assessment Review*, 29, 147–156. doi:10.1016/j.eiar.2008.10.002.

Taylor, E., Duveskog, D., and Friis-Hansen, E., 2012. Fostering transformative learning in non-formal settings: Farmer-field schools in East Africa. *International Journal of Lifelong Education*, 31 (6), 725–742. doi:10.1080/02601370.2012.713035.

16 Using empowering methods to research empowerment?

Peer research by girls and young women in Kinshasa, Democratic Republic of Congo

Lyndsay McLean, Triphène Mpongo,
Suzanne-Melissa Sumaili and
Naomie Tshiyamba Kabangele

Introduction

Between 2015 and 2017, the UK's Department for International Development supported a programme called *La Pépinière*, which aimed to support the empowerment of girls and young women aged 10–24 in Kinshasa, Democratic Republic of Congo (DRC). Kinshasa is a challenging urban context marked by the long-term absence of state services, corruption, high rates of unemployment, poverty, violence and gender inequalities, for example, relating to healthcare, educational attainment and decision-making power (DRC 2014; UNDP 2009, 2019). About half of Kinshasa's inhabitants are under the age of 20, and the population has grown rapidly in recent years owing to rural exodus and conflict (UNDP and UN Women 2014). The city has been documented as a precarious, sometimes violent, environment in which the majority of Kinshasa's inhabitants exercise multiple and creative forms of '*débrouille*' (resourcefulness) to survive on a daily basis (Ayipam 2014).

La Pépinière translates broadly as 'incubator' or 'greenhouse' in the sense of nurturing plants to grow healthy and strong. As part of this programme, a Girl-Led Research Unit – or *L'Unité des Fille Chercheuses* in French – was established, comprising young women researchers who were recruited, trained and mentored to participate in and lead research and project design activities. The term *fille* (or girl) was chosen by the researchers and in this context is commonly applied to young unmarried women and is not seen as pejorative. When *La Pépinière* was set up, the focus of most research and aid funding was on conflict and sexual violence in Eastern DRC and there was little information about the lives of girls and women in Kinshasa. The initial phase of the programme therefore focused on conducting research on the everyday realities of girls and young women and the factors that enabled or constrained their economic and social empowerment. This research was intended to influence the policies and programmes of government, donors and civil society organisations (CSOs) to reflect the priorities expressed by young women.

This chapter describes the process of developing the Girl-Led Research Unit. It then examines the benefits and challenges of peer research in a fragile context in which girls and young women have to navigate precarious circumstances to survive.

A girl-led peer methodology

The development of the Girl-Led Research Unit was informed by literature on participatory research methods with children in non-Western contexts, such as the 'children's movement' approach (Asselin and Doiron 2016) which advocates for girls and young women to have a central role in designing and conducting research about them. The first author and her Congolese counterpart (the programme's Capacity Development Manager) believed that – if recruited from a diversity of backgrounds and locations – girls and young women working as peer researchers would access a wider diversity of research participants, be better placed than adult researchers to interview them about the realities of their lives (Porter 2016; Vaughn et al. 2018), and could benefit from the process themselves in terms of their own life journeys.

With support from local community-based organisations (CBOs) working with women and young people in four districts in Kinshasa province (Kimbanseke, Gombe, Bandalungwa and Kisenso), girls and young women interested in becoming researchers were identified. Following initial pre-selection days facilitated by these CBOs in each neighbourhood, 25 girls aged 16–24 were invited to an agenda-setting workshop in late May 2015 and engaged in a process to develop *La Pépinière*'s research priorities and questions. This workshop also supported the recruitment of an initial team of 16 researchers – four from each district – on the basis of their engagement and participation in the workshop, their availability to conduct the research and their access to diverse peer networks.

These 16 researchers reflected a diversity of backgrounds and life experience: four were aged 16–19, and 12 were aged 20–24; four were university students, nine were in secondary school and three were not in, or had never been to, school; five had jobs, working as a seamstress, a hairdresser and in small trading (*petit commerce*); eight were able to read and write in French and Lingala, three could speak and write Lingala and speak (but not write) limited French, and five were illiterate in both languages (could not read or write) and spoke Lingala only; two had children; 11 lived with one or both parents, and five lived with a sibling, cousin, aunt or other relative. The three co-authors of this paper are three of the girl researchers who took part in this process.

Training took place during a series of workshops – co-facilitated by the first author and the Capacity Development Manager – with the aim of engaging these young researchers in the full research cycle 'in meaningful ways such as formulating the research questions, planning the methodology, collecting and/or analysing data, drafting recommendations and disseminating findings' (Coad and Evans

2008, p. 43). Two initial workshops – each lasting three days – focused on brainstorming concepts, agreeing research questions, formulating interview guides, training the researchers in qualitative interviewing skills, discussing participant recruitment strategies and agreeing ethical protocols.

During the first workshop we co-developed interview guides covering themes such as the socio-economic circumstances of girls and young women (e.g. education, income generation); their decision-making power relating to education, work, home life and relationships; the influence of family, friends, organisations and role models in their lives; understandings of 'empowerment' and social and contextual factors that facilitate and impede these processes; and life aspirations. We also worked together to determine purposive sampling and appropriate data collection methods for research participants. We decided that the girl researchers would each conduct a series of 12 one-to-one semi-structured interviews over a four-week period. They each undertook a participatory analysis of their social networks to identify interviewees including younger girls, peers of a similar age, and adult men or women who were influential in the lives of girls within their local communities.

The second workshop focused on interview practice and ethical considerations. Practice interviews were recorded and collectively analysed to identify and reflect on problems with how questions were asked and opportunities for improved probing and cross-checking. We then undertook a pilot round of interviews with girls and young women and followed the same process. During a participatory risk analysis exercise, girl researchers brainstormed potential risks to themselves and others and we jointly devised mitigation strategies and ethical approaches to dealing with anticipated problems and difficulties.

Data collection took place after these two workshops, supported by a mentoring system whereby each team of four girl researchers was assigned an adult mentor – either from the University of Kinshasa or a local CSO – with a background in research and working with girls and young women. Working in pairs, four researchers met weekly with their assigned mentor to listen to and discuss interviews; receive coaching on how to further improve their interviewing technique; undertake and document (on paper or via audio recordings) initial analysis of interviews. During these meetings, the mentors led a group reflection process and documented weekly notes on the progress of each girl researcher, the key findings by theme and the group discussion.

In total, interviews were conducted with 117 young women aged 12–24 and 60 influential adults (e.g. teachers, religious and community leaders, members of community-based organisations, and local business-women). Through a purposive sampling strategy, we reached a diversity of girls and young women, including those in education, work, combining the two, or struggling to earn an income; those living with parents, other family members or friends (rare) and those stigmatised because they engaged in sex work, transactional sex or were *fille-mères* (girl mothers). Interviews lasted 45–90 minutes, were conducted in Lingala (the majority language) or French, audio-recorded on smartphones, and took place in private, quiet locations in homes, community spaces and cafés.

All interviews were transcribed and translated into French by two of the researchers (literate in French and Lingala) and the mentors. They were then double-coded – informed by a coding framework derived from the interview discussion guides and additional inductive codes identified from the data – by the first author and a junior researcher, with support from the Capacity Development Manager. Thematic analysis was then undertaken and further cross-referenced with the weekly analysis forms/audio from each girl researcher and the weekly notes from the research mentors to identify commonalities and discrepancies.

At this stage, the girl researchers participated in another two further three-day participatory data analysis workshops, with support from the mentors, first author and Capacity Development Manager. The first workshop focused on training the girl researchers in data analysis skills, and engaged them in a systematic process of reviewing, checking and synthesising findings and discussing their implications for policy and practice. The second workshop focused on validation whereby the girl researchers presented the findings to the wider La Pépinière team. Thereafter, a study report was written (McLean-Hilker et al. 2016) and the girl researchers presented findings to representatives of government, donors and CSOs, and to community members in their neighbourhoods.

Several strategies were employed to ensure the full inclusion of all girl researchers in the process irrespective of differing literacy levels: the training and analysis workshops employed visual methods and were conducted in French and Lingala; the interview guides were produced in audio versions; and smartphones were used to record interviews. Each girl researcher understood and signed a formal letter of engagement, and received an appropriate daily stipend and subsistence for participation in the workshops, and a stipend per interview conducted. They were also given a monthly phone credit voucher and gifted the smartphone.

Peer research findings

Detailed research findings and recommendations are documented elsewhere (McLean and Modi 2016; McLean-Hilker et al. 2016). Here we identify and reflect on those findings which would have been especially difficult to identify without the use of a peer research approach.

Understanding 'empowerment'

While much debated, the term 'empowerment' can broadly be understood as a process during which individuals or groups experience enhanced social, political and economic power, agency or access to resources (Kabeer 1999; Lutrell et al. 2009). The word does not translate directly into French (*autonomisation* does not have the same meaning), nor Lingala. It was therefore important to understand local notions and ideas about empowerment in Kinshasa according to girls' and young women's own definitions.

Understandings of empowerment among girls and young women were multifaceted and not aligned with English or French definitions. During the research processes we identified and interrogated five terms in Lingala which were variously used to signify women with 'autonomy', 'agency', 'independence' and 'power'. The first, *mwasi malonga*, referred to a woman who was valued and respected in society as she had succeeded economically and socially, supported herself and others, and conformed with predominant social norms. *Mwasi amikoka*, on the other hand, referred to a woman who was capable, independent and economically self-sufficient. *Grande dame* referred to a woman with high status and profile, and who was capable, admired and valued. *Mwasi elombe* depicted a capable, ambitious and autonomous woman, who was self-sufficient, supporting herself and others. Finally, *elombe mwasi* referred to a dynamic, capable and physically powerful woman, who did not necessarily conform to social norms and was not necessarily well-respected by others.

Most girls and young women interviewed aspired to become a *mwasi malonga* who had economic self-sufficiency, independence from men and societal recognition as a capable, 'useful' and respected woman. Social integration and recognition were perceived to be as important as economic autonomy, and these required conforming to dominant social expectations about women's behaviour. We found that interviewees with some economic autonomy had mostly received social support to achieve this: some had been helped by their family to study and had started working alongside their studies around the time of puberty; others had received start-up capital usually from a family member; and/ or had received support from an older woman to 'socialise' them into a trade and associated networks.

Social norms and pressures

Interviewees described the social pressures they felt associated with the close policing of their behaviour, sexuality and fertility from the onset of puberty, both by their families and wider society. They described being categorised as either 'good girls' or 'bad girls', with a girl's life chances dependent on being *bien vu* (well regarded) in society. Good girls were seen as polite, respectful, 'serious' and *soumise* (submissive) to family and community expectations. They dressed conservatively; spent time productively studying, working or praying; avoided boys and pre-marital sex; married well; and became good wives and mothers by supporting their family economically and contributing to society.

A girl could quickly get a reputation as a bad girl if she was impolite, disrespectful and *légère* (easy), if she dressed in tight clothes, spoke her mind, was seen with boys, or gave birth to a child outside marriage:

> They always think badly of girls. If they see you chatting with boys, they expect you to get pregnant and stop your studies …. My paternal uncle can come to the house and if he sees me in shorts or a mini-skirt, he thinks that I have started love affairs with men.
>
> (Girl interviewee, 14 years old)

Girls that are said to be less serious include *mitu etoka nzinzi* [those with flies in their heads], *bana boya toli* [those who refuse advice], *likolo likolo* [in the air, in the air]. Those who dress badly – short dress, bare back, belly button on the outside …transparent neckline, underwear showing, bad characters, impolite…

(Man interviewee, 34 years old)

It was variously assumed – whether true or not – that a bad girl was having sexual relationships with many men to earn money, spending her time unproductively or in the wrong type of work. Such girls experienced unkind gossip, rejection by their friends and family and, sometimes, exclusion from community spaces such as schools and churches.

Girls and young women are perceived as personally responsible for meeting or falling short of dominant expectations. However, these expectations are out of step with a social reality in which many young women are expected to contribute money to households once they reach puberty; where men and boys pressure young women to have sexual relations and often use money and gifts to persuade them, and where sexual and reproductive health services are simply not accessible to unmarried girls and women. Few adult interviewees recognised how such social and economic pressures influenced young women's lives and the challenges, risks and obstacles young women face in trying to meet social expectations.

Precarious life experiences

Research findings suggested that most young women in their teenage years were ambitious about their future. Girls variously aspired to find a 'good job' as a doctor, businesswoman, lawyer, seamstress or journalist; to become 'rich and famous'; and/ or be 'useful' and help others in society. Yet interviewees aged over 18 described how their self-confidence could plummet after the completion of their studies and the pressure they felt to get married. While most girls and young women aspired to marry – and gain the social status associated with being a married woman – many feared constraints on their time, mobility and decision-making power, as well as the violence and lack of partner support that marriage could bring.

It is the possessive man … the man who sees the woman as a baby maker, a housewife … not someone who can look him in the eyes and say 'not this'. My aunt, for example, has a car and wants to learn to drive, but her husband insists on taking a chauffeur as he does not want to see her at the wheel …. Why? He does not want to see an emancipated woman who can take the steering wheel and go anywhere without him knowing …. It is men who are a brake on women's emancipation.

(Young woman interviewee, aged 24)

In this respect, it was striking that few of the older women role models the interviewees referred to as 'empowered' and 'successful' were married.

Young women's accounts also described the precarious nature of life for girls and young women in Kinshasa where there were few social or economic safety nets. Even for those who appeared to be progressing socially and economically, life chances could change rapidly as the result of the loss of a parent, illness in the family (and the associated medical expenses), becoming pregnant, or having their money or goods stolen.

Reflections on the peer research process

New skills and competencies for researchers

A core focus of this project was to help girls to develop new skills and competencies (see Porter 2016; Vaughn et al. 2018). In collaboration with each young woman, we therefore developed individual capacity development plans – covering personal and research skills and capacities – which were reviewed on a regular basis by the research mentors. Examples included organisational skills (e.g. the ability to plan interviews and manage time, and participate in agreed training and mentoring sessions); problem solving skills (e.g. the ability to manage unexpected circumstances and adapt to local realities); communication and social skills (e.g. communicating and maintaining good relationships with research participants and colleagues); and qualitative research skills (e.g. semi-structured interviewing, understanding and applying ethical guidelines, and data analysis).

Audio and video testimonies were collected from the girl researchers at various stages of the process – after research training, following the completion of this first study, and at the end of the first phase of *La Pépinière* project two years later. These demonstrated that positive changes in researchers' personal and professional capacities (McLean-Hilker et al. 2016), including in organisational skills, research and listening skills, self-awareness, confidence to participate in group discussions; relationship-building and collaborative skills; and open-mindedness towards others of different backgrounds and views. The names of girl researchers below are pseudonyms.

> The project has helped me to know the lives of other girls. I might have had my own ideas, but now I understand their own ideas .... I also learned how to ask good questions, how to put people at ease.
>
> (Evelyne, 16 years old, November 2015)

> By becoming a girl researcher, I also learn a lot myself and this helps me to progress today, tomorrow, or in the future. It has helped be to become more knowledgeable ... and I now know what I am capable of by myself.
>
> (Trinité, 24 years old, November 2015)

Wider economic and social impact on peer researchers

In September 2018, we collected further testimonies from several girl researchers about how their involvement in the peer research and *La Pépinière* programme had affected their lives. The testimonies demonstrate how involvement in peer research work can contribute to longer-term positive changes.

In addition to receiving a small stipend during this first study, the researchers were supported by their mentors and the Capacity Development Manager to invest these funds into specific projects which they felt could help them economically and/or socially. Some paid secondary school or university fees for themselves or a sibling; one set up a small stall selling food and joined a *likelemba* group savings and loans group; two others began to trade in clothing, bags and shoes, or jewellery; one started selling telephone credit and one expanded her hairdressing business.

> Beforehand, I did a little small trading, but I didn't save ... with *La Pépinière*, I started to understand how to save ... now I have opened a shop where I sell playstations and telephones .... I see that I am autonomous now. I have decision-making power. If I say no, it's no .... I am saving for doing more studying .... I want to restart university .... *La Pépinière* really trained me ...
> (Dévine, 23 years old, September 2018)

In line with the vision to ensure the participation of girls and young women throughout the programme, 15 girl researchers also continued their involvement with *La Pépinière* beyond this first study. This included roles as co-researchers and research assistants on other studies conducted by the programme, for example, with a Congolese partner research organisation, CERED-GL. Several researchers also took on roles in the monitoring and support teams for the pilot empowerment projects undertaken by the programme. One girl researcher eventually secured a job with CERED-GL:

> Professionally, I gained competencies that I did not have before ... now I have a job with CERED-GL. I learned about writing reports and how to explain their purpose to others .... I learned so many things from *La Pépinière* which have made me who I am today.
> (Rita, 26 years old, September 2018)

In September 2018, eight of the girl researchers were working to establish their own organisation to offer advice to Congolese and international organisations on programmes and policies for girls and young women. Each was paying a small amount into a core fund from their own income generating activities to support the set-up process. They were in the process of setting up an advisory board, had already been engaged to support two projects and were regularly consulted by NGOs and donor agencies.

> At the start, I didn't know anything about my capacities and how I could earn for myself .... Then I realised I could do this work and develop professional

capacities at the same time as studying …. I have continued to progress …. I was hired for one project to accompany children through a research process …. I have been invited to many trainings …. People want my opinion now …. I have been consulted many times … sometimes voluntary, sometimes paid.

(Prudence, 21 years old, September 2018)

Socially, within family and friendship networks, researchers reported changes in the ways they were perceived by others.

I now have a team of sisters …. I can call them if I have a problem …. I can count on them … a sort of family has been created …. In my [own] family, now I am considered highly …. My father now calls me as well as my brothers to ask advice …. This never happened before …. With my friends, they see that I work, they see my pictures on Facebook …. I get respect …. My uncle has changed how he speaks to me – he now speaks with respect …. At the personal level, I have learned how to manage my time …. I improved my Lingala …. I can now talk in front of a crowd …. I have no fear to approach someone and talk to them.

(Betty, 25 years old, September 2018)

One researcher – Félicité (pseudonym) – could not read or write and spoke Lingala and no French when we recruited her in May 2015. Her father had died when she was young and at the start of the project she was living with her mother in a poor area of Kinshasa and working as a hairdresser to earn income. Despite these challenges, Félicité proved to be one of the best peer researchers and by the end of the initial three-month research period – with the support of other members of the group – she had already started to read and write a little and speak some French. She then used her stipends to pay for a training course in sewing and set up a successful business. When we met her again in 2018, she had increased her income and reflected:

Before *La Pépinière*, I didn't know who I was and what I could do in life … then I learned that even if I was a 'girl-mother', my life was not ruined and I could still do something …. I became an example for other girls in my family and my neighbourhood …. I was on TV and showed other girls and other people what was possible even for a girl-mother and this gave hope …. Through *La Pépinière*, I developed my capacities to be a role model and a mentor for other girls …. I developed my business and looked after my brothers and sisters …. In the neighbourhood, many families send their girls to me for advice and mentoring …. I also work in the neighbourhood, so women know their rights.

(Félicité, 23 years old, September 2018)

Managing research 'quality'

Concerns about the reliability, validity and credibility of data collected and analysis carried out by people who are not qualified researchers are well documented (e.g. Vaughn et al. 2018). In this study, we used a number of approaches to enhance research quality.

First, the process of training the researchers and piloting interviews was intensive, comprising a step-by-step participatory process as described above. Second, weekly mentoring during the data collection process helped to troubleshoot problems, answer questions, hone and improve the researchers' interviewing and analysis skills on an ongoing basis. Girl researchers could also call their research mentor at any time to get support and advice. Third, the data analysis process was multi-stage and multifaceted. The scripts were double coded by the first author, a junior researcher and the Capacity Development Manager and analysed separately by the girl researcher teams with their mentors. During the coding process, the team discounted or treated with caution any responses to leading questions and any inconsistent findings. In the two data analysis workshops, the first author, Capacity Development Manager and mentors co-analysed data patterns and key findings and worked with the girl researchers to check for inconsistencies and negative cases which did not fit emerging trends.

Undertaking these steps to enhance the quality of data when using a peer research approach does entail relatively intensive support to the researchers, including a degree of on-the-job learning through mentoring and support. However, as with any research study, care is required to design the training, data collection methodology and analysis processes to minimise sources of bias and maximise validity of study findings and conclusions.

In this case, the authors are confident that the peer research approach was vital to this study – to the nature, depth and quality of the data collected, the contextual interpretation of the findings, and the recommendations formulated. Without the girl researchers, it would have been difficult to access a diversity of girls and young women – especially those hard-to-reach and social excluded such as sex workers. Moreover, in this context, it is unlikely that girls and young women would have talked so openly about sensitive issues around intimate relationships and sexual and reproductive health with adults or people they did not know.

Managing risk

Peer research approaches are not free of risk. Becoming a 'peer researcher' can shift an individual's sense of who they are, according them new powers and privileges, and affect their relationships with friends, families and communities (Devotta et al. 2016; Porter 2016). We attempted to anticipate this through a participatory risk assessment with the researchers during the second research training workshop.

One risk identified was linked to each researcher having a smartphone to record interviews and communicate with the rest of the team. The phones provided were not expensive, but in the milieu where many researchers lived, they were luxury items girls would not normally have access to. The girls predicted that their possessing such a phone might trigger questions and gossip about their involvement in a research project involving outsiders – in particular white Europeans. They said that family and community members might assume that they were being paid a lot of money and start to pressure them. We therefore undertook some safety training around how the researchers could talk about their involvement in *La Pépinière*, and when and how they would conduct interviews and safely use their smartphone. For example, they agreed never to use their phones in public spaces in the neighbourhood, to only conduct interviews in their home, cafés or community spaces.

Despite this, during the pilot work, a researcher – Marie – had her smartphone stolen by her mother's boyfriend and when she tried to retrieve it, he smashed it and threatened her. Marie's mentor – a trained support worker from the local CBO – learned that Marie regularly suffered abuse from her mother and boyfriend and helped connect her to support services. Despite this, Marie realised that her involvement in the project would worsen her situation and opted to withdraw.

Félicité's story also illustrates the jealousies and pressures a peer researcher can be subjected to as a result of a change in personal situation. Her experiences as a peer researcher attracted the interest of an international organisation that was making a TV series about courageous young women. Félicité was invited to tell her story as part of the series:

> Due to the TV programme, I had some problems. The people who had testi-fied about me thought that I was paid for that but I wasn't …. They thought I had earned money and not given them anything …. These people even went to the police to accuse me of taking all the money without thinking of them …. They wouldn't believe that I volunteered for this …. They even got law-yers involved … and I had to move to a different commune to get away from the harassment …. I tried to find the cameramen who had filmed so they could testify for me, but they weren't in Kinshasa any more …. I stayed away from the neighbourhood a long time and just now I am moving back again.

We asked her if she wished that she had not got involved with the peer research:

> Despite this, if I had the opportunity again, I would not refuse to do it …. I would do it again, over and over again. It has changed my life for the better.

Testimonies such as these show how an individual's involvement in peer research can affect their life in both positive and negative ways. They highlight key ethical responsibilities during a peer research process and suggest that risk management processes could also be supplemented by engaging with family and community members of young researchers to prepare the ground for their involvement.

Longer-term impacts of peer research

The peer research process and research outputs have led to positive impacts which reach beyond the lives of the girl researchers themselves. Over the 30-month project, we witnessed how *La Pépinière's* researchers became change agents in their families, communities and wider societies. Their work enabled Congolese and international organisations to recognise girls and young women as capable, skilled and resilient actors, acknowledge the specific situation and needs of this demographic, and develop new initiatives, policies and programmes to support them. A senior ministry official, for example, said:

> I saw the development of the Girl-Led Research Unit from the onset .... I was really impressed by the capacities of these adolescent girls and young women, especially those who were illiterate. The programme did an amazing job of training them and building their capacities. These girls showed that even if they could not read or write, that they could learn how to do research and do good research .... I saw these girls develop their self-confidence. There were some who were afraid to speak at the beginning and then, through the training, learned to do research, analyse issues and express themselves and stand up in front of government officials and donors and talk about the lives of girls in Kinshasa .... They did really good research, showing us the difficulties that young girls face in their lives, how much pressure they are under, but also how hard they work .... It really changed things for many people in government to see young girls stand up and give their analysis so confidently .... We realised that they were a really important group to consult.
> (Senior official, Ministry of Gender, Family and Children, DRC)

Following the initial peer research and the dissemination of the research findings in different fora in Kinshasa, international and local organisations started to engage the girl researchers, as well as other girls and young women, in their programme teams and approaches. For example, a Save the Children project was informed by the peer research approach and results of *La Pépinière*, and it recruited four of the girl researchers to train and mentor 10–14 year olds to conduct peer research on sexual and reproductive health for one of their programmes. A local NGO called Search for Common Ground engaged girl researchers to design a new programme for young people in Kinshasa with a focus on social and political empowerment.

In 2017, as a result of the research, the Ministry of Gender consulted the project's researchers and other girls and young women on the priorities for the new Government of DRC National Action Plan on Security Council Resolution 1325 (Women, Peace and Security) leading to a development of a special annex to the plan on girls and young women.

> I was so impressed with the capabilities of these young women from *La Pépinière* .... So I invited five girl researchers and other young women to a consultative workshop to work on the new National Action Plan on 1325. We developed a special annex on the need and priorities of girls and women and then managed to put some objectives and language in the main National

Action Plan. This is the first National Action Plan in Africa to explicitly refer to the needs of girls and young women.

(Senior official, Ministry of Gender, Family and Children, DRC)

Conclusion

Over the last decade, there has been growing recognition of the important role that girls and young women can play as researchers and advisors in the development of new policies and programmes. Although lauded for their focus on women's and girls' capacities, some approaches have also been subject to substantial critique, including the way they can instrumentalise, pressure and disempower girls and young women (see Batliwala 2007; Gonick et al. 2009; Koffman and Gill 2013).

The risks and challenges experienced by some of the peer researchers in this study reinforce the need to work with peer researchers to carefully develop ethical and practical procedures to enhance the safety of their participation. These should ensure young people employed in research roles are aware of the potential risks and benefits of their involvement, are given the opportunity to make their own choices, and are supported to participate safely, develop new skills and enhance career opportunities through the research.

Experience with the *La Pépinière* project has demonstrated that, with adequate training and mentoring, girls and young women – including those with limited literacy skills – can co-lead research design, data collection and data analysis processes, and produce good quality, credible qualitative research findings. Moreover, it shows that peer research approaches can access data that would be difficult to obtain through other study designs, enabling access to hard-to-reach groups and in-depth interviewing about sensitive subjects. Finally, peer research approaches can have a significant positive impact on the lives of those trained as peer researchers, as well as others around them, be these family and community members or individuals and organisations with the power to change policy and practice.

References

Asselin, M. and Doiron, R., 2016. Ethical issues facing researchers working with children in international contexts. *Canadian Children*, 41 (1), 24–35.

Ayipam, S., 2014. *Economie de la débrouille à Kinshasa: Informalité, commerce et réseaux sociaux*. Paris: Karthala.

Batliwala, S., 2007. Taking the power out of empowerment: An experiential account. *Development in Practice*, 17 (4/5), 557–565.

Coad, J. and Evans, R., 2008. Reflections on practical approaches to involving children and young people in the data analysis process. *Children & Society*, 22, 41–52.

Democratic Republic of Congo (DRC), 2014. *Demographic and Health Survey 2013–2014*. Ministère du Plan et Suivi (Ministry of Planning) et Ministère de la Santé Publique (Ministry of Public Health), MEASURE DHS, ICF International, Rockville, MD, U.S.A.

Devotta, K., et al., 2016. Enriching qualitative research by engaging peer interviewers. *Qualitative Research*, 16 (6), 661–680.

Gonick, M., et al., 2009. Rethinking agency and resistance: What comes after girl power? *Girlhood Studies*, 2 (2), 1–9.

Kabeer, N., 1999. Resources, agency, achievements: Reflections on the measurement of women's empowerment. *Development and Change*, 30 (3), 435–464.

Koffman, O. and Gill, R., 2013. 'The revolution will be led by a 12 year old girl': Girl power and global biopolitics. *Feminist Review*, 105, 83–102.

Lutrell, C. and Quiroz, S., with Scrutton, C. and Bird, K., 2009. *Understanding and Operationalising Empowerment*. London: ODI.

McLean, L. and Modi, A.T., 2016. 'Empowerment' of adolescent girls and young women in Kinshasa: Research about girls, by girls. *Gender & Development*, 24 (3), 475–491.

McLean-Hilker, L., Jacobson, J., and Modi, A.T., 2016. *The Realities of Adolescent Girls and Young Women in Kinshasa: Research about Girls, by Girls*. Kinshasa: La Pépinière. Available from: http://www.sddirect.org.uk/media/1700/la-pep-glru-full-report-english.pdf [Accessed 8 March 2020].

Porter, G., 2016. Reflections on co-investigation though peer research with young people and older people in sub-Saharan Africa. *Qualitative Research*, 16 (3), 293–304.

UNDP, 2009. *Province de Kinshasa: Profil Resumé: Pauvreté et conditions de Vie Des Ménages*. Available from: https://www.undp.org/content/dam/dem_rep_congo/docs/povred/UNDP-CD-Profil-Ville-Kinshasa.pdf [Accessed 8 March 2020].

UNDP and UN Women, 2014. *Profil du genre dans la Ville-Province de Kinshasa: Draft 1*. Kinshasa: UNDP and UN Women.

UNDP, 2019. *Human Development Report 2019*. Available from: http://hdr.undp.org/en/2019-report [Accessed 8 March 2020].

Vaughn, L.M., et al., 2018. Partnering with insiders: A review of peer models across community-engaged research, education and social care. *Health and Social Care in the Community*, 26 (6), 769–786.

17 Lessons learned from Australian case studies of sex workers engaged in academic research about sex worker health, well-being and structural impediments

Roanna Lobo, Kahlia McCausland, Julie Bates, Linda Selvey, Jesse Jones, Elena Jeffreys, Judith Dean and Lisa Fitzgerald

Introduction

Any consideration of the challenges for sex workers, current or past, working with academic teams in sex work-related research needs to also consider the hopes, desires and ongoing support necessary to advance policy change. I consider myself an 'accidental' researcher. I learned very early in my activist life that to get anywhere with policy change and funding for the representation of marginalised communities, it was essential to provide evidence on the structural impediments to full and healthy lives. My overarching preoccupation in any activity to do with sex work is to challenge myths and prejudice while encouraging new allies and forming new alliances in support of policy change and person-centred approaches to care and support. So began a partnership of sorts with clinicians, researchers and academic teams to gather and present findings of evidence-based research to government inquiries and legislative debates on law reform. My role and motivations as a sex worker engaging in academic research are not unique. What is unique is arriving at a time and place in life where disclosure is no longer a consideration in terms of impact on my now adult children and other family members or career paths. The challenge for academic teams is in translating research findings into reforms that honour the hopes, dreams and labour of peers involved in the project and find ways and means of funding and supporting the necessary advocacy needed to advance policy change.

(Julie Bates, AO)

The term 'sex work' is now used widely in academia, since its use was first acknowledged by the World Health Organization in the early 1990s and UNAIDS in 2000 (Jeffreys 2015). Importantly, the majority of people who provide sexual services – whether as a chosen career, for short-term income earning or to supplement other low paying jobs – prefer the term 'sex worker' and that their labour is defined as work. The more pejorative terms 'prostitute' or 'prostitution' are demeaning, stigmatising and detract from the position that sex work is legitimate and valued work to be afforded all of the necessary human, legal and labour rights protection the rest of society expects.

In this chapter, we draw on two Australian case studies that employed sex workers as peer researchers to discuss the impact of the sex work research on policy and practice. We seek to expose tensions associated with power dynamics in research partnerships, and outline lessons from our work to support future sex work-related research that puts sex workers, current and past, at the heart of the research to maximise impact.

Researching for, about and with sex workers

Sex work is not a risky practice in and of itself. The harms to health and well-being associated with sex work are generally deemed to be caused by structural impediments in policy, policing and allied health and support services. The criminalisation of aspects of sex work in many countries, including the majority of Australian states and territories (Donovan et al. 2012), is a structural impediment that contributes to sex workers' experiences of stigma and discrimination (McCausland et al. 2020). Sex work research that contributes evidence to advocate for legislative change in this area is therefore highly valued by sex workers. The legacy of the successful Australian response to the HIV epidemic in the 1990s (Bates and Berg 2014; Fitzgerald et al. 2019) is evident as sex workers remain actively engaged in community mobilisation, fighting stigma and discrimination, and challenging draconian laws (Aroney and Crofts 2019). When researching any aspect of sex work and sex workers' health and well-being, best practice identifies the importance of engaging sex workers as equals and not speaking for them (Jeffreys 2010). It is imperative that sex workers' voices, whether current or past, be heard in any research related to their rights or labour.

The term 'peer researcher' is a commonly used descriptor to designate the meaningful participation of members (peers) of the community under investigation in research (Vaughn et al. 2018), and has been defined as 'members of the target population who are trained to participate as co-researchers' (Roche et al. 2010, p. 4). In the context of sex work research in academic settings, peers joining a research team can include persons not formally employed in universities who are recruited for their lived experience of sex work, and persons formally employed with a lived experience of sex work, who may or may not be 'out' (i.e. openly disclosing their peer experience to academic colleagues, key stakeholders and other sex workers). Not all sex workers are out due to experiences of stigma and discrimination (Ahearne 2015; Heineman 2016).

Collaborative research with sex workers has previously received criticism from sex worker communities for limiting sex workers' roles to that of a 'gatekeeper' used to obtain access to participants, recruiting peers too late in the project, and restricting peer researcher positions to the simplest forms of collaboration rather than leadership (Jeffreys 2010). When research about sex work is undertaken by sex workers, the hostilities that may exist between the researcher and the researched are alleviated by the united aims of both parties. The risks of unwanted research – being over-researched or investing time and resources in research that does not result in changes to practice and policy – are also reduced. Employing sex workers as peer researchers ensures a more equal power relationship between the data collector and participant (Kim and Jeffreys 2013). Like many marginalised populations, sex workers have historically been treated as the subjects of research by academics and policymakers with limited opportunities to design and guide research. A paradigm shift is needed whereby participant-driven collaborations with researchers become the norm and 'the direction of expertise flows not from but to the researcher' (Bowen and O'Doherty 2014, p. 70).

Peer-based sex worker organisations are key advocates of participatory research and through their tenacity have had some success in shaping research processes and outcomes (Harrington 2017). Research for and about sex workers that involves sex workers as 'peer' or 'insider' researchers is not a new phenomenon and has been conducted to gain insight into diverse sex worker populations globally. There are several notable examples of best practice in peer-based sex work research internationally. In Australia, the national peak peer-based sex worker organisation, Scarlet Alliance, has conducted insider-led migrant sex work research in response to research undertaken by 'outsiders' that fails to understand and accurately present migrant sex workers' views, and policy that fails to recognise migrant sex workers as self-determining agents (Kim and Jeffreys 2013). In an effort to respond to existing gaps in HIV prevention and policy in Canada, community-based prevention research projects, such as the Maka Project Partnership, have been developed with, and implemented by, sex workers to investigate the health-related harms, service barriers, and impact of current harm reduction and prevention strategies among women working in survival sex work in Vancouver (Shannon et al. 2007).

Sex workers are best placed to represent the interests of sex worker communities while conceptualising, negotiating and discussing a research project with funders and potential outreach partners, disseminating findings, and advocating for structural and social change. Sex workers therefore should be consulted and involved in every stage of the research process (Kim and Jeffreys 2013). This consultative and engagement process imparts benefits including maintaining the integrity of the project; accounting for a range of perspectives among sex workers; facilitating unparalleled access to sex workers and workplaces, particularly migrant workers and unlicensed and/or illegal brothels; and enhancing efficiency through the use of established networks and intimate knowledge of the issues and intricacies affecting sex workers (Kim and Jeffreys 2013). The experience of being trained as a peer researcher can be empowering. It builds the capacity of sex worker communities by validating existing skills and introducing new knowledge and support in developing new skills, and bestows peers with a sense of value from having a central role in the production of knowledge and outcomes of significance to their community (O'Neill et al. 2017; Lobo et al. 2020).

Sex worker peer research practice

Trans and Male Sex worker (TaMS) project

This first case study describes work undertaken by Respect Inc, the lead peer-based sex worker organisation in Queensland, Australia, as part of the 2018 Trans and Male Sex worker (TaMS) project. This community participatory project involved a collaboration between Respect Inc and The University of Queensland, investigating the sexual health experiences and needs of trans and male sex workers in Queensland. Findings from it highlight the importance of peers driving research and critical points of leadership and participation across all aspects of research.

This qualitative study included semi-structured interviews – undertaken by two peer researchers – with 35 transgender and male sex workers from across Queensland to explore identified topics including work experiences, stigma, healthcare experiences and desired changes to improve sex workers' well-being. Data were analysed by one of the peer researchers in collaboration with The University of Queensland researchers to identify trends and themes. In the project, to overcome power imbalances between university and sex worker stakeholders, the research partners developed a collaboration embedded in mutual respect and acknowledgment of the rights and responsibilities of all, outlined in a memorandum of understanding.

Universities typically hold grant or research money. In the TaMS study, the grant signatories were Respect Inc and The University of Queensland. Significantly, Respect Inc drove project spending and other major decisions. A TaMS steering committee, involving peers and academics and led by the lead peer investigator, directed and monitored all research activity, from study design and data collection to analysis, reporting and presentation. Peers also led the authorship of the TaMS Report (Jones et al. 2018) and this case study. Peers represented the project in the public sphere – including at the International AIDS Conference in Amsterdam (2018) and the Australasian HIV&AIDS Conference in Sydney (2018) – reinforcing the importance of sex workers leading project outcomes.

Research underpinned by a community participatory approach enables peers to develop research skills. Peer researchers received training from the academic partners in interviewing, data collection, qualitative analysis and reporting. These are core skills that may create longer-term career opportunities for peers. In the TaMS project, peer researchers drove recruitment and completed all interviews, gaining access to participants that a mainstream project never could, such as in unlicensed brothels.

To date, much funding for sex work research has been associated with the promotion of sexual health, with an emphasis on HIV and sexually transmissible infections (STI). This can result in a blinkered, singular focus on the pathologisation of sex work. Trans people (primarily trans women but also trans men and others) are often combined with cis men as research participant groups. This conflation of intersecting yet discrete communities is a recognised problem in the HIV and STI sectors. In the TaMS project, the funder's priorities meant that cis male and trans workers were again merged into one project, demonstrating that collaborative research faces the same problematic trends as any other and is not immune to their potential pitfalls.

TaMS results identified that most participants described stigma and discrimination as barriers to accessing health services, however, these experiences differed between transgender and male sex workers. In particular, cis male workers spoke of the impact of homophobia but not as a specific barrier to access. Trans workers experienced transphobia and described how this combined with a lack of appropriate transgender affirming healthcare was a key barrier to accessing sexual health services. These differences highlight the problem with merging two very separate populations in a research project, even when all are sex workers.

The challenges of merging discrete populations, which is often driven by funders' priorities rather than community needs, raises the question of how to be critical in defining the topics pursued. Understanding HIV and STI issues must include exploration of general well-being and human rights. What peers wanted from the TaMS project was advocacy for decriminalisation, as a step towards improving sex worker health and well-being. How, then, could the TaMS project advance decriminalisation of sex work?

The research analysis identified themes relating to human rights, privacy, police abuse, stigma and marginalisation resulting from the law. This provided evidence of systemic obstacles of relevance to sex worker communities. As such, although decriminalisation was not specifically addressed in the research interview questions, it was an overarching theme and was presented in the final report as a determinant of sex worker health.

In the case of the TaMS project, the main output was a report to State government, with the sex worker peer researchers as lead authors. The report was presented to the State Health Minister, but the government has not provided funding to implement the project's key recommendations. Respect Inc has prioritised work identified by the TaMS outcomes, in particular sustainable, ongoing peer education led by trans and male sex workers. However, once the research was complete, and without follow-up funding, there was no ethical way to reorient service provision and institute identified recommendations, short of cancelling other activities. Problems often arise in short-term or brief activities targeting marginalised communities. TaMS identified that a longer-term commitment is required for project work to be fair, equitable and genuine. Nonetheless, the report has provided guidance for short-term work.

Engagement between the peer and academic researchers did not end with the TaMS report. The University of Queensland team and Respect Inc forged a relationship during TaMS that continues today. Activities by the university researchers include media involvement and lobbying for sex work decriminalisation, support within the health sector to raise the profile of sex worker issues, speaking at joint events, and discussion of trends and issues. The University of Queensland and Respect Inc workers are in the same sector and can harness academic and health practitioner credibility in support of decriminalisation, ensuring that sex worker demands receive attention in ways that sex workers alone cannot achieve. Messages from sex workers may be taken more seriously coming from academics, raising the issue of how to achieve that balance without academics taking over. The TaMS relationship has built trust between these groups.

Law and Sex worker Health (LASH) 2.0 study

The Law and Sex worker Health (LASH) study conducted in 2006 was a comparative study of the impact of different sex work legislation on the health and welfare of female sex workers in three Australian states, from prohibition in Western Australia, to legalisation/licensing in Victoria and decriminalisation in New South Wales (Donovan et al. 2012). One decade later, the Western Australian Department of Health commissioned the LASH 2.0 study (Selvey et al. 2017). A quantitative survey (paper-based and online) and in-depth interviews were used to examine changes in the sex industry in Western Australia; the impact of legislation on sex worker health and safety; and the intersections between sex workers, service providers and police. The study recruited 354 sex workers of all genders living in urban and regional areas.

Sex workers' expertise critically informed the design and conduct of both LASH studies. A member of the academic research team who was also a sex worker peer and long-term activist for the human and legal rights of sex workers was a key participant in both studies. With peer colleagues, she developed and implemented recruitment and training protocols for peer researchers, and engaged with owners of sex work businesses and other stakeholders. A project advisory group with representatives from the Western Australian sex worker support and advocacy organisations supported and guided the research. For example, highlighting the need for confidentiality, they recommended participants provide consent by ticking a box (no name required).

Eight sex workers, diverse in age, gender, sexual orientation, socio-economic status, culture, ethno-racial identity and sex industry experience were employed as peer researchers to undertake the fieldwork component of the study. Specific tasks were outlined in a job description and peer researchers were employed for their skills in health promotion, peer outreach, social research, knowledge of sex work businesses (i.e. including brothels, massage parlours, private and street-based sector, and escort agencies), and/or ability to speak Thai, Korean or Chinese. The academic research team provided research training for peer researchers, focusing on ethical considerations, data collection, recruitment, and fieldwork protocol and policies. See Lobo et al. (2020) for further details of the collaborative processes adopted.

Six months after the project ended, the peer researchers were invited to reflect on their experiences as peer researchers through semi-structured interviews which provided an opportunity to debrief and to identify lessons learned. Seven peers agreed to participate and through their reflections, several key issues were raised, of which some are discussed here.

Peer researchers believed their experience as sex workers, and knowledge of the sex industry enabled them to recruit survey participants for the study, as a result of existing relationships and empathy within the community. Recruitment included accessing male and trans sex workers, people who used illicit drugs, and those offering sexual services in venues where people may be 'cruising' for sex partners. However, peer researchers can still experience challenges in accessing study populations despite being peers (Roche et al. 2010). Gaining access to sex workers of Asian background in the LASH 2.0 study presented difficulties despite employing Asian peer researchers and translating the survey instrument into Korean, Chinese and Thai languages. Recruitment difficulties may have reflected the challenges experienced by Asian sex workers in Western Australia. These included social isolation, fear of disclosure, stress, and uncertainty about their legal standing, especially for those sex workers who had worked in other jurisdictions, leading to fear of authorities, including researchers (Selvey et al. 2018).

Peer researchers also experienced challenges when hearing study participants' views about sex work and legislation that were inconsistent with their own perspectives, or those of peer-based sex worker organisations, and discussed the difficulties of separating their roles as researchers and peers. Other insider research (Heslop et al. 2018) has also noted challenges related to role duality. The credibility of the LASH 2.0 study required that the position of trust held by peer researchers and the broader sex worker community was not compromised during the research process, resulting in animosity from peers or additional challenges to future peer-based outreach programmes.

What drives changes to policy and practice?

Recognising the motivations, needs and roles of all research partners

As evidenced in both of the case studies discussed here, sex worker (current and past) peers have a diverse range of skills, experiences and qualifications, including academic qualifications, and can provide invaluable expertise and insights as part of the research team beyond their peer experience and as 'gatekeepers'. However, sex workers who engage in academic research may experience issues of role conflict as a result of their ties to research institutions. Keeping relationships stable and navigating social standing amongst peers both during and after a study is important, particularly if the research findings are not supportive of broader sex work advocacy.

Sex workers engaged as peer researchers were generally motivated to participate in research that results in outcomes that benefit their peers. Action-oriented research can bridge the gap between theory and practice, although recognising that the research process may be empowering for the researched can challenge traditional assumptions of objectivity in research and the need for academic distance (Hubbard 1999). The credibility of research may subsequently be discredited or diminished as a result of peers' roles in data collection and analysis. Providing research training, supervision and support for peer researchers reduces the potential for researcher bias and helps to ensure data integrity. Sex workers engaged as peer researchers in both the studies described here demonstrated the highest standards of conduct to avoid substantiating claims that they were unable to engage in high-quality academic research.

Academic researchers have opportunities for personal and professional growth as a result of their research activities, gaining higher degree qualifications, and promotion or building a track record leading to additional grant income. However, in the case of sex work research, there is also the potential for negative association. The stigma associated with sex work can be transposed to those researching sex work with implications for the discrediting of academic work as illegitimate, taboo or unworthy of study (Hammond and Kingston 2014). Without academics being willing to partner with sex workers in research, sex work research in academic settings cannot occur. The 'survival' of such academics through the delivery of traditional academic outputs is therefore critical. Such outputs can be slow to realise and the time taken to develop research findings that have tangible impacts on policy and practice change can be lengthy. While problematic, this situation is not dissimilar to the challenges involved in health promotion and prevention research where outcomes may not be seen for years (Jackson and Shiell 2017). Researchers motivated to work in this area can do so by building long-term, trusting relationships with sex workers. This enables researchers to act quickly and follow funding opportunities as they arise, often for small-scale pieces of research.

Power dynamics

The sources and processes of funding sex work research can present specific issues for the conduct of peer-based research. From an ethical perspective, engaging peers as research partners requires that the issues of interest to sex workers are considered equitably with those of academic staff and funding bodies. This is not always possible, even when the academic team and funders are supportive of a partnership approach. For example, the research aims and objectives of the LASH studies were established by the funding body and focused on the impact of legislation on sex worker health and well-being. Both studies provided opportunities to include broader issues of interest to sex workers, such as issues related to stigma and discrimination of sex workers (McCausland et al. 2020). While some data were collected on these important issues, the scope was limited, with priority being given to specific impacts of sex work laws on mental and physical health and well-being (Selvey et al. 2017, 2018). Furthermore, available funding offered limited capacity to engage peers in research translation activities, including wider knowledge dissemination, co-authored publications and advocacy once the research was completed. A peer-led study investigating issues of stigma and discrimination among sex workers would have been constructed quite differently, with greater scope to develop research questions focused solely on stigma and discrimination.

Among some funders it is common practice to award monies to academic institutions rather than peer-based sex worker organisations, even if the latter have demonstrated research capabilities and will be engaged in much of the 'heavy lifting' associated with recruitment and data collection. This is where partnerships with academic research bodies can come into play in that they can provide an advocacy role for sex worker organisations seeking government funding for peer-based research projects. The TaMS study demonstrated that the sharing of funding between academic and sex worker peer-based organisations, with the peer-based organisations controlling their own budget, deepened the collaborative relationship throughout the research process, strengthening the quality of research undertaken (Jones et al. 2018).

Evidence generated by academic research is afforded a high degree of credibility within the academic community and by the general public. Depending on their experience, this may not always be the view of communities most affected by or involved in the research. The principal investigator of a study has the power to make the final decisions about how the research will be conducted. These decisions may be well intentioned but are often driven by finite resources, the expectations of funding bodies, and practical logistical matters. The number of sex workers in principal investigator roles is hard to quantify due to the potential for stigma and discrimination relating to disclosure. Barriers to the participation of peers in the research may also be evident. For example, academic roles that require certain qualifications or research skills and experience may preclude the employment of sex worker peers in these roles who do not meet the minimum requirements, regardless of other valuable contributions that they may make. In the LASH studies, challenges arose for peer researchers such as lack of access to transport, necessary technology and/or technological support to conduct data collection, and the potential for being 'outed' publicly and the harms that this might cause. These significant personal and structural impediments to full participation in the research only came to light once the project was up and running through supervision sessions. However, in order to mitigate potential challenges, they must be identified, addressed and accommodated as part of the training protocols and budgetary considerations in any peer research.

Advocacy for sensible public policy

If opportunities for advocacy and the translation of research findings into action do not occur due to lack of funding allocated to such activities, what are the reciprocal benefits for peer researchers and are these equitable to those experienced by academic researchers? For research to inform policy and practice, research findings and recommendations *must* be used for advocacy purposes. Ideally, this work should augment/support existing advocacy activities or inform future advocacy needs (Abel et al. 2010). Peer-based research is more likely to reflect priorities for advocacy and therefore more likely to be used for this purpose. For the past three decades, decriminalisation of sex work has been a key driver for peer-based sex worker organisations across Australia, given that criminalisation of sex work has enormous impacts on sex worker well-being. The impacts of decriminalisation must also be supported by changes in the way society and some service providers engage with, treat and view sex workers and their industry. Therefore, anti-discrimination protections are essential to support better policy outcomes.

Unfortunately, evidence alone is rarely sufficient to achieve major change to structural impediments. What is certain is that policy change cannot happen in isolation from a range of factors, including having a strong advocacy network of peers and allies to make use of the research findings along with a willing government, and the empirical evidence to back change (Abel et al. 2010). Even when governments fund sex worker-led health and well-being support services and sex work-related research, and learn of the harms associated with criminalising any aspect of the sex industry, advances in better policy (decriminalisation) are not assured. In South Australia, the 13th attempt by sex workers and allies to affect policy change failed in 2019 with the opposition government party casting the dissenting votes. Earlier successful policy change to decriminalisation in New South Wales and New Zealand was driven and enabled by a combination of advocacy by peers and allies through representations made possible by government funding of peer-led sex worker organisations, government inquiries and research. Activism and research by the Australian Prostitutes Collective in New South Wales appear to have been influential in shifting policy directions from moralistic approaches to pragmatic responses informed by the lived experience of sex workers (Aroney and Crofts 2019).

In the case of the LASH 2.0 study, the impact of the law on sex worker health and well-being was a major focus of the project but the study was broadened because of the involvement of peers. The research was commissioned by the Western Australian Department of Health to build on the evidence from the original LASH study to support future policy decisions related to sex work legislation in Western Australia. The survey questions were shaped by input from peers resulting in a greater emphasis on stigma and discrimination than had originally been intended by the academic research team. Findings revealed the impact of criminalisation on stigma and discrimination directed towards sex workers (Selvey et al. 2017; McCausland et al. 2020), which would not otherwise have been the case. The LASH 2.0 study findings informed the Western Australian Department of Health's funding for Magenta, Western Australia's sex worker organisation. Recommendations included increased outreach of peer-based services to sole traders working privately, and to those from culturally and linguistically diverse backgrounds, particularly in rural areas, together with a range of health and support services.

The pressure on sex work activists and peers to engage in sex work research or advocacy to utilise research findings for policy change is immense. What happens though if activists are unable to continue advocacy due to lack of funding support or if sex work researchers in academic settings are unable to secure funding for future sex work research? The evidence base to date provides an advocacy tool to refute unsubstantiated claims that support harmful policies. Law reform is one priority. Ongoing advocacy and activism are critical to improving sex worker health and wellbeing. While research findings may not translate into direct and immediate local legislative reform, they can have a beneficial impact on service delivery and can inform better policing practices in jurisdictions where sex work continues to be criminalised. They can also be used by others mounting campaigns for legislative reform in other jurisdictions. Findings from the LASH studies have been used to advocate for law reform in South Australia, in submissions to the Greens party in New South Wales with their Bill for anti-discrimination protection for sex workers, and in Victoria in a review to make recommendations for decriminalisation of sex work. The findings have also been relevant for activists in the Northern Territory and Queensland to support their advocacy efforts for decriminalisation.

A single piece of research is unlikely to result in major legislative change unless there has been significant groundwork as well as a conducive political and social environment. It remains important to undertake high-quality research on the impacts of criminalisation on the health and safety of sex workers as well as other related topics to build a body of evidence to support change. Research concerning more nuanced questions is also required, informed by sex workers themselves. Translating the research findings into action then requires a dedicated team effort that is adequately resourced by funders of sex work research, to facilitate changes to policy and practice. This level of collaboration between researchers, sex workers and advocacy groups is both necessary and ethical for peer-based research.

Conclusion

No research involving sex workers should be undertaken to address questions that are not considered of high priority by sex workers. This is a significant ethical issue and is also one that affects the quality of the research and its effectiveness at influencing policy and practice. Research in which peers have had input into the research question(s), study design, data collection and analysis will be more likely to address questions of concern to sex workers themselves. It will likely be of better quality because of the reduced risk of misinterpretation and outcomes will also be used more constructively to inform policy and practice. By themselves, studies and advocacy alone will not necessarily result in policy change. What is required is a supportive sociopolitical environment and a substantial body of evidence. How this evidence is used to stimulate and support further advocacy and leadership by example in best practice sex worker-led research, will determine its impact on public policy and practice over time.

References

Abel, G., et al., 2010. *Taking the Crime Out of Sex Work: New Zealand Sex Workers' Fight for Decriminalisation*. Bristol: Bristol University Press.

Ahearne, G., 2015. Between the sex industry and academia: Navigating stigma and disgust. *Graduate Journal of Social Science*, 11 (2), 28–37.

Aroney, E. and Crofts, P., 2019. How sex worker activism influenced the decriminalisation of sex work in NSW, Australia. *International Journal for Crime, Justice and Social Democracy*, 8 (2), 50–67.

Bates, J. and Berg, R., 2014. Sex workers as safe sex advocates: Sex workers protect both themselves and the wider community from HIV. *AIDS Education and Prevention*, 26 (3), 191–201.

Bowen, R. and O'Doherty, T., 2014. Participant-Driven Action Research (PDAR) with sex workers in Vancouver. In: C. Showden and S. Majic, eds. *Negotiating Sex Work: Unintended Consequences of Policy and Activism.* Minneapolis, MN: University of Minnesota Press, 53–74.

Donovan, B., et al., 2012. *The Sex Industry in New South Wales: A Report to the NSW Ministry of Health.* Sydney: Kirby Institute, University of New South Wales.

Fitzgerald, L., Mutch, A., and Herron, L., 2019. Responding to HIV/AIDS: Mobilisation through partnerships in a public health crisis. In: J. Luetjens, M. Mintrom, and P. `t Hart, eds. *Successful Public Policy: Lessons from Australia and New Zealand.* Canberra: ANU Press, 29–58.

Hammond, N. and Kingston, S., 2014. Experiencing stigma as sex work researchers in professional and personal lives. *Sexualities*, 17 (3), 329–347.

Harrington, C., 2017. Collaborative research with sex workers. In: M. Spanger and M. Skilbrei, eds. *Prostitution Research in Context: Methodology, Representation and Power.* Abingdon: Routledge, 85–100.

Heineman, J., 2016. *Schoolgirls: Embodiment Practices among Current and Former Sex Workers in Academia.* Thesis (PhD), University of Nevada.

Heslop, C., Burns, S., and Lobo, R., 2018. Managing qualitative research as insider-research in small rural communities. *Rural and Remote Health*, 18 (3), 4576.

Hubbard, P., 1999. Researching female sex work: Reflections on geographical exclusion, critical methodologies and 'useful' knowledge. *Area*, 31 (3), 229–237.

Jackson, H. and Shiell, A., 2017. *Preventive Health: How Much Does Australia Spend and is It Enough?* Canberra: Foundation for Alcohol Research and Education.

Jeffreys, E., 2010. Sex worker-driven research: Best practice ethics. *Challenging Politics: Critical Voices.* Available at: https://www.nswp.org/resource/sex-worker-driven-research-best-practice-ethics [Accessed 29 September 2020].

Jeffreys, E., 2015. Sex worker politics and the term 'sex work'. *Research for Sex Work 14: Sex Work is Work*, 14, 1–5.

Jones, J., et al., 2018. *TaMS: Factors Influencing Trans and Male Sex Worker Access to Sexual Health Care, HIV Testing and Support Study (TaMS) Report.* Brisbane: Respect.

Kim, J. and Jeffreys, E., 2013. Migrant sex workers and trafficking – Insider research for and by migrant sex workers. *Action Learning Action Research*, 19 (1), 62–96.

Lobo, R., et al., 2020. Sex workers as peer researchers – A qualitative investigation of the benefits and challenges. *Culture, Health & Sexuality.* doi:10.1080/13691058.2020.1787520.

McCausland, K., et al., 2020. "It's stigma that makes my work dangerous": Experiences and consequences of disclosure, stigma and discrimination among sex workers in Western Australia. *Culture, Health & Sexuality.* doi:10.1080/13691058.2020.1825813.

O'Neill, M., et al., 2017. Peer talk: Hidden stories: A participatory research project with women who sell or swap sex in Teesside. *Project Report. A Way Out: Stockton-on-Tees.*

Roche, B., Guta, A., and Flicker, S., 2010. Peer research in action I: Models of practice. *Community based Research Working Paper Series.* Toronto: Wellesley Institute.

Selvey, L., et al., 2017. *Western Australian Law and Sex Worker Health (LASH) Study. A Summary Report to the Western Australian Department of Health.* Perth: School of Public Health, Curtin University.

Selvey, L., et al., 2018. Challenges facing Asian sex workers in Western Australia: Implications for health promotion and support services. *Frontiers in Public Health*, 6 (171), 4–6.

Shannon, K., et al., 2007. Community-based HIV prevention research among substance-using women in survival sex work: The Maka Project Partnership. *Harm Reduction Journal*, 4 (1), 20.

Vaughn, L., et al., 2018. Partnering with insiders: A review of peer models across community-engaged research, education and social care. *Health & Social Care in the Community*, 26 (6), 769–786.

18 The lasting impact of peer research with Indigenous communities of Guyana, South America

Jayalaxshmi Mistry, Andrea Berardi, Elisa Bignante, Deirdre Jafferally, Claudia Nuzzo, Grace Albert, Rebecca Xavier, Bernie Robertson, Lakeram Haynes and Ryan Benjamin

Introduction

Between September 2011 and March 2015, we were researchers on a European Commission-funded project titled *Local solutions for future challenges: Community Owned Best practice for sustainable Resource Adaptive management in the Guiana Shield, South America (COBRA)*. Project COBRA aimed to turn the tables on representations of Indigenous people as poor, backwards and requiring help, a deficit model that is prevalent with decision makers and undermines already existing local solutions for environmental challenges. Our aim was to investigate how Indigenous community owned solutions have the potential to act as show-cases for the world to maximise ecological sustainability and social justice. The research partnership comprised of academic institutions, civil society organisations and Indigenous associations, and the majority of the community research was carried out by five Guyanese Indigenous peer researchers (GA, RX, BR, LH and RB). They were recognised members of the North Rupununi Indigenous communities with whom research was taking place, but were also 'peers' in their kinship, ties and alliances to other Indigenous people both within Guyana and more widely in the Guiana Shield region where the research took place.

Three years after the end of Project COBRA, video interviews were conducted with the Guyanese Indigenous peer researchers, community members and wider government and non-governmental stakeholders, to evaluate the project's benefits and legacy. In this chapter, we draw on the findings of these interviews and reflect on the lasting impacts of peer research – for individuals and communities, as well as for policy and practice – beyond project implementation.

Background

Indigenous peoples manage or have tenure rights over land that intersects about 40% of all terrestrial protected areas and ecologically intact landscapes (Garnett et al. 2018), highlighting how the maintenance of a healthy planet depends significantly on the institutions and actions of Indigenous peoples. Traditional livelihood practices, such as subsistence rotational farming, fishing and hunting, within secure tenured land, form the basis of maintaining ecological integrity within Indigenous territories. These practices depend on traditional knowledge, a knowledge that is deeply woven into land, as well as the spiritual and more than human aspects of the landscape. For Indigenous peoples, culture and biodiversity are intricately connected. Yet, of the 370 million Indigenous people worldwide, many do not have adequate access to basic services such as health and education, and Indigenous people account for about 15% of the world's extreme poor (World Bank 2019). Customary values, practices and knowledge have eroded at alarming rates, with the legacy of colonialism and the ongoing struggle for land and recognition of their rights rendering Indigenous peoples among the most marginalised on the planet.

This domination has not only been of the body, but also of the mind. Indigenous knowledges have been viewed as unsophisticated, anecdotal, illegitimate and needing of validation through scientific methods. As Indigenous scholar Pualani Louis (2007, cited in Clement 2019, p. 280) states,

> We have been pathologised by Western research methods that have found us deficient either as genetically inferior or culturally deviant for generations. We have been dismembered, objectified and problematised via Western scientific rationality and reason. We have been politically, socially, and economically dominated by colonial forces and marginalized through armed struggle, biased legislation, and educational initiatives and policies that promote Western knowledge systems at the expense of our own.

This undermining of Indigenous knowledges is not a thing of the past. Indigenous people are still represented as deprived, backwards and requiring help in contemporary popular discourse. This deficit model all-too-often prevails across academia as well as policy- and decision-making arenas, meaning that scientific approaches to conservation and sustainable development are generally designed and implemented by external 'experts' (Olsson and Folke 2001; Black 2003), who not only impose generic interventions that can undermine local solutions that already exist, but also continue to maintain a narrative of Indigenous peoples as dependent, naive and ignorant (Kaplan 2000).

Thus, research with Indigenous peoples should not only be focused on recording content or information/data derived from Indigenous knowledge. Emphasis also needs to be placed on process – through methods of engagement that build on Indigenous ways of knowing, are empowering, reinforce rather than undermine Indigenous identity, and make interventions more relevant to the communities they seek to support (Fu et al. 2012; Smith 2012; Mistry et al. 2019). This premise informed the methodological approach of Project COBRA. We used participatory video and participatory photography – audio-visual methods that allow people to explore issues and showcase their own solutions through storytelling, while taking collective action through cycles of planning, acting, observing and evaluating (Bignante 2010; Mistry 2013). Over the three and a half years of the project, participatory video and participatory photography were led by the five Indigenous peer researchers from the North Rupununi, Guyana. The aim was to use a System Viability framework – defined as the processes and structures a system develops to guarantee its survival in the long term in response to environmental opportunities and challenges (Berardi et al. 2015) – to identify and evaluate a wide cross-section of community practices and then record, through iterative cycles of participatory video and participatory photography, the most successful community owned solutions present in their villages (Mistry et al. 2016). These visual outputs were then shared with other Indigenous communities in Guyana, Suriname, Brazil, Colombia, French Guiana and Venezuela, to assess whether these videos and photostories could inspire others to act on their own environmental and social challenges (Tschirhart et al. 2016). As peer researchers, this core team had two tasks – to train and facilitate participatory video and participatory photography with a small team of peer researchers in the nine Indigenous villages engaged in Project COBRA, and to oversee the overall production of the video and photography materials from all the nine villages.

It is clear that the peer researchers had considerable responsibility for the delivery of the research, and had to engage both with the Indigenous communities with whom they engaged on a day-to-day basis, as well as the wider academic team who visited every couple of months to build capacity, mentor, assess progress and evaluate findings. We reflect on the ethical challenges of a local research team working in a participatory research project within their own Indigenous communities of the Guyanese interior elsewhere (Mistry et al. 2015). We show how complex issues of trust, relationships and positionality in relation to other community members meant that the peer researchers had to confront frequent comments, criticisms and jealousies, yet also benefitted by gaining access and logistical help for the research. We also highlight the inherent tensions for peer researchers trying to navigate research on the ground within their communities while also managing the expectations of academic knowledge and 'rigour'. Overall, we argue that despite the inherent difficulties of peer research, the Indigenous community researchers were a powerful conduit for authentic Indigenous voices and we offer some pragmatic solutions to counter ethical challenges.

Project COBRA finished with a conference at the European Commission in Brussels where three of the peer researchers presented their research and participatory videos to an international audience of policymakers, practitioners and academics. That the project progressed mostly in a positive direction led us to the assumption that there were beneficial impacts from peer research. At the same time, a general trend emerged where a range of institutions at all levels of governance began to support peer research approaches and more 'horizontal' models of capacity building, showing capacity to instil positive change and to empower a wide range of community members (Fukuda-Parr and Lopes 2003; McFarlane 2006). Although there are studies looking at the ethical issues and benefits arising from peer research (Patel and Mitlin 2002; Wahbe et al. 2007; Reed et al. 2014), few studies focus on the longer-term impact of projects or inventions where peer researchers have played a significant role in actually leading a research intervention. Our aim in this chapter, therefore, is to investigate if and what were the lasting impacts of Project COBRA, for individuals and communities, as well as for policy and practice beyond project implementation.

Methods

In order to assess the legacy of the project, we undertook video interviews in Guyana with the peer researchers, community members and wider government and non-governmental stakeholders in May 2018, three years after the project had ended. In total, interviews comprised five Indigenous peer researchers, twelve community members that participated in the project, three Indigenous leaders, two non-Indigenous civil society organisation managers, one non-Indigenous Indigenous rights activist and one official from the Ministry of Indigenous Peoples' Affairs.

Interviews were done through video as one of our objectives was to share the findings in visual form with interviewees and other interested stakeholders. Before the interviews occurred, a consent process with interviewees was done where the purpose of the interviews was clearly explained and an outline of how the videos would be analysed and distributed was provided. Interviews lasted between 30 and 60 minutes and revolved around the skills and knowledge gained during the project, the approach and methodologies, and achievements of the project at different scales.

Interviews were transcribed for data analysis, which took place using inductive coding to identify key themes from the data. These included changing worldviews and self-perceptions, increased capacity of individuals and communities, changing worldviews of decision makers, and sustaining impact. The video footage was also summarised into a series of short films.[1] Each key theme was then associated with relevant quotes from interviewees. Quotes were used to elicit discussion among the authors on the project's peer research approach, on its strengths, limits and challenges, and to reflect on how using a peer research approach allowed us to uncover health and social development issues within the communities. It was also useful to elicit and share our self-perceptions of the peer research approach, in terms of what it meant to us and how it affected us.

Findings

Changing worldviews and self-perceptions

This theme highlights lasting changes in worldviews and self-perception within the peer researchers and the wider community. The interviewees described how, prior to the project, there was an expectation that solutions to their challenges would be provided by external experts. There was a tacit understanding that their own practices were the cause of many of their challenges, or, at the very least, inadequate. However, interviewees' role in identifying and promoting their own community solutions during Project COBRA changed those perceptions:

> I think the communities have changed their mindset. At first, they were asking why you want information from me, but then they learn about finding own solution without waiting for the government.
>
> (female peer researcher)

> We feel we have this authority and we feel much more comfortable. We think we have a body that can solve it here, while when people come and then leave, many time the problem is still there. We have the power to solve it in the community!
>
> (male community member)

Interviewees attributed this change of mindset to the Project COBRA approach in calling up communities to face and address their own strengths and weaknesses:

> The local knowledge are hidden in the communities and need to be show. COBRA Project help to do that.
>
> (male community member)

> [The] COBRA project was useful because there were so many other project here in the region, but none of them was looking deeper in helping communities to find owns solution to everyday life. This project was a special project, took the communities to another level.
>
> (male peer researcher)

Peer researchers also reflected on how this changing worldview extended beyond Project COBRA itself:

> I was involved in the women group [since Project COBRA], little organisation. Cassava [focus of organisation]. When we face a challenge, we try to handle in different way, we from our level we try to find our own solutions in our own way.
>
> (female peer researcher)

Increased capacity of individuals and communities

This theme identified how peer researchers and community members felt empowered to initiate interventions, rather than being passive spectators of unfolding crises within their communities. Capacity was built in individuals to work on community development:

> To be more open minded to speak with people and to speak at an international level gave me the confidence to deal with my community. To be able to do presentations for the ministry, at NRDDB [North Rupununi District

Development Board] level, it was all because of the confidence that I have gained with COBRA project.

(male peer researcher)

I feel more confident ... COBRA project has given me time, discipline and initiative, and training. I deal with things instead of waiting for someone telling me what to do. Since the COBRA project finished I was engaged in a community development project and the skills and knowledge that I gained in Project COBRA allow me to lead the current project.

(female peer researcher)

This was particularly important for female peer researchers and it emerged both from a national and local perspective:

The role of young women leading in the project was something new. Young people taking part in the training in photography, script writing, interviews, in the general meeting of people and taking this message across.

(male government decision maker)

I am a resource person for documenting. I don't see it as personal thing but as a resource for my community. Since COBRA project ended, I involve myself not as a personal thing but in the communities as development of my women's group.

(female peer researcher)

At the same time, the project helped people in their everyday lives and for personal career progression:

[The] COBRA project has opened my eyes on personal capacity in building relationships. I have now a method of approach, the systematic approach of facing challenges step 1–2–3 in a simple way.

(male Indigenous leader)

Since [the] COBRA project ended, I have done so many things especially with NGOs, using the COBRA handbook and the same approach of COBRA. Photography and videography turned into a business for me. I am bringing more PV in the communities and also it turns in a business that is going well.

(male peer researcher)

Peer researchers showed that they have reflected on the approach and made it their own, each in their own personal way:

I don't use the [COBRA] handbook page by page but I use the approach. Also as leader in my village, it is very useful.

(male peer researcher)

The handbook is a guide. How do you do a workshop, how do you give a training, how do you do PV, how do you develop a scenario of an activity. A list of things that tell you step by step the process of doing things. You can apply it in personal life too.

(male peer researcher)

In part, this change was the result of the introduction of new visual means of communication. Prior to Project COBRA, communication within communities, and the maintenance of Indigenous knowledges, was mainly through face-to-face oral means, while there was an expectation that communication with decision makers had to be in written form in order to be effective. What the project achieved was to demonstrate how visual communication could play a strong role in both maintaining and enhancing Indigenous knowledges, while also being respected by decision makers. Interviewees highlighted the increased ability of Indigenous communities to use participatory video and participatory photography collectively to document and raise awareness of Indigenous issues and solutions:

Before COBRA came here, was difficult to make our report. Now we take pictures and videos of wildlife, we can show what we see in the field. We also use photostories that we learned from COBRA when we have meeting with the communities. People take more attention to the pictures.

(male community member)

This project brought a new method to find solutions using participatory video and photos. Communities were able to participate by involving themselves collectively to deal with issues. That was something that never happen before.

(male peer researcher)

Making videos in our communities and showing it to people at a different level it would be great benefit. It is not every day people will be in our community but if we can do a video and send it out and they [decision makers] can have a better look at it.

(female community member)

Changing worldviews of decision makers

Changes in self-perception were enhanced by changes in attitudes that peer researchers identified in policymakers and decision makers when engaging with communities:

I think the policymakers have changed their attitudes, because the communities have come up with their own solutions now.

(female peer researcher)

For decision makers, I believe that they have seen that communities can bring their own solutions and they can support in different ways, with projects, financially and developing their ideas together.

(male peer researcher)

Awareness of the importance of community owned solutions and visual methods of communication became more apparent in the decision makers themselves. Participants reported benefits associated with longevity of impact and the engagement of certain populations, such as young people, who are not typically involved in community decision making:

Promoting community owned solutions is the only way to go in terms of development that is genuine that would have ongoing impact and future references. I think that COBRA did a very good job with empowering and encouraging these sorts of things to happen.

(female non-Indigenous activist)

The benefit of promoting community owned solutions is very important if you are talking about communities taking the lead, especially in conservation. It is better that the solutions come from communities because it is important to have a lasting impact. Community owned solutions as a tool. Do you want to have long-term solution owned by communities? That's the best way!

(female non-Indigenous civil society
organisation manager)

It is very empowering and useful. Capacity building. Especially young people put forward questions and even solutions. It creates this opportunity of discussion that is needed in any community development. Especially in the hinterland it is very, very useful.

(male government decision maker)

Besides acknowledging the relevance of Project COBRA's community owned solutions approach, some institutions went further and decided to adopt it themselves in other projects:

The use of community owned solutions is very important for WWF. COBRA project helped WWF. We involved a community called Chenapau next to Kaieteur National Park. We used the COBRA community owned solutions approach to train this community. They were very welcome to learn and they still use this approach to express what they feel about the national park and how they want to participate in the management of national park.

(female non-Indigenous civil society
organisation manager)

Sustaining impact

Sustaining the impact of Project COBRA has its own challenges. These were identified as weak leadership, or a leadership comfortable with maintaining the status quo:

> There is some form of impact that is visible clearly, but unfortunately some community leaders are not taking up the instance, as leaders and communities members struggle.
>
> (male peer researcher)

Community researchers felt that although Project COBRA had an impact on themselves and the most marginalised community members, especially women and youth, more work needed to be carried out to build the capacity and change the worldviews of those in positions of leadership:

> Confidence in leadership. I think our leaders should have the skills. Leaders should be visionaries looking into the future sustainability. The unification of our communities.
>
> (male government decision maker)

It was felt that community leaders were still focusing their attention on using scarce community resources to pursue expensive external solutions rather than investing in further promoting community owned solutions:

> The challenge for North Rupununi was the funding. We were only able to work with some communities. Collecting indicators from forest villages and savanna villages. Limited human resources, we needed more staff.
>
> (male Indigenous leader)

There was still a certain mindset among some community leaders that now that Project COBRA was over, the whole approach can be forgotten about, and attention could now be focused on the next lucrative development or research project, whatever that may be. Yet, community peer researchers continued to champion the process they had established:

> At the end of the project, people were wondering what is going to happen. We indicate that the project finish but the process is not going to end, it remained in any village. Leaders and group village can use it [community owned solutions approach].
>
> (male peer researcher)

They also felt that key governmental decision makers had other priorities, but were hopeful that a change of government could provide more opportunities for promoting community owned solutions:

I feel that there was not so much influence to the government because we were focus on processes, practices while they were focus on something else. The current government is different. I believe we could achieve more.

(male peer researcher)

Discussion

Our findings show that peer researchers were key to a process of self-reflection within individuals and communities, and a subsequent positive change in the narrative of Indigenous people towards pride, solutions and autonomy. Through the peer research approach, peer researchers and communities went through a process of self-empowerment.

The fact that people from the community carried out the research served as an example for the community members to try and look to themselves for local solutions already existing within the community. That these researchers came from the local communities was in itself a demonstration that solutions to community problems could already be present within the community.

Project COBRA was effective because it practised and demonstrated the effectiveness of community ownership and capability by building capacity and empowering Indigenous researchers to lead the research process. It did not consist of someone from outside coming to tell them to identify their best practices. Instead, it involved local people who shared their problems and fears, and who were trying to face them by figuring out their own solutions to addressing the challenges of the complex research process. It took time, as the quotes show, but first community researchers and then communities became progressively more confident that they already had solutions to sustain their social and cultural development, or that the existing solutions could be improved and strengthened. Various experiences – such as realising they did not have to depend on external researchers to undertake research, understanding the project was about bringing up solutions that already existed in the community and working on these, acknowledging that they owned those solutions – contributed in making participants proactive in bringing up their views, experiences and ideas on health, social and environmental practices which were already being applied within the community successfully.

As community members became progressively more confident in the peer researchers' work, they became more confident in looking at some of the community practices with renewed eyes. As stated by one male peer researcher, 'Communities were able to participate by involving themselves collectively to deal with issues. That was something that never happen before.' Participatory video and participatory photography methods were important in this process. Since the project brought wider awareness of community owned solutions, it gave village leadership ideas of how they could use these solutions for the betterment of their villages, using the videos and photostories as a catalyst to move their solutions forward. For example, one community started a cultural group to promote knowledge transmission to youth, which encouraged its senior councillor to budget for the community to build a *benab* (traditional meeting space) where they could practise and hold events. Peer researchers noted that, while in the past people took photos with limited capacity on how to weave these into a powerful and purposeful communication strategy, now they take pictures with the intention of telling stories that carry important messages.

In the case of rotational Indigenous farming, peer research showcasing it as a best practice helped to change the narrative about the practice. Indigenous farming is often looked at in terms of productivity, as something archaic and not efficient, less advanced than more intensive mechanised forms of farming. Identifying rotational farming as a best practice – highlighting its potential in land regeneration, preservation of forest habitats, mutual community work and promoting healthy physical and eating practices – shows how Indigenous communities viewed their practices without being influenced by external perceptions of what might be classified as best practice. In addition, researching farming made people think more about safeguarding their staple crop, cassava. Highlighting that having many varieties of cassava was a good way of having options, in light of crop failures, climate change and healthy diets, has led to people making a move to ensure that cassava varieties are planted on appropriate lands and stored properly for continuity.

Peer researchers using their newly acquired skills for career progression, to work within local community development, and in their everyday lives, shows how peer research approaches are able to create new mindsets and proactive attitudes. One of the main challenges communities face is lack of cohesion. The peer research approach helped to increase personal capacity in building relationships, with community members working together and facilitating constructive and productive discussions. They were able to rely on themselves to find creative solutions, rather than waiting for help to come from outside, to enhance their well-being and the well-being of their communities. As stated by one female peer researcher, 'I deal with things instead of waiting for someone telling me what to do.' Peer researchers, as stated by one of them, feel their role is not 'a personal thing', but 'a resource for the community'. This role is something, as they state, that did not end with the project, but has kept going through other projects and through personal enterprise.

The increasing confidence of peer researchers in engaging with other communities and with actors at different levels, was very important in making the work of Project COBRA more visible and genuine to decision makers. On the one hand, ministries and civil society organisations have realised the effectiveness of videos and photostories to get their information to the communities, showing more videos rather than printed materials which many could not read, while long presentations were found to be boring and not understandable to all. On the other hand, despite some difficulties experienced by women peer researchers – including security issues, and social and cultural norms (Mistry et al. 2015) – having a diverse and young team of Indigenous researchers presenting their own findings at high-level platforms such as ministerial meetings and the European Commission, prompted people to stop and listen. Indigenous society in Guyana is strongly patriarchal, both in terms of age and gender, and voice and wisdom are generally attributed to elders, particularly males. Peer researchers showed that they could navigate cultural norms, respecting the opinions and knowledge of elders while at the same time representing that knowledge in policy arenas as younger members and future leaders of those communities. The significance of communicating through the detached medium of an intermediary artefact was key in this respect (Shaw 2015). Young people and women are often intimidated when speaking publicly in front of powerful and older men, who consequently tend to dominate discussions in important public debates and decision-making processes. However, through video and photography, youth and women had a propensity to be able to say what they knew and felt. The participatory video and photography processes allowed marginalised voices to provide the visual evidence to support their statements. These visual artefacts could then be shared in public and with decision makers, thus encouraging a wider appreciation of the significant issues and solutions raised by youth and women.

A major challenge of most development and conservation interventions is sustaining impact. Peer researchers identified this as an issue. In the case of Project COBRA, turn around in local leaders and political affiliations meant that some new village leaders were not keen on championing initiatives proposed or started by previous (and politically rival) leaders, even if these were beneficial for the community. The region also suffers from a common development ailment of new donors and projects coming in and basically either replicating or undermining previous work, rather than evaluating the situation and building on what has worked. Indigenous communities are looking for funds and will not say no to any offers. Thus, project sustainability can be undermined. Nevertheless, having peer researchers embedded in the communities can help mitigate some of these issues. In our case, post Project COBRA, the peer researchers have gone on to set up businesses focused on participatory video and photography, worked on other projects and community initiatives using their acquired skill sets, trained other young people in the communities, and become leaders in their own villages. One peer researcher's business is now a nationally recognised technology centre by the Ministry of Indigenous Peoples' Affairs and other organisations, and has been a great help for the North Rupununi communities, offering participatory video and photography training, information technology training and social services like helping with job applications. Four of the peer researchers became part of a new project aimed at integrating Indigenous knowledge within conservation policy and practice, thus continuing to build their skills and to improve their leadership capability. In this way, the peer researchers continue the legacy of Project COBRA. COBRA has become a recognisable name in the region, and no matter what they may be visiting the communities for, the peer researchers are still referred to as the 'COBRA team'!

Conclusions

> In order to be performed in an effectively decolonizing way, geographical research from/with Indigenous epistemologies needs to respect minimal requirements, namely to be respectful of Indigenous communities, values, knowledges, and customs, to exclude an 'extractive' attitude leading to collecting information for the exclusive interest of academic centres, to acknowledge that not all Indigenous knowledges are meant for a general audience, and to ensure that the production of new geographical knowledge will benefit Indigenous peoples.
>
> (Clement 2019, p. 290)

Despite increasing calls to recognise the important role of Indigenous peoples and their knowledge in environmental management and governance (e.g., Brondizio and Le Tourneau 2016; Mistry and Berardi 2016), there has been little in-depth discussion of ways of engaging with this knowledge in a respectful and self-governing way. From our experiences in Project COBRA, we have found that impact was achieved due to a combination of four interrelated aspects: a peer research approach; a community owned solutions paradigm; a holistic framework (system viability) that enabled a wide cross section of community practices to be explored; and use of participatory video and participatory photography as the key tools of communication. Each nurtured the other. The system viability framework, participatory video and participatory photography facilitated peer researchers' interactions with the community, and helped to identify and share community owned solutions. The peer research approach allowed community owned solutions to come to the surface; it would have been much harder (and arguably unethical) with external researchers carrying out the research. Also, the identified community owned solutions were sustained after the project thanks to the peer research approach empowering community researchers. They became strategic actors in the communities, they shared the acquired relational skills with others, and kept alive the community owned solutions within their communities. It was their project, their communities and their chance to improve their situation. After the project ended, the Indigenous peer researchers and other former researchers of Project COBRA, including authors of this paper, established the Cobra Collective CIC – a social enterprise with a mission for social innovation by empowering marginalised communities to identify, record, promote and practise community owned solutions.[2] Through the work of the Cobra Collective, we aim to continue working with peer researchers and establishing peer research processes in future projects.

Acknowledgements

We thank the communities of the North Rupununi, Guyana, for their active and enthusiastic participation in Project COBRA. Project COBRA was funded by the Environment Programme, Management of Natural Resources, DG Research and Innovation, European Commission 7th Framework.

Notes

1 These videos are available at: https://vimeo.com/channels/communityownedsolutions.
2 See www.cobracollective.org.

References

Berardi, A., et al., 2015. Applying the system viability framework for cross-scalar governance of nested social-ecological systems in the Guiana Shield, South America. *Ecology and Society*, 20 (3), 42.

Bignante, E., 2010. The use of photo elicitation in field research: Exploring Maasai representation and use of natural resources. *EchoGéo*, 11, 1–18.

Black, L., 2003. Critical review of the capacity-building literature and discourse. *Development in Practice*, 13 (1), 116–120.

Brondizio, E.S. and Le Tourneau, F.-M., 2016. Environmental governance for all. *Science*, 352 (6291), 1272–1273.

Clement, V., 2019. Beyond the sham of the emancipatory enlightenment: Rethinking the relationship of Indigenous epistemologies, knowledges, and geography through decolonizing paths. *Progress in Human Geography*, 43 (2), 276–294.

Fu, Y., et al., 2012. Climate change adaptation among Tibetan pastoralists: Challenges in enhancing local adaptation through policy support. *Environmental Management*, 50 (4), 607–621.

Fukuda-Parr, S. and Lopes, C., eds., 2003. *Capacity for Development. New Solutions to Old Problems*. London: Routledge.

Garnett, S.T., et al., 2018. A spatial overview of the global importance of Indigenous lands for conservation. *Nature Sustainability*, 1, 369–374.

Kaplan, A., 2000. Capacity building: Shifting the paradigms of practice. *Development in Practice*, 10 (3–4), 517–526.

McFarlane, C., 2006. Knowledge, learning and development: A post-rationalist approach. *Progress in Development Studies*, 6 (4), 287–305.

Mistry, J., 2013. Commentary on participatory video. *J-Reading: Journal of Research and Didactics in Geography*, 1, 119–123.

Mistry, J., et al., 2015. Between a rock and a hard place: Ethical dilemmas of local community facilitators doing participatory projects. *Geoforum*, 61, 27–35.

Mistry, J., et al., 2016. Community owned solutions: Identifying local best practices for social-ecological sustainability. *Ecology and Society*, 21 (2), 42.

Mistry, J. and Berardi, A., 2016. Bridging indigenous and scientific knowledge. *Science*, 352 (6291), 1274–1275.

Mistry, J., et al., 2019. Indigenous knowledge. In: A. Kobayashi, ed. *Encyclopaedia of Human Geography*, 2nd ed., vol. 7. Amsterdam: Elsevier, 211–215.

Olsson, P. and Folke, C., 2001. Local ecological knowledge and institutional dynamics for ecosystem management: A study of Lake Racken Watershed, Sweden. *Ecosystems*, 4 (2), 85–104.

Patel, S. and Mitlin, D., 2002. Sharing experiences and changing lives. *Community Development Journal*, 37 (2), 125–136.

Reed, M.S., et al., 2014. Five principles for the practice of knowledge exchange in environmental management. *Journal of Environmental Management*, 146, 337–345.

Shaw, J., 2015. Re-grounding participatory video within community emergence towards social accountability. *Community Development Journal*, 50 (4), 624–643.

Smith, L.T., 2012 [1999]. *Decolonizing Methodologies: Research and Indigenous People.* London/Dunedin: Zed Books/Otago University Press.

Tschirhart, C., et al., 2016. Learning from one another: The effectiveness of horizontal knowledge exchange for natural resource management and governance. *Ecology and Society*, 21 (2), 41.

Wahbe, T.R., et al., 2007. Building international indigenous people's partnerships for community-driven health initiatives. *EcoHealth*, 4 (4), 472–488.

World Bank, 2019. *Understanding Poverty: Indigenous Peoples.* Available from: http://www.worldbank.org/en/topic/indigenouspeoples [Accessed 2 May 2019].

Index

For Product Safety Concerns and Information please contact our EU
representative GPSR@taylorandfrancis.com
Taylor & Francis Verlag GmbH, Kaufingerstraße 24, 80331 München, Germany

www.ingramcontent.com/pod-product-compliance
Lightning Source LLC
Chambersburg PA
CBHW060448240326
41598CB00088B/3953

9 780367 766634